T0289762

Parkinson's Disease: Diagnosis and Clinical Management

Parkinson's Disease: Diagnosis and Clinical Management

Editor: Aubrey Walsh

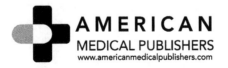

AMERICAN
MEDICAL PUBLISHERS
www.americanmedicalpublishers.com

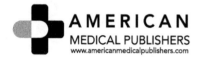

AMERICAN
MEDICAL PUBLISHERS
www.americanmedicalpublishers.com

Cataloging-in-publication Data

Parkinson's disease : diagnosis and clinical management / edited by Aubrey Walsh.
    p. cm.
Includes bibliographical references and index.
ISBN 979-8-88740-362-5
1. Parkinson's disease. 2. Parkinson's disease--Diagnosis. 3. Parkinson's disease--Treatment.
4. Brain--Diseases. I. Walsh, Aubrey.
RC382 .P373 2023
616.833--dc23

American Medical Publishers,
41 Flatbush Avenue,
1st Floor, New York,
NY 11217, USA

ISBN 979-8-88740-362-5 (Hardback)

Contents

Preface

Parkinson's disease (PD) is a neurodegenerative condition characterized by bradykinesia, rigidity and resting tremor. This disease has motor and non-motor symptoms. Some of the common symptoms of this disease are trembling of hands, inadequate balance and coordination, and low movement. Individuals with Parkinson's disease may experience melancholy, sleep issues, or difficulty in chewing, etc. In early stages, symptoms appear slowly and usually to one side of the body and as the disease progress, effects can be seen on both sides of body. Parkinson's disease occurs when the nerve cells in the brain fails to construct sufficient dopamine. A wide range of medications can occasionally improve symptoms of this disease. In critical cases of Parkinson's disease deep brain stimulation (DBS) and surgery can be beneficial. This book unravels the recent studies on the diagnosis and management of Parkinson's disease. It can be used by physicians, researchers, and neuroscientists who want to learn more about this disease. The book is appropriate for those seeking detailed in this area.

This book unites the global concepts and researches in an organized manner for a comprehensive understanding of the subject. It is a ripe text for all researchers, students, scientists or anyone else who is interested in acquiring a better knowledge of this dynamic field.

I extend my sincere thanks to the contributors for such eloquent research chapters. Finally, I thank my family for being a source of support and help.

Editor

Pathophysiology of L-Dopa Induced Dyskinesia — Changes in D1/D3 Receptors and Their Signaling Pathway

Sacnité Albarran Bravo, Claudia Rangel-Barajas and
Benjamín Florán Garduño

1. Introduction

Parkinson's disease (PD) is a neurodegenerative disorder characterized by the progressive loss of dopaminergic mesencephalic neurons. The most used and successful therapy for this condition is L-3, 4 dihydroxyphenylalanine (L-DOPA), a precursor in the synthesis of dopamine. However long-term treatment leads to disabling abnormal involuntary movements known as L-DOPA-induced Dyskinesia (LID), which are uncontrolled and repetitive movement in the axis, arms, legs and oro-facial zone [1-2]. The LID is a serious limitation in the usage of L-DOPA and it can be thought that solving the diskinesia by new therapeutic targets could extend the time of treatment with L-DOPA in the parkinsonian patients with an acceptable quality of life. To propose new alternatives is necessary to know the pathogenesis and pathophysiology of this phenomenon.

According with the classical basal ganglia model [3], PD is the result of an imbalance in the motor networks that stimulate and/or inhibit the initiation of movements. There are two main pathways that have been studied in the basal ganglia. The direct pathway, which is associated with D1-like dopamine receptors, and the indirect pathway that it has been related with D2-like dopamine receptors. The adequate balance between the direct (stimulatory) and indirect (inhibitory) networks facilitates the execution of movements [4]. In PD the loss of dopaminergic control leads to a hyperactivity of the inhibitory pathway, which produces bradykinesia the main symptom of this disease [5]. The restoration of dopamine with L-DOPA counteract the unbalance of the two pathways, nevertheless several cellular and molecular changes caused by L-DOPA move the system toward the opposite side, producing a hyperactivity of the direct pathway and originating the dyskinesia phenomenon [5]. Many changes in basal ganglia circuitry have been associated with dyskinesia [6]; one of the most studied is the hyperactivity of direct pathway that produces an increased GABAergic neurotransmission on striato-nigral neurons, which are controlled by dopamine D1 receptors, and it seems to be the most relevant finding. The dopamine D_3 receptors have been involved in dyskinesia since was reported that L-DOPA treatment increases its expression in basal ganglia [7], suggesting the use of ligands of these receptors as a target for dyskinesia, but the neurobiological basis of these changes and the site of action is not well understood since conflicting results in experimental assays have been reported [8-12]. The recent finding of co-existence and interaction between D_1 and D_3 dopamine receptors in the direct pathway [13-16] could contribute to solve this question.

The aim of this review is provide a global view of the pathophysiology of dyskinesia based on the changes reported in animal models and parkinsonian patients that involve the direct pathway and the dopamine D_1 and D_3 receptors, the understanding of this changes could result in a potential novel therapeutic approaches to treat the dyskinesia.

2. Basal ganglia, the control of movement and Parkinson's disease

Basal ganglia are organized in four segregated circuits: motor, oculo-motor, limbic and associative [17]. In PD the motor loop is altered in these structures. The basal ganglia circuit originates in glutamatergic cortical neurons from motor and premotor areas that project to caudate (C) and putamen (P), the striatum in rats (Str). The main phenotype of striatum is the GABAergic medium-size spiny neurons (MSNs), which projects to the direct and indirect pathways. The substance P/Dynorphyn positive MNSs GABAergic neurons project to substantia nigra pars reticulata (SNr) and/or to the internal segment of globus pallidus (GPi), the entopeduncular nucleus (EPn) in rats. SNr and GPi is the output nucleus of the motor loop to the thalamic glutamatergic nucleus, which in turn stimulates the motor cortex; this network is called the direct pathway. While the striatal enkephaline positive MNSs GABAergic neurons project to the external segment of the globus pallidus (GPe), pallidal GABAergic neurons which in turn project their axons to the glutamatergic neurons of the Subthalamic nucleus (Sth) and this neurons project to the output nuclei forming the indirect pathway [17]. (See Fig. 1).

Neurons of the thalamic relay nucleus are subject to a tonic inhibitory control from GABAergic GPi/SNr neurons, the removal of this control leads to the activation of thalamus that in consequence activates the motor cortex facilitating the movement. The activity of GPi/SNr neurons is maintained by a tonic stimulatory action of the Sth controlled reciprocally by the GPe. Stimulation of the MNSs GABAergic striatal neurons by the cortex in the direct pathway produces inhibition of the output nucleus through the release of GABA. The remotion in the inhibition of the thalamus toward to the cortex turns in the initiation of the movement, thus the activation of the direct pathway allows the movement. In contrast the activation of MNSs GABAergic neurons from the indirect pathway inhibits GPe neurons, which removes the tonic inhibitory action on Sth, the increased activity of the glutamatergic neurons stimulates the output nuclei, producing inhibition of thalamus and in consequence inhibit the motor cortex, which means that the activation of the indirect pathway inhibits the movements.

Simultaneous activation of the direct and indirect pathway will produce an antagonistic action on movement. The adequate balance between direct and indirect pathway is maintained by dopamine. The Substantia nigra pars compacta (SNc) is the source of dopamine in the basal ganglia since SNc neurons project to all the basal ganglia nuclei (Fig.1A) in normal conditions [18].

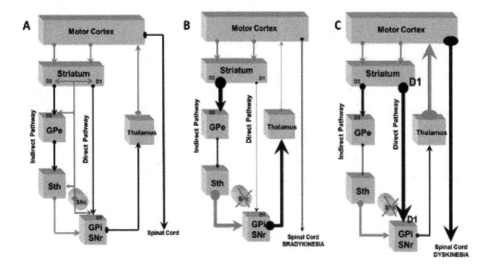

Figure 1. The basal ganglia motor circuits in normal (A), parkinsonism (B) and L-DOPA-induced dyskinesia (C). GPe, external globus pallidus; Sth, subthalamic nucleus; GPi, internal globus pallidus; SNr, substantia nigra pars reticulata; SNc, substantia nigra pars compacta, D1, dopamine D1 receptor and D2, dopamine D2 receptor.

Two families of receptors mediate the action of dopamine through the basal ganglia, D1-like (D$_1$ and D$_5$ subtypes) and D2-like (D$_{2short}$, D$_{2long}$ D$_3$ and D$_4$ subtypes). D1-like receptors are expressed predominantly in substance P/Dynorphyn positive MNSs GABAergic neurons and their activation increases the firing rate at soma and also the GABA release in the terminals [19-22]. It have been reported that some population of striato-nigral neurons also expresses D$_3$ receptors [14, 23]. While the dopamine D2-like receptors are associated to striatal enkephalin positive MNSs GABAergic neurons and their activation decreases the firing at soma and the GABA release at the terminals [20, 24-26]. Some population of striato-palidal neurons also expresses D$_5$ receptors [23]. Dopamine via D1-like receptors potentiates the stimulation of the direct pathway, while via D2-like receptors decreases indirect pathway activity, synergizing the activity of both pathways and facilitating movement [17]. Other association of dopamine receptors subtypes with neuronal elements of these circuits occurs [27-32], however the role of their function in the integral circuitry is not well understood.

The progressive loss of dopaminergic neurons of the SNc causes the neurodegenerative dis-order called Parkinson's disease. The loss of dopamine has serious consequences in the bal-ance of direct and indirect pathways, in fact a hyperactivity of the indirect pathway with a decrease in the activity of the direct pathway coexists and that explains the hypomotility or bradykinesia observed in patients and in animal models of PD (Fig. 1B) [17].

3. Pathophysiology of L-DOPA-induced dyskinesia (LID)

Dopamine replacement therapy with L-DOPA restores the lack of the neurotransmitter in the basal ganglia [33]. It has been shown that L-DOPA (a precursor in dopamine synthesis, Fig. 2) is transformed to dopamine in the central nervous system by decarboxylation via cen-tral aromatic acid decarboxilase (DCAA) [34]; also it has been proposed that remaining dop-aminergic neurons (Fig. 2) and/or serotoninergic neurons are host candidates for transformation of L-DOPA [35], mediating an ectopic and false transmitter release [36] in fact any cell that express DCAA can eventually transform L-DOPA into dopamine. The dop-amine synthesized from L-DOPA activates D1-like and D2-like family of receptors. Howev-er it has been also suggested the existence of DOPAergic receptors [37], since direct effects of L-DOPA on dopamine receptors have been reported [19, 38 -39] but also effects are mediat-ed by either L-DOPA or their metabolites [39, 40-41] that could participate in their therapeu-tic or side effects including dyskinesia [42-43]. Probably the effectiveness of L-DOPA over dopamine receptor agonist is due to a variety of actions in the central nervous system [44].

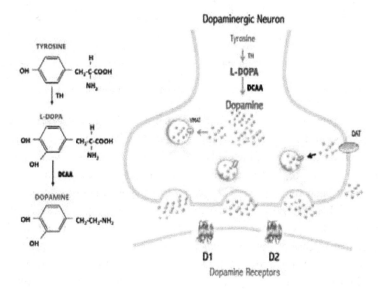

Figure 2. Synthesis of dopamine from L-DOPA in the dopaminergic nerve terminals. DCAA, aromatic acid decarboxy-lase; DAT, dopamine transporter, TH, Tyrosine Hydroxylase; D1, D1-like dopamine receptor; D2, D2-like dopamine re-ceptor.

During L-DOPA treatment the activation of dopamine receptors restores the movement in PD patients and the locomotor activity in experimental animal models. L-DOPA treatment produces a priming effect where the brain is sensitized to L-DOPA after chronic administration and finally produces dyskinesia as main side effect [45] with a prevalence of 30-45% in patients [46]. However early age of Parkinsonism onset and severity of disease have been classified as risk factors in the development of LID [47] and more recently the nigral-associated pathology has been related with early onset of LID [48]. It has been shown that pharmacokinetic properties of L-DOPA are also related with the onset of dyskinesia with phenomenological differences in the altered movements. When the higher plasma levels of L-DOPA are reached the maximum antiparkinsonic effect can be achieved. In contrast dyskinesia occurs at intermedium L-DOPA plasma levels either when bioavailability is increasing or decreasing due to metabolism of L-DOPA, interesting when the lower L-DOPA plasma levels are reached generalized dystonic postures occurs [49].

The dyskinesia also has been observed in experimental models of PD under chronic L-DOPA treatment [50], the effect is dose and species dependent, since different population with high and low dyskinesia score have been reported [51-52].

The mechanism of the genesis of dyskinesia is essentially unknown. Initial studies suggested that L-DOPA or metabolites could be responsible of the side effects, however the inhibition of L-DOPA decarboxylation, does not correlate with LID scores [53]. Plenty evidence has been published recently showing that several compensatory effects occur after dopamine denervation and LID.

The changes in nuclear function of striato-nigral and striato-pallidal neurons have been related with denervation, most of them are associated with proteins involved in the dopamine receptors signaling and in the regulation of glutamatergic transmission by dopamine [54], it can be though that L-DOPA therapy should restore these parameters. However that is not the case since the major alterations related to LID occur on these cellular systems [52, 55-60].

It has been reported alteration in gene expression during L-DOPA therapy particularly on transcription factors. Early gene expression which are markers of neural activity has been studied and increased expression of the transcription factor ΔFosB has been associated with L-DOPA induced dyskinesia in rats and related with sensitization process [61-64], while accumulated ΔJunD has been shown drop the severity of LID in monkeys without reduction of antiparkinsonian effects [63]. Also zif-268 has been related with a persistent stimulation of D1 receptors by L-DOPA and has been proposed like a potential marker for the onset of the dyskinetic phenomena [65]. On the other hand histone activation mediated by D1 receptors it has also been related with dyskinesia [66-67] suggesting that changes in gene transcription factors are altered, then is plausible suggest that many alterations in signaling molecules activated by dopaminergic receptors could contribute to the leading of motor disabilities. The resulting changes of the altered activity culminates with expression of proteins related with the activity of D1-associated neurons like the increased expression of prodynorhin, glutamic acid decarboxylase, adenylyl cyclase, PKA, DARPP-32 and CDk5 [52, 54-60].

Nevertheless LID can be also pathophysiologically explained by a change in the balance of the direct/indirect pathway. In this condition an increase in the activity of the direct pathway that facilitates movements can explain the phenomena (Fig. 1C) [5]; since the direct pathway stimulates movement, dyskinesia can be considered a pathologic condition with over-activation of this pathway generated by pulsatile activity of striato-nigral neurons. In fact experimental data supports this idea; a higher release of GABA in SNr/EP has been shown in experimental models of LID [52,68], which in turns facilitates the inhibition of the output neurons and removes the inhibition of premotor nuclei leading activation of the movement.

The role of the indirect pathway and dopamine D2-like receptors is less understood and explored. An over-activity of the GPe is associated with LID [55], and dopamine D2 receptors [69- 71]; however pallidotomy does not modify significantly LID in hemiparkinsonian monkeys [72]. Some D2-like agonist has beneficial effect on L-DOPA induced dyskinesia [73], but the genetic inactivation of dopamine D_2 receptor expression in striatum does not modify the development of LID [66]. On the other hand D_2 dopamine receptor agonist treatment in PD models produce lower LID compared with D_1 receptor agonist treatment suggesting a predominantly role of dopamine D_1 receptors [65,74]. Interesting recent reports have shown that L-DOPA restores spine density in D2-expressing striatal neurons of LID mice [75], suggesting an undefined role of striato-pallidal in the dyskinetic phenomenon. On the other hand adenosine A_{2A} receptors are selectively expressed in the indirect pathway and an increased expression of these receptors was found in patients with LID [76], the A_{2A}/D_2 receptor heterodimer interaction has been suggested is modified during LID in the indirect pathway [77]. All this data suggested a role of the indirect pathway in LID development; however further studies are needed to clarify the role of D_2 receptor and the indirect pathway in the dyskinesia phenomenon.

Other non-dopaminergic alterations have been involved in LID, which contributes to this phenomenon. The idea of a role of the glutamatergic system in LID comes from the use of amantadine in Parkinson's disease and as an adjuvant in the management of LID [78], in fact amantadine increases extracellular dopamine from L-DOPA in parkinsonian rats [79]. Dopaminergic denervation decreases the expression and phosphorilation of NR1 subunit of the NMDA receptor without change in NR2 subunit. L-DOPA restores the expression of the subunit but also increases the phosphorilation level of the NR2A subunit with a consecutive high activity of the NMDA channel [80-81]. It has been shown also that D1-like receptors increase the phosphorylation of the channel subunits through the PKA signaling pathway [82-83]. Furthermore D1 receptor promotes the expression of NMDA in membrane [80] and can interact at the level of protein [84], in consequence if a generalized hypersensitivity of D1-like receptor activity occurs, the NMDA receptor activity will also be potentiated [80, 85]. Dopamine modulates long-term potentiation (LTP) of the glutamatergic system, in consequence in dyskinesia, L-DOPA could contribute to the prolongation of this effects [78, 86]. It has been shown in dyskinetic rats an increased levels of PSD-95 and SAP97 proteins of the postsynaptic density, those proteins are involved in the interaction of NMDA and AMPA receptors in the membrane, but their participation in the phenomenon has not been completely determined [87-89]. The consequence in all these alterations of the glutamatergic system is a higher excitatory transmission to the direct pathway. An interesting review on the role of D1/NMDA interaction and LID is found in Fiorentini et al., 2008 [90]. Changes in synaptic plasticity induced by L-DOPA also occur in the output nuclei [91].

The role of the serotoninergic system on LID comes from the hypothesis of conversion of L-DOPA to dopamine in serotoninergic neurons and nerve terminals within the basal ganglia [92, 93]. It has been suggested a false-transmitter release of dopamine from this neurons [36, 94], in consequence a higher dopaminergic activity would be the responsible of LID. According with this hypothesis the role of serotonin system in LID is related with effects on dopamine formed in the terminals. Some studies indicates that increasing serotonin levels suppress LID, the effect seem to be mediated by 5-HT$_{1A}$ receptors [95], since these receptors are also located at cortico-striatal glutamatergic terminals is plausible that blockade of D$_1$ receptor activity explains the therapeutically effect [96]. Moreover blockade of serotonin transporter also attenuates LID suggesting that a reduce turnover [95] and activation of serotonin receptors is involved in its beneficial effect.

Dopamine denervation and L-DOPA treatment increases mRNA codifying opioid precursors pro-enkephaline A and B, which correlates with the development of dyskinesia [55, 97]. This effect has been observed in striato-nigral neurons [98] and has been postulated participate in LID due to an enhanced coupling of opioid receptors to G protein [99]. However the blockade of these receptors in dyskinetic rats does not prevent symptoms and in fact there is an increase in the dyskinesia score [100, 101]. It seems that the over-expression is just consequence of denervation, recent studies have been shown that modification of δ-opiod receptor modify dyskinesia in hemiparkinsonian rats [102], but the role of opioids in LID remains unclear and needs further study. Finally the role of noradrenergic system in LID is poorly studied but it has been suggested that an increased norepinephrine transmission in Str could be related with dyskinesia since the blockade of norepinephrine receptors reverts LID [103].

Since the direct pathway of the basal ganglia and D$_1$ receptors activity is associated with dyskinesia, the research has been focusing on changes in these neurons, their activity, neurochemical tracers and their receptors particularly dopamine D$_1$ and D$_3$ receptors, in order to propose alternatives to the therapeutic management of the Parkinson patients.

4. The dopamine D1-like receptors signaling in the direct pathway

D1-like family of dopamine receptors includes D$_1$ and D$_5$ subtypes. D$_1$ has 466 amino acids and D$_5$ has 477 with a homology of 80% located mainly in the transmembrane domains [104]. D$_1$ and D$_5$ receptors have a differential distribution in the central nervous system; moreover there is a controversy of their signaling pathway. Initially was proposed that both receptors stimulate adenylyl cyclase; however some dopamine effects on PLC activity seem to be mediated by the D$_5$ type [105].

Dopamine D1 receptors are members of the G protein coupled receptors family (GPCRs) stimulates adenylyl cyclase trough Gα_{olf} or Gα_s proteins [106]. In the D1-like receptors associated to the striato-nigral neurons, the subunit $G\alpha_{olf}$ interacts with the catalytic domain of adenylyl cyclase V [107], increasing the activity and therefore cAMP formation [108]. It have been reported $G\alpha_{olf}$ is expressed in the direct pathway and the level of expression can change after dopamine denervation [52].

The cAMP formed by D1 receptor activation stimulates PKA, and recent studies suggested the activation of the GEF (nucleotide interchange factor) EPAC and the consequence activation of Rap1 a low weight G protein that activates MAPK [109]. The activation of PKA phosphorylates several substrates that include: Na^+, voltage depending K^+ and GIRKs channels, producing inhibition; whereas Ca^{2+} L, N, P, Q, NMDA, AMPA and $GABA_A$ channels are stimulated by the phosphorylation. PKA also phosphorylates DARPP-32 at threonine 34, DARPP-32 phosphorylated inhibits protein phosphate 1 (PP1). Phosphorilation of NMDA channels by D1 receptor signaling through DARPP-32, synergize their stimulatory action, whereas by the same pathway attenuates $GABA_A$ inhibitory currents. PP1 has several substrates such as Ca^{2+} L, N, P and AMPA channels (for references see Udieh, 2010 [105]).

D1 receptors also induce activation of anti-apoptotic signals. PKA phosphorylates Akt (also known like PKB), which phosphorylates CREB that translocate to the nucleus inducing gene expression related with cellular survival. D1 receptors interact with other receptors, ionic channels and cytoskeleton proteins. Protein-protein interaction between NMDA at the level of NR1 subunit produces signaling via PI3K, interaction with NR2 subunit decreases NMDA current [105]. D1 receptors form heterodimers with adenosine A1 receptors producing decrease in GABA release [110], while D_5 receptor interacts with $GABA_A$ channels decreasing Cl^- current [111]. Neurofilament M, COP gamma and DIRP78 are cytoskeleton proteins related with expression, sensitization, and transport of D1 receptors [105].

D1 receptor interactions with other dopamine receptors have been described. Dimmers between D_1-D_2 receptors induce an increased intracellular Ca^{2+} probably mediated by the $G_{\alpha q}$ $\rightarrow$PLC pathway [112]. It has also been reported the interaction of dopamine D_1/D_3 receptors, here we will discuss latter the role of this dimmer in PD and LID.

The adenylyl-cyclase$\rightarrow$PKA stimulated by D1-like receptors induces GABA release in the Str and SNr [19, 22, 113] and increases the firing rate MNSs [21], mechanism that has been related with the facilitation of movement in the direct pathway. Dopamine D1 receptor effects on firing rate and GABA release are mediated by DARPP-32 and PP1 [21, 83, 113, 114]. The effects on firing rate and release have been associated to modulation of L-type and P/Q calcium channels [21, 113-116].

5. Mechanisms of D1 dopamine receptors sensitization in PD and LID: Changes in signal transduction pathways

As we discuss before the loss of dopamine innervation induces molecular and signal transduction changes in the neurons of the basal ganglia attributed to a compensatory response. Most of the experimental studies have been assessed using toxins to induce experimental models of PD like 6-hydroxydopamine (6-OHDA) for rats or 1-metyl-4-phenyl-1,2,3,6 tetra-hydropyridine (MPTP) for mice or non-human primates, because their ability to induce the degeneration of dopaminergic neurons [117-118]. The changes after dopamine denervation have been studied in particular on striato-nigral (direct pathway) and pallido-nigral (indirect pathway) neurons and plenty evidence shows that cellular and functional changes occurs, this phenomenon is called supersensitivity to dopamine denervation [119, 120]. The supersensitivity has been shown in expression levels of mRNA for enkephalins, substance P and dynorphins [121] but also up-regulation of more than 30 genes including zif 268, c-fos, c-jun and MAPK-1, most of them related with neuronal activity [54, 122]. Interesting several of those genes and changed proteins convey to D1 dopamine receptors and their signal transduction pathways [54].

Perhaps one of the most studied effects of denervation is the altered expression of dopamine receptors in the basal ganglia [20]. D2-like dopamine receptors increase in number, sensibility and consistently with that the mRNA in the striato-palidal neurons[20], which explain the hypomotolity. In contrast despite some contradictory results [56, 123], there is evidence that not only the mRNA of D1-like dopamine receptors decreases in the striatal neurons [20] but also the expression [124-125], with no changes in the affinity studied by radioligand binding techniques in SNr [125]. Proteasome altered activity observed in L-DOPA treatment produces an altered D1-like receptor abnormal trafficking that might be responsible for this changes [126]. Contrary to the decrease of D1-like dopamine receptors an increased response to their activation is observed in the striatum [120, 122, 127], and also a substantial increase in GABA release in the striato-nigral terminals [68, 125]. However despite the supersensitivity phenomenon the lack of endogenous dopamine in PD to activate the receptors explains the poor activation of basal ganglia pathways and therefore the hypomotility.

The activation of dopamine receptors would be the target in order to restore the balance in the circuit of the basal ganglia. The gold-standard therapy in PD is L-DOPA, because is converted to DA, or even can activate dopamine receptors directly increasing firing rate in striatal neurons and inducing GABA release in SNr. In addition the activation of D1 receptors leads an increase of GABA release in striato-nigral terminals promoting the activation of the direct pathway related with the movement, which is the main purpose of the pharmacological approach to treat PD.

It can be thought that replacement of DA with L-DOPA should restore the number, sensitivity and response of the activation of dopamine receptors observed in experimental conditions. Nevertheless that is not the case, chronic L-DOPA treatment only produces a partial recovery of D1-like dopamine receptors [125], whereas increases even more the biological response to their activation, producing a very high level of GABA release in the striato-nigral terminals than occurred only with dopamine denervation in hemiparkinsonian rats [125, 128-129]. An analysis of D1 receptor expression in striatum in L-DOPA treated rats indicates that D1-like receptors activity does not go back to healthy conditions in LID [126]. During L-DOPA treatment the expression of early genes like c-fos, c-jun and zif 268 is increased more than observed in dopaminergic denervation [55]. Furthermore the effect was mimetized [122] and synergized by D1 dopamine receptor agonists [130]. This suggested that the DA converted by L-DOPA treatment, activates D1 dopamine receptors producing high gene expression and translation, causing an overstimulation of the direct pathway [119]. The high activity of D1 dopamine receptors is also supported by the high expression of substance P and dynorphin both markers of direct pathway neurons [55].

The abnormal activation of the direct pathway with increased GABA release in SNr (related with the activation of the movement) could be occurring during LID as we mention before. The changes in GABA transmission is supported by studies in which has been shown altered metabolic activity measured by 2-deoxyglucose during LID in striato-nigral terminals [131] but also the increased expression of the enzymes responsible of synthesize GABA [132]. The mechanism underlying the increased GABA release in the striato-nigral neurons during LID has been studied by several groups of investigation [125, 128, 132-133] and some hypothesis has been proposed.

First was postulated that the increased GAD_{65} and GAD_{67} expression observed in denervation and L-DOPA treatment, induces an enhanced synthesis of GABA, which is available for the release [132, 134]. However the fact that GABA contents in SNr is not altered by denervation [135] indicates that the synthesis of GABA is not a simple cause-effect relationship.

Then, studies of D1 dopamine receptors signaling in the striato-nigral terminals turned to be the most studied and strong hypothesis. Since the level of expression of D1 dopamine receptors was contradictory and the down-regulation does not explain the hyperactivity of direct pathway, their signal transduction pathways had been dissected. Cai and coworkers (2002) [123] showed an increased coupling between D1 dopamine receptors and $G\alpha_{olf}$ proteins in hemiparkinsonian rats, but the level of protein expression of $G\alpha_{olf}$ remained unchanged. In contrast studies in postmortem patients with PD showed increased expression of $G\alpha_{olf}$ proteins [136] and the effect was also observed in hemiparkinsonian rats, interesting the effect was reverted by chronic but not acute L-DOPA treatment [134], which was also demonstrated in either mild or severe dyskinetic rats after chronic L-DOPA treatment [52]. Recent studies have shown a persistent increase in $G\alpha_{olf}$ expression in dyskinetic mice [59] however the reason for this discrepancy is unknown and requires more study.

In next steps downstream the activation of D1 receptors induces the activity of adenylyl cyclase isoform V by coupling of $G\alpha_{olf}$ protein, which in turn induces the production of a second messenger cAMP in striato-nigral neurons and PKA activation, supersensitivity of D1 receptors could be in these proteins. Since cAMP modulates firing rate and GABA release in striatum and SNr [113-114] and stimulates the protein kinase activated by cAMP (PKA) which in turn can produce several effects that are related with GABA release, a higher expression/or activity of adenylyl cyclase, PKA and DARPP-32 signaling was related with LID [54]. Consequent with the activation of D1 receptors Ras-mTOR-ERK induced altered mRNA translation was found in the nucleus striatum [57-58, 67, 120, 137]. However other studies have been suggested that ERK hypersensitivity is not related with cAMP/PKA signaling and this is a condition is needed for the development of LID, whereas hypersensitivity of cAMP/PKA has a permissive role [59]. Recent studies suggested that Shp-2 phosphatase is the link between D1 receptor activation and ERK, and that is persistent activated in LID [60]. Probably ERK supersentivity is related with control of the expression of proteins related with cAMP/PKA pathway supersensitivity. The activation of cAMP/PKA is the mechanism that conduces to the increased GABA release in the striato-nigral terminals of the direct pathway of basal ganglia since GABA release is highly sensitive to cAMP (Fig. 3) [114, 125] and the increased activity through the direct pathway is a necessary condition to produce the involuntary movements.

Rangel-Barajas and coworkers (2011) [52] have shown that a persistent increase in activity and expression of adenylyl cyclase V/VI occurs in LID animals without changes in activity of PKA of striato-nigral terminals. This change on the adenylyl cyclase V/VI is correlated with an increased GABA release in SNr in severe dyskinetic rats and did not happened in mild dyskinesia. It was also suggested an increased phosphorylation of DARPP-32 in Thr34 found in denervation and LID, this change cannot been associated exclusively with higher GABA release since not all GABA released in striatum by D1 receptor stimulation is related with DARPP-32, inferred from DARPP-32 know-out mice studies [138] and it's likely that the increased activity of adenylyl cyclase V could mediate the phosphorylation and therefore activation of DARPP-32 via PKA [139]. Thus a higher expression/activity of adenylyl cyclase seems to have a central role in the LID. Probably several beneficial effects that helps in experimental therapies to control LID can be related with antagonistic actions on adenylyl cyclase for example, $5HT_{1A}$ receptor activation, which modulates negatively AC by $G\alpha_i$ proteins reducing LID [96, 140], CB1 receptor also coupled to $G\alpha_i$ proteins decreased LID and PKA activation [141] and finally mGlu4 receptors modify also LID [142]. According with a recent study showed by single exon sequencing, that the only gene codifying for adenylyl cyclase V was mutated in a familiar form of dyskinesia [143]. Further *in vivo* studies are needed to targeting adenylyl cyclase V in LID, to asses if the therapeutic is plausible, since adenylyl cyclase V has a wide distribution and also plays an important role in cardiac function [144], anxiety modulated by D1 dopamine receptors [145] and depression [146]. This data suggested that the indirect modulation of the activity of adenylyl cyclase could be effective in LID.

In summary LID could represent an exaggerated supersitivity of D1 receptor response to the denervation induced by L-DOPA treatment leading to a pulsatile and high GABA release on striato-nigral terminals through the sensitization of adenylyl cyclase activity.

6. Role of D_3 dopamine receptors in Parkinson's disease

The D_3 dopamine receptors are expressed mostly in limbic system, islands of Calleja, olfactory bulb, and the pituitary intermediate lobe, with a low but significant expression in basal ganglia structures [147]. The amino acid sequence homology for the helical transmembrane spanning (TMS) segments of the D_2 and D_3 dopamine receptor subtypes was found to be 75-80%. Since the TMS regions are involved in the construction of the orthosteric-binding site, the pharmacologic profiles of D_2 and D_3 receptors are very similar [148-150]. Probably that is the reason why in PD the role of D_3 dopamine receptors were poorly studied. The pharmacological approach to treat PD besides L-DOPA was because D2-like dopamine agonist showed effectiveness to treat bradykinesia [151]. In the past two decades with advanced pharmacological and molecular tools, the role of D_3 dopamine receptors became a potential field of study in PD and LID animal models.

With very good agreement is known that during denervation, the D2-like dopamine receptors are up-regulated in pallido-nigral neurons of the basal ganglia [20], then it was unclear whether or not the D_3 dopamine receptors subtype was participating in the supersentitivity by dopamine denervation, however their low expression in striatum made focus the attention in D2 dopamine receptors [152]. It was pointed out that in the basal ganglia, the segregation of the expression of D1-like and D2-like dopamine receptors in the direct and indirect pathways respectively was not precisely accurate, but a relative low abundance of D_3 receptors were expressed also in the direct pathway [23]. Probably disease conditions enhance their expression, according with that; recently it has been shown that D_3 dopamine receptors are up-regulated in caudo-putamen and SNc in Lewy Body disease and Parkinson disease Dementia [153].

Bordet and coworkers (1997)[7] showed that mRNA codifying to D_3 dopamine receptors remains unchanged during dopamine denervation, but the L-DOPA treatment induces a remarkable increase in dynorphin positive striatal neurons, which project to the SNr where D_3 dopamine receptors normally has moderate expression. Interesting the binding for D_3 dopamine receptors was decreased in hemiparkinsonian rats [148,154] but up-regulated when animals were treated with L-DOPA [7]. Since then, the ectopic over-expression of D_3 dopamine receptors has been related with L-DOPA induced behavioral sensitization in hemiparkinsonian rats [119], and several studies support the idea that D_3 dopamine receptors can attenuate the LID by normalizing their function [8, 11, 120]. However the location of D_3 receptor sensitized by L-Dopa treatment is not clear. On the other hand D_3 dopamine receptors interact with proteins and/or form heterodimers with other receptors that can change signal pathways and responses, e.g. D_2/D_3, D_1/D_3 heterodimers [14-16]. Recently it has been shown that the up-regulation of D_2 dopamine receptors in denervated striatum is probably mediated by D_3 receptors through Ca^{2+} channels [155]. All these finding together shown that several changes in D_3 receptor expression and function can be related with Parkinson Disease and L-DOPA treatment.

7. D_1/D_3 dopamine receptors interaction in LID like a novel therapeutic target

D_3 receptors are members of the D2-like receptors are coupled to $G\alpha_i$ proteins [106]. It has been shown classical $G\alpha_i$ responses mediated by these receptors: inhibition of adenylyl cyclase, blockade of Ca^{2+} channels, open of K^+ channels etc [106]. However interaction with D1 receptors produces an antagonistic and synergistic response [14, 156]; that depends of the nuclei studied. In the antagonist interactions, D_3 receptors prevent D1 receptor stimulatory effects by the inhibition of adenylyl cyclase stimulated by D1 receptor, an interaction explained by cross-talk inhibition the AC activity. In the synergistic interaction D_3 receptors potentiates D_1 effects, and this interaction seems to be more complex and explained in terms of heterodimerization, where D_3 receptor induces an increased sensitivity of D1 receptor for dopamine, potentiating cAMP formation and stabilizing them in the membrane (Fig. 3) [15-16]. This synergistic interaction occurs at the striato-nigral pathway and it's regulated by CAMKIIα during neural activity [13-14].

D_3 receptors have been associated with different elements of the basal ganglia. The mRNA codifying for D_3 receptors have been shown in dopaminergic neurons [147], subthalamo-nigral neurons [30] and striato-nigral neurons [23]. In dopaminergic neurons D_3 receptors controls the firing rate and dopamine release [157] and has neurotrophic effects [158]; probably the decreased expression in D_3 receptors observed in dopaminergic denervation [148, 154] occurs by the degeneration of the dopaminergic neurons. Several studies have pointed out the importance of these receptors in nigral neurogenesis [158], neuro-protection and re-pair in PD [160] and other cognitive conditions related to PD [153].

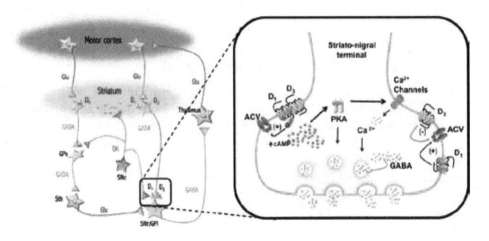

Figure 3. Synergistic and antagonistic interaction between D_1 and D_3 dopamine receptors in the striato-nigral neu-rons. Glu, glutamate; DA, dopamine; GPe, external globus pallidus; Sth, subthalamic nucleus, SNr, substantia nigra pars reticulata, GPi, internal globus pallidus; ACV, adenylyl cyclase V; PKA, protein kinase activated by cAMP.

In subthalamo-nigral neurons D_3 receptors are probably controlling the firing rate and gluta-mate release that have been attributed to members of the D2-like receptor family [31-32]. Since during denervation subthalamic neurons shown high activity rates and contribute to hypomotility, the D2-like agonist used in the control of Parkinson disease like pramipexole or ropirinole are able to decrease neuronal firing or glutamate release leading a clinical im-prove of symptoms. Interesting these D_3-preferring agonists decrease the dyskinesia.

As we mention D_3 receptors interact with D_1 receptors at striato-nigral neurons. The syner-gistic interaction has been shown in striatum [15-16] and substantia nigra on nerve terminals [14]. In the interaction D_3 receptors increases D_1 receptor affinity for dopamine, increasing cAMP formation and GABA release in striato-nigral terminals, this effect is very important since the higher release of GABA seems to mediate LID. Co-precipitation in native tissue and studies using transferred energy like FRET and BRET in heterologous expression system indicate that the heterodimerization is the cause for the observed effects [13-16].

The D_1/D_3 dopamine receptors interaction is important in dopaminergic denervation and L-DOPA treatment? The expression of D_3 receptors in the striato-nigral and subthalamo-nigral neurons leads the speculation that D_3 receptors are involved in the motor control by potentiation of GABA release stimulated by D1 receptors and inhibition of glutamate release leading to a decreased activity of the output neurons and increased activation of motor cortex. These effects are expected occur by the administration of L-DOPA and explain their powerful therapeutic effect; however the role of D_3 receptors in subthalamo nigral and D_1/D_3 interaction at striato-nigral neurons during denervation and L-DOPA treatment is unknown. However behavioral experiments suggested that D_3 dopamine receptor agonists potentiate the D1 receptor-induced rotation in hemiparkinsonian rats only after L-DOPA treatment [161] suggesting that the D_1/D_3 interaction persist.

Chronic L-DOPA therapy sensitizes D_3 receptor expression, which has been related with LID development and the therapeutic management was experimentally evaluated. Two current opinions are in literature, one proposed that the normalizing D_3 function decreases LID with partial agonists [8, 12], another one propose that antagonist also are able to do that [10-11] while other suggested that antagonist does not modify LID [9].

The mechanisms through D_3 dopamine receptors selective compounds can help to LID is still unclear, but recent studies have suggested that it could be due to a modulation of D1 dopamine receptors or direct actions on D_3 receptors. Albarran and coworkers [162] reported that activation of D_3 receptors in hemiparkinsonian dyskinetic rats prevents the D1 dopamine receptor stimulation of GABA release at striato-nigral terminals and the effect is mediated by an antagonist interaction between the receptors explained by a cross-talk as previously described [156]. This change in the D_1/D_3 relationship observed in dyskinesia with respect normal conditions could explain why D_3 receptor agonist prevents dyskinesia in L-DOPA treatment models, antagonizing adenylyl cyclase stimulated by D1 receptors and in consequence GABA release. This observation also suggested that the maintenance of the dyskinesia is due to the sensitization of the D1 receptor signaling pathway in the direct pathway that has been related with the LIDs [52]. If the heterodimeric interaction between D1 and D_3 receptor is modified by L-DOPA remains unclear and more studies are needed to clarify it. The effect of antagonist in LID need to be also clarified since current basal ganglia models does not predict the effect observed, also the wide expression of D_3 receptors in other brain areas can contribute to the observed effect. However all the studies suggest that the use of D_3 receptors ligands on LID is promising.

8. Conclusion

The D1 dopamine receptors supersensitivity in striato-nigral neurons are closely related with LID with a central role of adenylyl cyclase, co-expression of D_3 receptors with D1 receptors and the modifications of their interaction during experimental Parkinson and LID suggested a promissory therapeutical alternative in the management of motor disabilities related with L-DOPA administration.

Acknowledgements

The work was supported by a grant (152326) from CONACyT (México) to BF.

Author details

Sacnité Albarran Bravo[1], Claudia Rangel-Barajas[2] and Benjamín Florán Garduño[1]

1 Departamento de Fisiología, Biofísica y Neurociencias. Centro de Investigación y de Estudios Avanzados del Instituto Politécnico Nacional, Mexico

2 Department of Pharmacology & Neuroscience. University of North Texas Health Science Center, Fort Worth, USA

References

[1] Cotzias GC, Papavasiliou PS, Gellene R. L-dopa in parkinson's syndrome. N Engl J Med. 1969. p. 272.

[2] Yahr MD, Duvoisin RC. Medical therapy of Parkinsonism. Mod Treat. 1968. p. 283-300.

[3] Penney J, Young A. Speculations on the functional anatomy of basal ganglia disorders. Annual review of neuroscience. 1982. p. 73–94.

[4] Albin R, Young A, Penney J. The functional anatomy of basal ganglia disorders. Trends in neurosciences. 1989. p. 366–75.

[5] Obeso J, Rodríguez-Oroz M, Rodríguez M, Lanciego J, Artieda J, Gonzalo N, et al. Pathophysiology of the basal ganglia in Parkinson's disease. Trends in neurosciences. 2000. p. S8–19.

[6] Barroso-Chinea P, Bezard E. Basal Ganglia circuits underlying the pathophysiology of levodopa-induced dyskinesia. Frontiers in neuroanatomy. 2009.

[7] Bordet R, Ridray S, Carboni S, Diaz J, Sokoloff P, Schwartz J. Induction of dopamine D3 receptor expression as a mechanism of behavioral sensitization to levodopa. Proceedings of the National Academy of Sciences of the United States of America. 1997. p. 3363–7.

[8]   Bézard E, Ferry S, Mach U, Stark H, Leriche L, Boraud T, et al. Attenuation of levodo-
       pa-induced dyskinesia by normalizing dopamine D3 receptor function. Nature medi-
       cine. 2003. p. 762–7.

[9]   Mela F, Millan M, Brocco M, Morari M. The selective D(3) receptor antagonist,
       S33084, improves parkinsonian-like motor dysfunction but does not affect L-DOPA-
       induced dyskinesia in 6-hydroxydopamine hemi-lesioned rats. Neuropharmacology.
       2010. p. 528–36.

[10] Kumar R, Riddle L, Griffin S, Chu W, Vangveravong S, Neisewander J, et al. Evalua-
       tion of D2 and D3 dopamine receptor selective compounds on L-dopa-dependent ab-
       normal involuntary movements in rats. Neuropharmacology. 2009. p. 956–69.

[11] Kumar R, Riddle L, Griffin S, Grundt P, Newman A, Luedtke R. Evaluation of the D3
       dopamine receptor selective antagonist PG01037 on L-dopa-dependent abnormal in-
       voluntary movements in rats. Neuropharmacology. 2009. p. 944–55.

[12] Riddle L, Kumar R, Griffin S, Grundt P, Newman A, Luedtke R. Evaluation of the D3
       dopamine receptor selective agonist/partial agonist PG01042 on L-dopa dependent
       animal involuntary movements in rats.Neuropharmacology. 2010. p. 284–94.

[13] Avalos-Fuentes A, Loya-López S, Flores-Pérez A, Recillas-Morales S, Cortés H, Paz-
       Bermúdez F, et al. Presynaptic CaMKIIα modulates dopamine D3 receptor activation
       in striatonigral terminals of the rat brain in a Ca2+ dependent manner. Neurophar-
       macology. 2013. p. 273–81.

[14] Cruz-Trujillo R, Avalos-Fuentes A, Rangel-Barajas C, Paz-Bermúdez F, Sierra A, Es-
       cartín-Perez E, et al. D3 dopamine receptors interact with dopamine D1 but not D4
       receptors in the GABAergic terminals of the SNr of the rat. Neuropharmacology.
       2013. p. 370–8.

[15] Fiorentini C, Busi C, Gorruso E, Gotti C, Spano P, Missale C. Reciprocal regulation of
       dopamine D1 and D3 receptor function and trafficking by heterodimerization. Mo-
       lecular pharmacology. 2008. p. 59–69.

[16] Marcellino D, Ferré S, Casadó V, Cortés A, Le Foll B, Mazzola C, et al. Identification
       of dopamine D1-D3 receptor heteromers. Indications for a role of synergistic D1-D3
       receptor interactions in the striatum. The Journal of biological chemistry. 2008. p.
       26016–25.

[17] Alexander GE, Crutcher MD.Functional architecture of basal ganglia circuits: neural
       substrates of parallel processing. Trends Neurosci. 1990. p. 266-71.

[18] Prensa L, Cossette M, Parent A. Dopaminergic innervation of human basal ganglia.
       Journal of chemical neuroanatomy. 2000. p. 207–13.

[19] Floran, B., Aceves, J., Sierra, A. & Martinez-Fong, D. Activation of D1 dopamine re-
       ceptors stimulates the release of GABA in the basal ganglia of the rat. Neurosci Lett.
       1990. p. 136-40.

[20] Gerfen CR, Engber TM, Mahan LC, Susel Z, Chase TN, Monsma FJ Jr, Sibley DR. D1 and D2 dopamine receptor-regulated gene expression of striatonigral and striatopallidal neurons. Science. 1990. p. 1429-32.

[21] Hernández-López S, Bargas J, Surmeier DJ, Reyes A, Galarraga E. D1 receptor activation enhances evoked discharge in neostriatal medium spiny neurons by modulating an L-type Ca2+ conductance. J Neurosci. 1997. p. 3334-42.

[22] Radnikow G, Misgeld U. Dopamine D1 receptors facilitate GABAA synaptic currents in the rat substantia nigra pars reticulata. J Neurosci. 1998. p. 2009-16.

[23] Surmeier D, Bargas J, Hemmings H, Nairn A, Greengard P. Modulation of calcium currents by a D1 dopaminergic protein kinase/phosphatase cascade in rat neostriatal neurons. Neuron. 1995. p. 385–97.

[24] Hernandez-Lopez S, Tkatch T, Perez-Garci E, Galarraga E, Bargas J, Hamm H, et al. D2 dopamine receptors in striatal medium spiny neurons reduce L-type Ca2+ currents and excitability via a novel PLC[beta]1-IP3-calcineurin-signaling cascade. The Journal of neuroscience: the official journal of the Society for Neuroscience. 2000. p. 8987–95.

[25] Floran B, Floran L, Sierra A, Aceves J. D2 receptor-mediated inhibition of GABA release by endogenous dopamine in the rat globus pallidus. Neuroscience letters. 1997. p. 1–4

[26] Cooper A, Stanford I. Dopamine D2 receptor mediated presynaptic inhibition of striatopallidal GABA(A) IPSCs in vitro. Neuropharmacology. 2001. p. 62–71.

[27] Ariano M, Wang J, Noblett K, Larson E, Sibley D. Cellular distribution of the rat D4 dopamine receptor protein in the CNS using anti-receptor antisera. Brain research. 1997. p. 26–34.

[28] Acosta-García J, Hernández-Chan N, Paz-Bermúdez F, Sierra A, Erlij D, Aceves J, et al. D4 and D1 dopamine receptors modulate [3H]GABA release in the substantia nigra pars reticulata of the rat. Neuropharmacology. 2009. p. 725-730.

[29] Gasca-Martinez D, Hernandez A, Sierra A, Valdiosera R, Anaya-Martinez V, Floran B, Erlij D, Aceves J. Dopamine inhibits GABA transmission from the globus pallidus to the thalamic reticular nucleus via presynaptic D4 receptors. Neuroscience. 2010. p. 1672-1681.

[30] Flores G, Liang J, Sierra A, Martínez-Fong D, Quirion R, Aceves J, et al. Expression of dopamine receptors in the subthalamic nucleus of the rat: characterization using reverse transcriptase-polymerase chain reaction and autoradiography. Neuroscience. 1998. p. 549–56.

[31] Ibañez-Sandoval O, Hernández A, Florán B, Galarraga E, Tapia D, Valdiosera R, et al. Control of the subthalamic innervation of substantia nigra pars reticulata by D1 and D2 dopamine receptors. Journal of neurophysiology. 2006. p. 1800–11.

[32] Shen K-Z, Johnson S. Regulation of polysynaptic subthalamonigral transmission by D2, D3 and D4 dopamine receptors in rat brain slices. The Journal of physiology. 2012. p. 2273–84.

[33] Anderson E, Nutt J. The long-duration response to levodopa: phenomenology, potential mechanisms and clinical implications. Parkinsonism & related disorders. 2011. p. 587–92.

[34] Lopez A, Muñoz A, Guerra M, Labandeira-Garcia J. Mechanisms of the effects of exogenous levodopa on the dopamine-denervated striatum. Neuroscience. 2000. p. 639–51.

[35] Tanaka H, Kannari K, Maeda T, Tomiyama M, Suda T, Matsunaga M. Role of serotonergic neurons in L-DOPA-derived extracellular dopamine in the striatum of 6-OHDA-lesioned rats. Neuroreport. 1999. p. 631–4.

[36] Navailles S, Bioulac B, Gross C, De Deurwaerdère P. Serotonergic neurons mediate ectopic release of dopamine induced by L-DOPA in a rat model of Parkinson's disease. Neurobiology of disease. 2010. p. 136–43.

[37] Misu Y, Goshima Y, Ueda H, Okamura H. Neurobiology of L-DOPAergic systems. Progress in neurobiology. 1996. p. 415–54.

[38] Silva I, Cortes H, Escartín E, Rangel C, Florán L, Erlij D, et al. L-DOPA inhibits depolarization-induced [3H]GABA release in the dopamine-denervated globus pallidus of the rat: the effect is dopamine independent and mediated by D2-like receptors. Journal of neural transmission. 2006. p. 1847–53.

[39] Yue J, Nakamura S, Ueda H, Misu Y. Endogenously released L-dopa itself tonically functions to potentiate postsynaptic D2 receptor-mediated locomotor activities of conscious rats. Neuroscience letters. 1994. p. 107–10.

[40] Nakamura S, Yue J, Goshima Y, Miyamae... T. Non-effective dose of exogenously applied l-DOPA itself stereoselectively potentiates postsynaptic D2 receptor-mediated locomotor activities of ... 1994.

[41] Nakazato T, Akiyama A. Behavioral activity and stereotypy in rats induced by L-DOPA metabolites: a possible role in the adverse effects of chronic L-DOPA treatment of Parkinson's disease. Brain research. 2002. p. 134–42.

[42] Alachkar A, Brotchie J, Jones O. Locomotor response to L-DOPA in reserpine-treated rats following central inhibition of aromatic L-amino acid decarboxylase: further evidence for non-dopaminergic actions of L-DOPA and its metabolites. Neuroscience research. 2010. p. 44–50.

[43] Fisher A, Biggs C, Eradiri O, Starr M. Dual effects of L-3,4-dihydroxyphenylalanine on aromatic L-amino acid decarboxylase, dopamine release and motor stimulation in the reserpine-treated rat: evidence that behaviour is dopamine independent. Neuroscience. 1999. p. 97–111.

[44] Mercuri N, Bernardi G. The "magic" of L-dopa: why is it the gold standard Parkinson's disease therapy? Trends in pharmacological sciences. 2005. p. 341–4.

[45] Nadjar A, Gerfen C, Bezard E. Priming for l-dopa-induced dyskinesia in Parkinson's disease: a feature inherent to the treatment or the disease? Progress in neurobiology. 2009. p. 1–9.

[46] Müller T, Woitalla D, Russ H, Hock K, Haeger D. Prevalence and treatment strategies of dyskinesia in patients with Parkinson's disease. Journal of neural transmission. 2006. p. 1023–6.

[47] Sharma J, Bachmann C, Linazasoro G. Classifying risk factors for dyskinesia in Parkinson's disease. Parkinsonism & related disorders. 2010. p. 490–7

[48] Cerasa A, Salsone M, Morelli M, Pugliese P, Arabia G, Gioia C, et al. Age at onset influences neurodegenerative processes underlying PD with levodopa-induced dyskinesias. Parkinsonism & related disorders. 2013.

[49] Guridi J, González-Redondo R, Obeso J. Clinical features, pathophysiology, and treatment of levodopa-induced dyskinesias in Parkinson's disease. Parkinson's disease. 2011. p. 943159.

[50] Iderberg H, Francardo V, Pioli E. Animal models of L-DOPA-induced dyskinesia: an update on the current options. Neuroscience. 2012. p. 13–27.

[51] Johnston T, Lane E. Experimental Models of l-DOPA-Induced Dyskinesia. International review of neurobiology. 2010. p. 55–93.

[52] Rangel-Barajas C, Silva I, Lopéz-Santiago L, Aceves J, Erlij D, Florán B. L-DOPA-induced dyskinesia in hemiparkinsonian rats is associated with up-regulation of adenylyl cyclase type V/VI and increased GABA release in the substantia nigra reticulata. Neurobiology of disease. 2010. p. 51–61.

[53] Buck K, Ferger B. Intrastriatal inhibition of aromatic amino acid decarboxylase prevents l-DOPA-induced dyskinesia: a bilateral reverse in vivo microdialysis study in 6-hydroxydopamine lesioned rats. Neurobiology of disease. 2008. p. 210–20.

[54] Napolitano M, Centonze D, Calce A, Picconi B, Spiezia S, Gulino A, et al. Experimental parkinsonism modulates multiple genes involved in the transduction of dopaminergic signals in the striatum. Neurobiology of disease. 2002. p. 387–95.

[55] Cenci M, Lee C, Björklund A. L-DOPA-induced dyskinesia in the rat is associated with striatal overexpression of prodynorphin- and glutamic acid decarboxylase mRNA. The European journal of neuroscience. 1998. p. 2694–706.

[56] Aubert I, Guigoni C, Håkansson K, Li Q, Dovero S, Barthe N, et al. Increased D1 dopamine receptor signaling in levodopa-induced dyskinesia. Annals of neurology. 2004. p. 17–26.

[57] Santini E, Valjent E, Usiello A, Carta M, Borgkvist A, Girault J-A, et al. Critical involvement of cAMP/DARPP-32 and extracellular signal-regulated protein kinase sig-

naling in L-DOPA-induced dyskinesia. The Journal of neuroscience⊚: the official journal of the Society for Neuroscience. 2007. p. 6995–7005.

[58] Lebel M, Chagniel L, Bureau G, Cyr M. Striatal inhibition of PKA prevents levodopa-induced behavioural and molecular changes in the hemiparkinsonian rat. Neurobiology of disease. 2010. p. 59–67.

[59] Alcacer C, Santini E, Valjent E, Gaven F, Girault J-A, Hervé D. Gα(olf) mutation allows parsing the role of cAMP-dependent and extracellular signal-regulated kinase-dependent signaling in L-3,4-dihydroxyphenylalanine-induced dyskinesia. The Journal of neuroscience⊚: the official journal of the Society for Neuroscience. 2012. p. 5900–10.

[60] Fiorentini C, Savoia P, Savoldi D, Barbon A, Missale C. Persistent activation of the D1R/Shp-2/Erk1/2 pathway in l-DOPA-induced dyskinesia in the 6-hydroxy-dopamine rat model of Parkinson's disease. Neurobiology of disease. 2013. p. 339–48.

[61] Pavón N, Martín A, Mendialdua A, Moratalla R. ERK phosphorylation and FosB expression are associated with L-DOPA-induced dyskinesia in hemiparkinsonian mice. Biological psychiatry. 2005. p. 64–74.

[62] Valastro B, Andersson M, Lindgren H, Cenci M. Expression pattern of JunD after acute or chronic L-DOPA treatment: comparison with deltaFosB. Neuroscience. 2007. p. 198–207.

[63] Berton O, Guigoni C, Li Q, Bioulac B, Aubert I, Gross C, et al. Striatal overexpression of DeltaJunD resets L-DOPA-induced dyskinesia in a primate model of Parkinson disease. Biological psychiatry. 2009. p. 554–61.

[64] Cao X, Yasuda T, Uthayathas S, Watts R, Mouradian M, Mochizuki H, et al. Striatal overexpression of DeltaFosB reproduces chronic levodopa-induced involuntary movements. The Journal of neuroscience. 2010. p. 7335–43.

[65] Carta A, Frau L, Pinna A, Morelli M. Dyskinetic potential of dopamine agonists is associated with different striatonigral/striatopallidal zif-268 expression. Experimental neurology. 2010. p. 395–402.

[66] Darmopil S, Martín A, De Diego I, Ares S, Moratalla R. Genetic inactivation of dopamine D1 but not D2 receptors inhibits L-DOPA-induced dyskinesia and histone activation. Biological psychiatry. 2009. p. 603–13.

[67] Santini E, Heiman M, Greengard P, Valjet E, Fisone, G. Inhibition of mTOR signaling in Parkinson's disease prevents L-DOPA-induced dyskinesia. Neuroscience. 2009.

[68] Mela F, Marti M, Bido S, Cenci M, Morari M. In vivo evidence for a differential contribution of striatal and nigral D1 and D2 receptors to L-DOPA induced dyskinesia and the accompanying surge of nigral amino acid levels. Neurobiology of disease. 2011. p. 573–82.

[69] Kovoor A, Seyffarth P, Ebert J, Barghshoon S, Chen C-K, Schwarz S, et al. D2 dopa-
      mine receptors colocalize regulator of G-protein signaling 9-2 (RGS9-2) via the RGS9
      DEP domain, and RGS9 knock-out mice develop dyskinesias associated with dopa-
      mine pathways. The Journal of neuroscience. 2005. p. 2157–65.

[70] Gold S, Hoang C, Potts B, Porras G, Pioli E, Kim K, et al. RGS9-2 negatively modu-
      lates L-3,4-dihydroxyphenylalanine-induced dyskinesia in experimental Parkinson's
      disease. The Journal of neuroscience. 2007. p. 14338–48.

[71] Yin L-L, Geng X-C, Zhu X-Z. The involvement of RGS9 in l-3,4-dihydroxyphenylala-
      nine-induced dyskinesias in unilateral 6-OHDA lesion rat model. Brain research bul-
      letin. 2011. p. 367–72.

[72] Blanchet PJ, Boucher R, Bédard PJ. Excitotoxic lateral pallidotomy does not relieve L-
      dopa-induced dyskinesia in MPTP parkinsonian monkeys. Brain Res. 1994. p. 32-9.

[73] Taylor J, Bishop C, Walker P. Dopamine D1 and D2 receptor contributions to L-
      DOPA-induced dyskinesia in the dopamine-depleted rat. Pharmacology, biochemis-
      try, and behavior. 2005. p. 887–93.

[74] Li L, Zhou F-M. Parallel dopamine D1 receptor activity dependence of l-Dopa-in-
      duced normal movement and dyskinesia in mice. Neuroscience. 2013. p. 66–76.

[75] Suárez L, Solís O, Caramés J, Taravini I, Solís J, Murer M, et al. L-DOPA Treatment
      Selectively Restores Spine Density in Dopamine Receptor D2-Expressing Projection
      Neurons in Dyskinetic Mice. Biological psychiatry. 2013.

[76] Calon F, Dridi M, Hornykiewicz O, Bédard P, Rajput A, Di Paolo T. Increased adeno-
      sine A2A receptors in the brain of Parkinson's disease patients with dyskinesias.
      Brain. 2004. p. 1075–84.

[77] Antonelli T, Fuxe K, Agnati L, Mazzoni E, Tanganelli S, Tomasini M, et al. Experi-
      mental studies and theoretical aspects on A2A/D2 receptor interactions in a model of
      Parkinson's disease. Relevance for L-dopa induced dyskinesias. Journal of the neuro-
      logical sciences. 2006. p. 16–22.

[78] Jenner P. Molecular mechanisms of L-DOPA-induced dyskinesia. Nature reviews.
      Neuroscience. 2008. p. 665–77.

[79] Arai A, Kannari K, Shen H, Maeda T, Suda T, Matsunaga M. Amantadine increases
      L-DOPA-derived extracellular dopamine in the striatum of 6-hydroxydopamine-le-
      sioned rats. Brain research. 2003. p. 229–34.

[80] Dunah A, Standaert D. Dopamine D1 receptor-dependent trafficking of striatal
      NMDA glutamate receptors to the postsynaptic membrane. The Journal of neuro-
      science®: the official journal of the Society for Neuroscience. 2001. p. 5546–58.

[81] Gardoni F, Picconi B, Ghiglieri V, Polli F, Bagetta V, Bernardi G, et al. A critical interaction between NR2B and MAGUK in L-DOPA induced dyskinesia. The Journal of
neuroscience. 2006. p. 2914–22.

[82] Blank T, Nijholt I, Teichert U, Kügler... H. The phosphoprotein DARPP-32 mediates
cAMP-dependent potentiation of striatal N-methyl-D-aspartate responses 1997.

[83] Flores-Hernandez J, Hernandez S, Snyder G, Yan Z, Fienberg A, Moss S, et al. D(1)
dopamine receptor activation reduces GABA(A) receptor currents in neostriatal neurons through a PKA/DARPP-32/PP1 signaling cascade. Journal of neurophysiology.
2000. p. 2996–3004.

[84] Lee F, Liu F. Direct interactions between NMDA and D1 receptors: a tale of tails. Biochemical Society transactions. 2004. p. 1032–6.

[85] Oh J, Russell D, Vaughan C, Chase T, Russell D. Enhanced tyrosine phosphorylation
of striatal NMDA receptor subunits: effect of dopaminergic denervation and L-
DOPA administration. Brain research. 1998. p. 150–9.

[86] Picconi B, Centonze D, Håkansson K, Bernardi G, Greengard P, Fisone G, et al. Loss
of bidirectional striatal synaptic plasticity in L-DOPA-induced dyskinesia. Nature
neuroscience. 2003. p. 501–6.

[87] Nash J, Johnston T, Collingridge G, Garner C, Brotchie J. Subcellular redistribution of
the synapse-associated proteins PSD-95 and SAP97 in animal models of Parkinson's
disease and L-DOPA-induced dyskinesia. FASEB journal: official publication of the
Federation of American Societies for Experimental Biology. 2005. p. 583–5.

[88] Gardoni F, Picconi B, Ghiglieri V, Polli F, Bagetta V, Bernardi G, et al. A critical interaction between NR2B and MAGUK in L-DOPA induced dyskinesia. The Journal of
neuroscience: the official journal of the Society for Neuroscience. 2006. p. 2914–22

[89] Gardoni F. MAGUK proteins: new targets for pharmacological intervention in the
glutamatergic synapse.Eur J Pharmacol. 2008. p. 147-52.

[90] Fiorentini C, Busi C, Spano P, Missale C. Role of receptor heterodimers in the development of L-dopa-induced dyskinesias in the 6-hydroxydopamine rat model of Parkinson's disease. Parkinsonism & related disorders. 2007. p. S159–64.

[91] Prescott I, Dostrovsky J, Moro E, Hodaie M, Lozano A, Hutchison W. Levodopa enhances synaptic plasticity in the substantia nigra pars reticulata of Parkinson's disease patients. Brain: a journal of neurology. 2009. p. 309–18.

[92] Arai R, Karasawa N, Geffard M, Nagatsu T, Nagatsu I. Immunohistochemical evidence that central serotonin neurons produce dopamine from exogenous L-DOPA in
the rat, with reference to the involvement of aromatic L-amino acid decarboxylase.
Brain Res. 1994. p. 295-9.

[93] Yamada H, Aimi Y, Nagatsu I, Taki K, Kudo M, Arai R. Immunohistochemical detection of L-DOPA-derived dopamine within serotonergic fibers in the striatum and the

substantia nigra pars reticulata in Parkinsonian model rats. Neuroscience research. 2007. p. 1–7

[94] Carta M, Carlsson T, Muñoz A, Kirik D, Björklund A. Involvement of the serotonin system in L-dopa-induced dyskinesias. Parkinsonism & related disorders. 2007. p. S154–8.

[95] Bishop C, George J, Buchta W, Goldenberg A, Mohamed M, Dickinson S, et al. Serotonin transporter inhibition attenuates l-DOPA-induced dyskinesia without compromising l-DOPA efficacy in hemi-parkinsonian rats. The European journal of neuroscience. 2012. p. 2839–48.

[96] Dupre K, Eskow K, Barnum C, Bishop C. Striatal 5-HT1A receptor stimulation reduces D1 receptor-induced dyskinesia and improves movement in the hemiparkinsonian rat. Neuropharmacology. 2008. p. 1321–8.

[97] Brotchie J. Adjuncts to dopamine replacement: a pragmatic approach to reducing the problem of dyskinesia in Parkinson's disease. Movement disorders⊚: official journal of the Movement Disorder Society. 1998. p. 871–6.

[98] Henry B, Duty S, Fox S, Crossman A, Brotchie J. Increased striatal pre-proenkephalin B expression is associated with dyskinesia in Parkinson's disease. Experimental neurology. 2003. p. 458–68.

[99] Chen L, Togasaki D, Langston J, Di Monte D, Quik M. Enhanced striatal opioid receptor-mediated G-protein activation in L-DOPA-treated dyskinetic monkeys. Neuroscience. 2004. p. 409–20.

[100] Klintenberg R, Svenningsson P, Gunne L, Andrén PE. Naloxone reduces levodopa-induced dyskinesias and apomorphine-induced rotations in primate models of parkinsonism. J Neural Transm. 2002. p. 1295-307.

[101] Samadi P, Grégoire L, Bédard PJ. Opioid antagonists increase the dyskinetic response to dopaminergic agents in parkinsonian monkeys: interaction between dopamine and opioid systems. Neuropharmacology. 2003. p. 954-63.

[102] Billet F, Costentin J, Dourmap N. Influence of corticostriatal δ-opioid receptors on abnormal involuntary movements induced by L-DOPA in hemiparkinsonian rats. Experimental neurology. 2012. p. 339–50.

[103] Buck K, Ferger B. Comparison of intrastriatal administration of noradrenaline and l-DOPA on dyskinetic movements: a bilateral reverse in vivo microdialysis study in 6-hydroxydopamine-lesioned rats. Neuroscience. 2009. p. 16-20.

[104] Wang Q, Jolly JP, Surmeier JD, Mullah BM, Lidow MS, Bergson CM, Robishaw JD. Differential dependence of the D1 and D5 dopamine receptors on the G protein gamma 7 subunit for activation of adenylylcyclase. J Biol Chem. 2001. p. 39386-93.

[105] Undieh A. Pharmacology of signaling induced by dopamine D(1)-like receptor activation. Pharmacology & therapeutics. 2010. p. 37–60.

[106] Neve KA, Seamans JK, Trantham-Davidson H. Dopamine Receptor Signaling. Journal of Receptor and Signal Transduction Research. 2004. p. 165-205

[107] Zhuang X, Belluscio L, Hen R. G(olf)alpha mediates dopamine D1 receptor signaling.J Neurosci. 2000. p. RC91.

[108] Tesmer JJ, Sunahara RK, Gilman AG, Sprang SR. Crystal structure of the catalytic domains of adenylyl cyclase in a complex with Gsalpha.GTPgammaS. Science. 1997. p. 1907-16.

[109] Chen J, Rusnak M, Lombroso PJ, Sidhu A. Dopamine promotes striatal neuronal apoptotic death via ERK signaling cascades. Eur J Neurosci. 2009. p. 287-306.

[110] Fuxe K, Ferré S, Zoli M, Agnati L. Integrated events in central dopamine transmission as analyzed at multiple levels. Evidence for intramembrane adenosine A2A dopamine D2... 1998.

[111] Yan Z, Surmeier D. D5 dopamine receptors enhance Zn2+-sensitive GABA(A) currents in striatal cholinergic interneurons through a PKA/PP1 cascade. Neuron. 1997. p. 1115–26.

[112] Perreault M, Hasbi A, O'Dowd B, George S. The dopamine d1-d2 receptor heteromer in striatal medium spiny neurons: evidence for a third distinct neuronal pathway in Basal Ganglia. Frontiers in neuroanatomy. 2010. p. 31.

[113] Arias-Montaño J-A, Floran B, Floran L, Aceves J, Young J. Dopamine D(1) receptor facilitation of depolarization-induced release of gamma-amino-butyric acid in rat striatum is mediated by the cAMP/PKA pathway and involves P/Q-type calcium channels. Synapse (New York, N.Y.). 2007. p. 310–9.

[114] Nava-Asbell C, Paz-Bermudez F, Erlij D, Aceves J, Florán B. GABA(B) receptor activation inhibits dopamine D1 receptor-mediated facilitation of [(3)H]GABA release in substantia nigra pars reticulata. Neuropharmacology. 2007. p. 631-7.

[115] Surmeier D, Bargas J, Hemmings H, Nairn A, Greengard P. Modulation of calcium currents by a D1 dopaminergic protein kinase/phosphatase cascade in rat neostriatal neurons. Neuron. 1995. p. 385–97.

[116] Sánchez L, Recillas S, Caballero R, Sierra A, Erlij D, Aceves J, Floran B. Dopamine modulates GABA release in striato-nigral, pallido-nigral and striato-pallidal terminals regulating L-type calcium chennels. Sc Neursc Abstr 470.01/GGG1. 2013.

[117] Blum D, Torch S, Lambeng N, Nissou M, Benabid AL, Sadoul R, Verna JM. Molecular pathways involved in the neurotoxicity of 6-OHDA, dopamine and MPTP: contribution to the apoptotic theory in Parkinson's disease. Prog Neurobiol. 2001. p. 135-72.

[118] Blandini F, Armentero MT, Martignoni E. The 6-hydroxydopamine model: news from the past. Parkinsonism Relat Disord. 2008. p. S124-9.

[119] Bordet R, Ridray S, Schwartz J, Sokoloff P. Involvement of the direct striatonigral pathway in levodopa-induced sensitization in 6-hydroxydopamine-lesioned rats. The European journal of neuroscience. 2000. p. 2117–23.

[120] Feyder M, Bonito-Oliva A, Fisone G. L-DOPA-Induced Dyskinesia and Abnormal Signaling in Striatal Medium Spiny Neurons: Focus on Dopamine D1 Receptor-Mediated Transmission. Front Behav Neurosci. 2011. p. 71.

[121] Sivam SP. Dopamine dependent decrease in enkephalin and substance P levels in basal ganglia regions of postmortem parkinsonian brains. Neuropeptides. 1991. p. 201-7.

[122] Berke JD, Paletzki RF, Aronson GJ, Hyman SE, Gerfen CR. A complex program of striatal gene expression induced by dopaminergic stimulation. J Neurosci. 1998. p. 5301-10.

[123] Cai G, Wang HY, Friedman E. Increased dopamine receptor signaling and dopamine receptor-G protein coupling in denervated striatum. J Pharmacol Exp Ther. 2002. p. 1105-12.

[124] Marshall JF, Navarrete R, Joyce JN. Decreased striatal D1 binding density following mesotelencephalic 6-hydroxydopamine injections: an autoradiographic analysis. Brain Res. 1989. p. 247-57.

[125] Rangel-Barajas C, Silva I, García-Ramírez M, Sánchez-Lemus E, Floran L, Aceves J, et al. 6-OHDA-induced hemiparkinsonism and chronic L-DOPA treatment increase dopamine D1-stimulated [(3)H]-GABA release and [(3)H]-cAMP production in substantia nigra pars reticulata of the rat. Neuropharmacology. 2008. p. 704–11.

[126] Berthet A, Bezard E, Porras G, Fasano S, Barroso-Chinea P, Dehay B, et al. L-DOPA impairs proteasome activity in parkinsonism through D1 dopamine receptor. The Journal of neuroscience. 2012. p. 681–91.

[127] Gerfen CR, Miyachi S, Paletzki R, Brown P. D1 dopamine receptor supersensitivity in the dopamine-depleted striatum results from a switch in the regulation of ERK1/2/MAP kinase. J Neurosci. 2002. p. 5042-54.

[128] Ochi M, Shiozaki S, Kase H. L-DOPA-induced modulation of GABA and glutamate release in substantia nigra pars reticulata in a rodent model of Parkinson's disease. Synapse. 2004. p. 163-5.

[129] Yamamoto N, Pierce R, Soghomonian J-J. Subchronic administration of L-DOPA to adult rats with a unilateral 6-hydroxydopamine lesion of dopamine neurons results in a sensitization of enhanced GABA release in the substantia nigra, pars reticulata. Brain research. 2006. p. 196–200.

[130] St-Hilaire M, Landry E, Lévesque D, Rouillard C. Denervation and repeated L-DOPA induce complex regulatory changes in neurochemical phenotypes of striatal neurons: implication of a dopamine D1-dependent mechanism. Neurobiol Dis. 2005. p. 450-60.

[131] Bezard E, Brotchie JM, Gross CE. Pathophysiology of levodopa-induced dyskinesia: potential for new therapies. Nat Rev Neurosci. 2001. p. 577-88.

[132] Katz J, Nielsen K, Soghomonian J-J. Comparative effects of acute or chronic administration of levodopa to 6-hydroxydopamine-lesioned rats on the expression of glutamic acid decarboxylase in the neostriatum and GABAA receptors subunits in the substantia nigra, pars reticulata. Neuroscience. 2004. p. 833–42

[133] Mela F, Marti M, Dekundy A, Danysz W, Morari M, Cenci MA. Antagonism of metabotropic glutamate receptor type 5 attenuates l-DOPA-induced dyskinesia and its molecular and neurochemical correlates in a rat model of Parkinson's disease. J Neurochem. 2007. p. 483-97.

[134] Carta AR, Fenu S, Pala P, Tronci E, Morelli M. Selective modifications in GAD67 mRNA levels in striatonigral and striatopallidal pathways correlate to dopamine agonist priming in 6-hydroxydopamine-lesioned rats. European Journal of Neuroscience. 2003. p. 2563-2572.

[135] Aceves J, Floran B, Garcia M. D1 Receptor Mediated Trophic Action of Dopamine on the Synthesis of GABA at the Terminals of Striatal Projections. Advances in Behavioral Biology. 1994. p. 421-427.

[136] Corvol J-C, Muriel M-P, Valjent E, Féger J, Hanoun N, Girault J-A, et al. Persistent increase in olfactory type G-protein alpha subunit levels may underlie D1 receptor functional hypersensitivity in Parkinson disease. The Journal of neuroscience®. 2004. p. 7007–14

[137] Subramaniam S, Napolitano F, Mealer R, Kim S, Errico F, Barrow R, et al. Rhes, a striatal-enriched small G protein, mediates mTOR signaling and L-DOPA-induced dyskinesia. Nature neuroscience. 2012. p. 191–3.

[138] Fienberg AA, Hiroi N, Mermelstein PG, Song W, Snyder GL, Nishi A, Cheramy A, O'Callaghan JP, Miller DB, Cole DG, Corbett R, Haile CN, Cooper DC, Onn SP, Grace AA, Ouimet CC, White FJ, Hyman SE, Surmeier DJ, Girault J, Nestler EJ, Greengard P. DARPP-32: regulator of the efficacy of dopaminergic neurotransmission. Science. 1998. p. 838-42.

[139] Nishi A, Kuroiwa M, Shuto T. Mechanisms for the modulation of dopamine d(1) receptor signaling in striatal neurons. Frontiers in neuroanatomy. 2010. p. 43.

[140] Ba M, Kong M, Ma G, Yang H, Lu G, Chen S, et al. Cellular and behavioral effects of 5-HT1A receptor agonist 8-OH-DPAT in a rat model of levodopa-induced motor complications. Brain research. 2007. p. 177–84.

[141] Martinez A, Macheda T, Morgese M, Trabace L, Giuffrida A. The cannabinoid ago-nist WIN55212-2 decreases L-DOPA-induced PKA activation and dyskinetic behav-ior in 6-OHDA-treated rats. Neuroscience research. 2012. p. 236–42.

[142] Bennouar K-E, Uberti M, Melon C, Bacolod M, Jimenez H, Cajina M, et al. Synergy between L-DOPA and a novel positive allosteric modulator of metabotropic gluta-mate receptor 4: implications for Parkinson's disease treatment and dyskinesia. Neu-ropharmacology. 2013. p. 158–69.

[143] Chen YZ, Matsushita MM, Robertson P, Rieder M, Girirajan S, Antonacci F, Lipe H, Eichler EE, Nickerson DA, Bird TD, Raskind WH. Autosomal dominant familial dys-kinesia and facial myokymia: single exome sequencing identifies a mutation in ade-nylyl cyclase 5. Arch Neurol. 2012. p. 630-5.

[144] Vatner SF, Park M, Yan L, Lee GJ, Lai L, Iwatsubo K, Ishikawa Y, Pessin J, Vatner DE. Adenylyl cyclase type 5 in cardiac disease, metabolism, and aging. Am J Physiol Heart Circ Physiol. 2013. p. H1-8.

[145] Kim KS, Lee KW, Baek IS, Lim CM, Krishnan V, Lee JK, Nestler EJ, Han PL. Adenyl-yl cyclase-5 activity in the nucleus accumbens regulates anxiety-related behavior. J Neurochem. 2008. p. 105-15.

[146] Krishnan V, Graham A, Mazei-Robison MS, Lagace DC, Kim KS, Birnbaum S, Eisch AJ, Han PL, Storm DR, Zachariou V, Nestler EJ. Calcium-sensitive adenylyl cyclases in depression and anxiety: behavioral and biochemical consequences of isoform tar-geting. Biol Psychiatry. 2008. p. 336-43.

[147] Levant B. Differential distribution of D3 dopamine receptors in the brains of several mammalian species. Brain Res. 1998. p. 269-74.

[148] Sokoloff P, Giros B, Martres MP, Bouthenet ML, Schwartz JC. Molecular cloning and characterization of a novel dopamine receptor (D3) as a target for neuroleptics. Na-ture. 1990. p. 146-51.

[149] Luedtke RR, Artymyshyn RP, Monks BR, Molinoff PB. Comparison of the expres-sion, transcription and genomic organization of D2 dopamine receptors in outbred and inbred strains of rat. Brain Res. 1992. p. 45-54.

[150] Chio CL, Lajiness ME, Huff RM. Activation of heterologously expressed D3 dopa-mine receptors: comparison with D2 dopamine receptors. Mol Pharmacol. 1994. p. 51-60.

[151] Worth PF. How to treat Parkinson's disease in 2013. Clin Med. 2013. p. 93-6.

[152] Prieto G, Perez-Burgos A, Fiordelisio T, Salgado H, Galarraga E, Drucker-Colin R, et al. Dopamine D(2)-class receptor supersensitivity as reflected in Ca2+ current modu-lation in neostriatal neurons. Neuroscience. 2009. p. 345–50.

[153] Sun J, Cairns NJ, Perlmutter JS, Mach RH, Xu J. Regulation of dopamine D3 receptor in the striatal regions and substantia nigra in diffuse Lewy body disease. Neuroscience. 2013. p. 112-126.

[154] Lévesque D, Martres MP, Diaz J, Griffon N, Lammers CH, Sokoloff P, Schwartz JC. A paradoxical regulation of the dopamine D3 receptor expression suggests the involvement of an anterograde factor from dopamine neurons. Proc Natl Acad Sci U S A. 1995. p. 1719-23.

[155] Prieto G, Perez-Burgos A, Palomero-Rivero M, Galarraga E, Drucker-Colin R, Bargas J. Upregulation of D2-class signaling in dopamine-denervated striatum is in part mediated by D3 receptors acting on Ca V 2.1 channels via PIP2 depletion. Journal of neurophysiology. 2011. p. 2260–74.

[156] Schwartz J, Diaz J, Bordet R, Griffon N, Perachon S, Pilon C, et al. Functional implications of multiple dopamine receptor subtypes: the D1/D3 receptor coexistence. Brain research. Brain research reviews. 1998. p. 236–42.

[157] Mercuri NB, Calabresi P, Bernardi G. The electrophysiological actions of dopamine and dopaminergic drugs on neurons of the substantia nigra pars compacta and ventral tegmental area. Life Sci. 1992. p. 711-8.

[158] Du F, Li R, Huang Y, Li X, Le W. Dopamine D3 receptor-preferring agonists induce neurotrophic effects on mesencephalic dopamine neurons. The European journal of neuroscience. 2005. p. 2422–30.

[159] Van Kampen JM, Robertson HA. A possible role for dopamine D3 receptor stimulation in the induction of neurogenesis in the adult rat substantia nigra. Neuroscience. 2005. p. 381-6.

[160] Joyce JN, Millan MJ. Dopamine D3 receptor agonists for protection and repair in Parkinson's disease. Curr Opin Pharmacol. 2007. p.100-5.

[161] Pilla M, Perachon S, Sautel F, Garrido F, Mann A, Wermuth CG, Schwartz JC, Everitt BJ, Sokoloff P. Selective inhibition of cocaine-seeking behaviour by a partial dopamine D3 receptor agonist. Nature. 1999. p. 371-5.

[162] Albarrán S, Ávalos-Fuentes A, Paz-Bermúdez F, Erlij D, Aceves J, Floran B. Dopamine D3 receptor prevents D1 receptor stimulation of [3H] GABA release in substantia nigra pars reticulata of hemiparkinsonian dyskinetic rats. Soc Neursc Abstr 240.06/M7. 2013.

2

The Potential of Targeting LRRK2 in Parkinson's Disease

F.Y. Ho, K.E. Rosenbusch and A. Kortholt

1. Introduction

Parkinson's disease (PD) is the second most common neurodegenerative disease that affects more than 5 million people, accounting to 1-2 % of the population worldwide. It is characterized by the loss of dopaminergic neurons in the substantia nigra associated with the formation of fibrillar aggregates that are composed of α-synuclein and other proteins [1]. PD is clinical characterized by four major symptoms; tremor, bradykinesia, rigidity and postural instability. Initially PD was considered sporadic, however genetic studies in patients families revealed mutations that are segregating with PD. Nowadays, in addition to environmental factors, mutations within 6 loci (SNCA, LRRK2, PRKN, DJ1, PINK1 and ATP13A2) have been clearly demonstrated to be causative to familial PD [2-4]. Among them, SNCA and LRRK2 mutations cause autosomal dominant forms of PD [5]. Human leucine-rich-repeat kinase 2 (LRRK2) has been found to be thus far the most frequent cause of late-onset PD [6, 7]. The identification of missense mutations in LRRK2 has redefined the role of genetic variation in PD susceptibility. The mutations are found in 5-6 % of patients with familial PD, and also have been implicated with sporadic PD [8]. LRRK2 mutations initiate a penetrant phenotype with complete clinical and neurochemical overlap with idiopathic PD (IPD). Penetrance is age-related, around 75 % mutation carriers showed PD symptoms at the age of 80 [9, 10]. Tremor is more commonly observed in LRRK2 mediated PD compared to IPD [11]. Although dementia and cognitive defects are not frequently present in patients with mutations in LRRK2, LRRK2 does associate with Lewy bodies in IPD and dementia [12-14].

LRRK2 belongs to the Roco family of proteins, which constitute a novel family of Ras-like G-proteins that have an unique domain architecture [15]. LRRK2 is a large and complex protein with multiple domains; Armadillo repeats (ARM), Ankyrin repeats (ANK), leucine-rich repeats (LRR), a Ras of complex (Roc), a C-terminal of Roc (COR), kinase domain and WD40 repeats (Fig. 1). Most of the PD mutations are accumulated around the central core of the protein, one is found in the LRR, two in the Roc domain (with multiple substitutions), one in

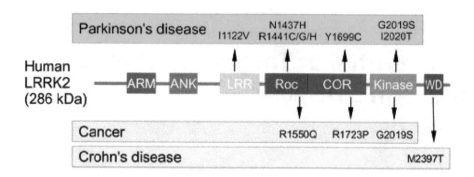

Figure 1. Domain topology of human LRRK2. The labels show the segregating mutations of LRRK2 in Parkinson's disease (green box), cancer associated mutations (blue box) and Crohn's disease (yellow box).

the COR and two in the kinase domain [16, 17]. The multiple disease-linked mutations in LRRK2 represent a unique opportunity to explore the activation mechanism of the protein and its miss-regulation in PD. In this chapter we will focus on the effects of LRRK2 on cellular signalling, the recent progress in elucidating the activation mechanism and discuss possible ways to therapeutically target LRRK2 mediated PD.

2. Cellular function of LRRK2

Although several potential LRRK2 mediated pathways and interaction partners have been identified, yet much about the cellular functions of LRRK2 and LRRK2 mediated progression of PD remains unknown [17]. Below we highlight the evidence for a role of LRRK2 in a wide variety of these cellular pathways and discuss a possible link to other PD-related genes.

2.1. Neurite development, outgrowth and branching

LRRK2 is directly linked to neurite outgrowth. Several studies have shown that primary neurons over-expressing mutant LRRK2 have significantly reduced neurite outgrowth and branching. However, the reported reduction varies and might only be significant in long term culture [18-20]. Adult neurogenesis and neurite outgrowth is impaired in mice overexpressing G2019S LRRK2 in the subventricular zone (SVZ) and hipppocampal denate gyrus [21]. This deficiency of neurite outgrowth can be rescued by inhibiting LRRK2 kinase activity with non-specific or more specific LRRK2 inhibitors, such as staurosporin [20] or G1023 [22], respectively. A recent study analysed LRRK2 expression in neonatal and postnatal mouse embryo and showed that LRRK2 expression can be detected in E10.5 of neural tissue. At the time of neurogenesis, prominent expression is found in the ventricular and SVZ of the telencephalon [23]. LRRK2 is also expressed in adult SVZ, where neural stem cells generate neurons in adult brain [24]. Both R1441G and G2019S LRRK2 impair development of neural stem cells [25-27], whereas LRRK2 deficient cells have increased neurite development [25, 28, 29]. Although the mechanisms are yet to be identified, these data show that LRRK2 is regulating neurite-, and neural development. Interestingly, LRRK2 is not only controlling neurite development via its kinase activity, also the LRRK2 G-domain and protein-protein interaction domains play a direct and important role. Tubulin, ArfGAP1, Rac1 and DVL family proteins bind to and/or are regulated by the G domain of LRRK2 and subsequently modulate the cytoskeleton [30-34]. Wnt signalling is essential for several steps in neural development, including presynaptic assembly, signal transduction at the postsynaptic cleft and adult neurogenesis [35, 36]. Overexpression of Wnt7a or inhibition of the Wnt signalling suppressor GSK3β promotes neuron differentiation and maturation [37, 38]. LRRK2 interacts with both the Wnt co-receptor low-density lipoprotein receptor-related protein 6 (LRP6) and the downstream DVL proteins, suggesting that LRRK2 might function as a scaffold for Wnt signalling proteins [39].

2.2. Autophagy

It is generally accepted that neurodegenerative diseases are associated with dysregulation of autophagy [40]. Autophagy is the regulated self-degradation of damaged organelle, ubiquiti-nated proteins and protein aggregates by lysosomes. Autophagy is an adaptive response which is stimulated by stress or unfavourable conditions, such as starvation, accumulation of aggregate-prone proteins, oxidative stress, and infection [41]. Autophagy is a double-edged sword; it can promote cell survival or lead to cell death [42]. Autophagy regulates the removal of protein aggregates, which are a common symptom in neurodegenerative diseases, and thereby promotes cell survival [43-45]. Protein aggregates such as α-synuclein [46], tau [47], and huntingtin [48] are cleared by autophagy. Disruption of the autophagy related genes *atg5* or *atg7* in mice, results in severe impairment autophagy and neurodegeneration [49, 50]. The purkinje cells of the mutant mice are characterized by axonal dystrophic swelling and degenerate within a few weeks after birth [51, 52]. Mice with conditional knockdown of *atg7* gene in the substantia nigra and cerebellum showed age-related loss of dopaminergic neurons and autophagy deficiency dependent accumulation of alpha-synuclein aggregates [53]. Expression of LRRK2 G2019S in retinoic acid differentiating SH-SY5Y neuroblastoma cells results in the accumulation of LRRK2 containing-autophagic vacuoles and shortens neuritic processes. Cells expressing wild-type LRRK2 show a similar but less severe phenotype. Disruption of *atg7* and microtubule-associated protein 1A/1B-light chain 3 (*lc3*) in these LRRK2 mutants completely rescues the phenotype [54]. Co-localization of LRRK2 with p62 and LC3 puncta in autophagic vacuoles is reported for human brain and by several other cell culture studies [55]. Not only overexpression of wildtype and mutant LRRK2 increases accumulation of autophagic vacuoles and the induction of autophagy [56-58], also knocking down LRRK2 activity by either RNAi or with specific LRRK2 inhibitors stimulates autophagy [59]. In addition, LRRK2 activity itself is regulated by macroautophagy and chaperon-mediated autophagy (CMA). LRRK2 inhibits CMA and hinders clearance of α-synuclein by CMA [60]. The complex role of LRRK2 in autophagy is not only playing a role in Parkinson's disease but has been linked to several other diseases as well (see below).

2.3. Mitochondrial disease

Mitochondrial dysfunction in the pathogenesis of PD has been studied extensively. Although the cellular mechanism remains largely unclear, LRRK2 seems to be important for proper mitochondrial regulation. Some reports suggest that LRRK2 partly localizes in mitochondria and several LRRK2 PD associated mutations results in impaired mitochondrial function [61]. Cells carrying the LRRK2 G2019S mutation display a general uncoupling of the oxidative phosphorylation [62]. The mitochondrial potential and intracellular ATP levels are reduced along with increased oxygen utilization [62]. Also shape and organization of the mitochondria are significantly affected as they appear elongated with an enhanced interconnectivity [63]. The increased kinase activity of LRRK2 G2019S leads to an increased AMP- activated protein kinase (AMPK) level [57]. Since, AMPK is an autophagy regulating protein, its enhanced activity results in an increased number of autophagosomes [57]. High levels of autophagy/ autophagic vacuoles lead, as described above, to a vulnerability and thus retraction and degeneration of neurons, one of the main characteristic features of PD [54]. Several other PD associated proteins, including α-synuclein, Parkin, DJ- 1, PINK1 and HTRA2 [64-66], show similar defects in mitochondria regulation, suggesting that LRRK2 and other PD associated proteins share common pathogenic pathways.

2.4. Common pathways for LRRK2 and other PD-relelated proteins?

Lewy bodies are protein aggregates found in degenerating dopaminergic neurons of PD patients. They are composed of many different proteins, including LRRK2 and α-synuclein [67, 68]. α-synuclein is a small protein (140 amino acids) that is located in presynaptic nerve terminal vesicles, plasma membrane lipid rafts and the nucleus [69-71]. Recent studies show that α-synuclein promotes SNARE-complex assembly [72, 73], and either overexpression or aggregation of α-synuclein interferes with vesicular trafficking [74-76]. Phosphorylation of α-synuclein is critical for aggregation and pathology. Since phosphorylation of α-synuclein serine residue 129 in HEK293T expressing LRRK2 is increased, it was initially proposed that α-synuclein is a direct substrate of LRRK2 [77]. However, phosphorylation of α-synuclein is normal in LRRK2$^{-/-}$ mice [78], suggesting that the rather weak effect of LRRK2 on α-synuclein S129 phosphorylation in cells is most likely indirect. Expression of LRRK2 and α-synuclein is co-regulated; increase of α-synuclein in mouse striatum results in increased LRRK2 transcription [79]. Both LRRK2 and α-synuclein interact with Rab5, which is important for vesicle trafficking [80, 81], suggesting LRRK2 and α-synuclein might share common pathways. Recessive mutations of Parkin, PINK1 and DJ-1 are causative to PD [82]. PTEN-induced kinase 1 (PINK1) is important for mitochondrial function and its deletion leads to increased susceptibility to oxidative stress [83, 84]. PINK1 is a cytosolic serine/threonine kinase under steady-state condition and its mitochondrial localization is stabilized by decreased mitochondrial membrane potential, an indicator of damaged mitochondria [85]. Parkin is an E3 ubiquitin ligase, which is phosphorylated and recruited to mitochondria by PINK1. The activated Parkin and PINK1 in conjugation clear damaged mitochondria via selective degradation and autophagy [85]. Co-expression of Parkin and LRRK2 G2019S in flies protects rotenone-induced neurodegeneration of dopaminergic neurons [86]. Expression of LRRK2 PD mutants in *pink1-*

null flies enhances the phenotype [87]. In human cells, LRRK2 is found to interact with Parkin, and co-expression of the two proteins increases LRRK2 containing aggregates. Altogether, this suggests that LRRK2 and PINK1/Parkin pathway are using similar pathways for the regulation of mitochondrial function. DJ-1 is a redox sensitive protein that is linked to a large variety of function, for example Ras-dependent cell transformation, neuroprotection, transcription, apoptosis suppression, P53 signalling, chaperon and protease [88]. It protects neurons from oxidative stress, by scavenging mitochondrial peroxide through oxidation of cysteine residues, and by binding metal ions like mercury and copper [89]. In cells that are exposed to oxidizing agents and mouse brains treated with rotenone, DJ-1 converts to more acidic isoforms [90, 91]. DJ-1 deficient cells, including cell lines and primary neurons, display altered mitochondrial morphology and an increase in autophagic flux [92]. PINK1 and Parkin overexpression can rescue the mitochondrial morphology of *dj-1*-null cells, but vice versa DJ-1 cannot rescue the defects of PINK1 and Parkin mutants. However, DJ-1 can protect PINK1 deficient neurons from oxidative stress induced by rotenone, suggesting DJ-1 may act both upstream and parallel to the PINK1/Parkin pathway [93]. In comparison to PINK1/Parkin, LRRK2 shows a less direct relation with DJ-1, albeit it still clearly exacerbate the eye phenotype of DJ-1 overexpression / loss in *Drosophila* [87]. As described previously, LRRK2 is important for autophagy in neurons, thus it is tempting to speculate that LRRK2 plays a role together with PINK1/Parkin and DJ-1 in regulating mitochondrial homeostasis.

2.5. LRRK2 and other diseases

Mutations in LRRK2 have been linked to several other diseases, including Crohn's disease and cancer. Carriers of LRRK2 G2019S mutation have an increased risk of non-skin cancer [94, 95]. Knock-down of LRRK2 in different cancer cell lines by RNAi, results in decreased stability of the 4E-BP1 protein [96]. Stability of 4E-BP1 protein is dependent on its phosphorylation state; it is a known downstream target of mTOR, inhibition of mTOR leads to accumulation of dephosphorylated 4E-BP and blocks cell transformation in a Kaposi's sarcoma model [97]. The PI3K/mTOR pathway is very frequently dysregulated in human cancer [98]. Previously, 4E-BP was identified as a direct LRRK2 kinase substrate (see section 3.3), suggesting LRRK2 might play a role in regulating 4E-BP stability and thus the oncogenic PI3K/mTOR pathway.

Genome wide association studies linked LRRK2 mutations to Crohn's disease (CD) and leprosy [99, 100]. CD associated mutations in the LRRK2 locus are located in non-coding regions, with an exception of the polymorphism rs3761863, which is leading to M2397T substitution in the WD40 repeats of LRRK2 [99]. CD is a chronic inflammatory disorder which primarily affects the gastrointestinal tract. Patients with CD have defective macrophages and neutrophils, resulting in a deficient innate immunity [101, 102]. LRRK2 is widely expressed in many organs and tissue, including brain, kidney and spleen. In the spleen, LRRK2 is highly expressed in CD19$^+$ B cells, whereas lower expression was detected in CD4$^+$ or CD8$^+$ T-cells, macrophages, and monocytes [103, 104]. In macrophages, LRRK2 expression is induced by activation of Toll-like receptors and viral transduction [103]. CD patients exhibit high concentrations of proinflammatory cytokines, including interferon-γ (IFN-γ), which induces LRRK2 expression in macrophages [105]. In cell-based reporter studies, LRRK2 is found to activate

NFκB and inhibit NFAT, which both are important transcription factors in the immune system [103, 106]. Interestingly this effect is independent of LRRK2 kinase activity, since expression of both wildtype and kinase dead LRRK2 result in a similar phenotype.

3. Intramolecular LRRK2 activation mechanism

LRRK2 has two bona-fide enzymatic activities from its Roc and kinase domain. It has been shown that both a functional Roc G-domain and kinase are essential for the pathogenicity of LRRK2. Importantly, several of the pathogenic mutations in LRRK2 result in decreased GTPase activity and enhanced kinase activity, suggesting a possible PD-related gain of abnormal function [107-109]. However the exact molecular mechanisms by which these mutations enhance LRRK2 catalytic activity are not completely resolved so far. Because of the lack of sufficient high quality recombinant LRRK2 protein, important understanding of the complex regulatory mechanism of LRRK2 has come from work with related Roco family proteins.

3.1. Homologous Roco proteins as model to study the mechanism of LRRK2 mediated PD

Roco proteins constitute a novel family of complex Ras-like GTPases that have an unique domain architecture [15]. Roco proteins are characterized by the presence of a Ras-like Guanine nucleotide binding domain, called Roc (Ras of complex proteins), followed by a COR domain (C-terminal of Roc), a conserved stretch of 300-400 amino-acids with no significant homology to other described protein domains (Fig. 2). The Roc and COR domains always occurs as a pair and so far no proteins are identified containing either the Roc or COR domain alone, suggesting that these two domains might function as one inseparable unit. Roco proteins were first identified in the social amoeba *Dictyostelium discoideum* and are found in prokaryotes, plants and metazoa, but not in *Plasmodium* and yeast. Based on domain topology, the family of Roco proteins can be divided into three groups, each containing at least one mammalian member. The first group is found in mammals (MASL1), plants and in prokaryotes. These proteins contain besides a Roc and COR domain always a N-terminal stretch of leucine-rich repeats (LRR), which are supposed to be involved in protein-protein interaction. The second group of Roco proteins is present in *Dictyostelium* and metazoa. In these proteins the Roc domain is again preceded by LRRs and the COR domain always succeeded by a kinase domain of the MAPKKK subfamily of kinases. A subset of Roco proteins contains the metazoan tumour suppressor death-associated protein kinases (DapK) domain, which is found in many proteins with apoptotic function [110]. Although there is a high variation in additional regulatory domains among the Roco proteins, previous studies have shown that the function and regulation of the catalytic core is conserved.

3.2. Dictyostelium Roco proteins to study the LRRK2 activation mechanism

Dictyostelium discoideum is a social, soil- dwelling amoeba that feeds on bacteria. The organism is genetically tractable with the ease of making gene disruptions and inducible expression, and at the same time it can be grown to large quantities for biochemical analyses [111]. Most

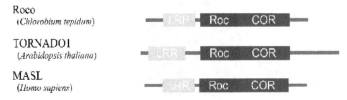

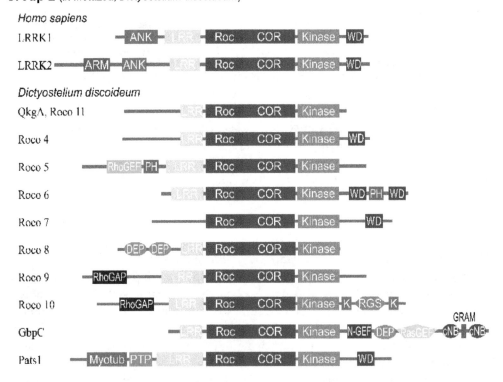

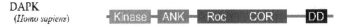

Figure 2. Domain architecture of the Roco family of proteins. The domains are leucine-rich repeat (LRR), Ras in complex domain (Roc), C-terminal of Roc domain (COR), ankyrin repeat (ANK), Kinase domain (Kinase), WD40 repeats (WD), armadillo repeat (ARM), Rho guanine nucleotide exchange factor domain (RhoGEF), Pleckstrin domain (PH), Dishevelled, Egl-10 and Pleckstrin domain (DEP), Rho GTPase activating protein domain (RhoGAP), Kelch motif (K), regulator of G protein signalling domain (RGS), N-terminal motif of RasGEF (N-GEF), Ras guanine nucleotide exchange factor domain (RasGEF), cyclic nucleotide binding domain (cNB), glucosyltransferases, Rab-like GTPase activators and myotubularins domain (GRAM), N-terminal myotubulin-related domain (myotub), protein tyrosine phosphatase domain (PTP) and death domain (DD).

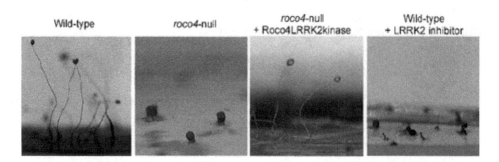

Figure 3. LRRK2 function and inhibition experiment with *Dictyostelium* cells. Wild-type, *roco4*-null and *roco4*-null cells expressing Roco4-LRRK2 kinase in which the kinase domain of Roco4 has been replaced with the kinase domain of LRRK2, were allowed to develop for 48 hours on nutrient-free agar. Pieces of agar were excised and photographed from the side. *roco4*-null cells fail to make a normal fruiting body due to defective synthesis of cellulose. The right panel shows a side view of the development of wild-type cells in the presence of the LRRK2-inhibitor H1152. Cells in the presence of 0.5 mM H1152 have the typical *roco4*-null phenotype. Figure modified with permission from Proc. Natl. Acad. Sci. USA, (Gilsbach et al., 2012).

importantly, many key pathways are conserved between *Dictyostelium* and human. Therefore, *Dictyostelium* offers unique advantages for studying fundamental cellular processes, as well as the molecular causes of human diseases [112]. Although *Dictyostelium* neither has a brain nor muscle, it is, as described below, an excellent model to study the molecular basis of LRRK2-mediated PD.

Dictyostelium contains eleven Roco family members, that all belong to the second subgroup of the Roco family. They are sharing the characteristic Roc, COR and kinase domains and in addition most also have LRR (Fig. 2, [15]). *Dictyostelium* Roco proteins are structurally more varied than the Roco proteins found in all the other species together; various domains are additionally fused to the conserved region. Roco proteins are most likely the result of recent gene duplications, and are very homologous to mammalian LRRK2 [113]. Disruption of *Dictyostelium* Roco genes leads to very different phenotypes, indicating that they are involved in multiple cellular processes. They participate in processes as diverse as chemotaxis, cell division, osmotic-stress-response and development [114]. The strong and diverse phenotypes of the *Dictyostelium* Roco disruption mutants therefore provide a strong tool to investigate the activation mechanisms of Roco proteins. Especially the studies with *Dictyostelium* Roco4 gave mechanistic insight into the regulation of LRRK2 [114, 115]. *Dictyostelium* Roco4 has the same domain architecture as LRRK2, but in contrast to LRRK2, Roco4 is biochemically and structurally more tractable [115]. Roco4 plays an important role in the late development stage of *Dictyostelium* [114]. During the vegetative growth stage, single *Dictyostelium* cells feed on bacteria and divide by simple mitotic divisions. In times of starvation, a developmental program is initiated, which is accompanied by major changes in gene expression. As a result, single cells are able to form aggregates via cAMP- dependent chemotaxis, resulting in the development of mobile multicellular forms, called slugs [111]. Eventually, the slugs will permanently settle down, culminate and generate fruiting bodies, which consist of a cellulose containing stalk and basal disc and end in a spore head [116]. Single cell amoebae are embedded in the spore head, which are resistant to extreme temperatures or drought and can be released upon germination under more favourable environmental conditions [111]. Cells lacking *roco4* undergo the characteristic streaming, aggregating and mound forming phases, however after 12 hours of starvation the cells start to display severe developmental defects. The formation of slugs and subsequent stalks and spore heads is severely delayed; 72 hours in the mutant cells, compared to 24 hours in wild-type [114]. Furthermore, *roco4*-null cells display aberrant fruiting body morphology as the spore heads are located on the agar surface due to a reduced cellulose level and thus instable stalks (Fig. 3, second panel). The strong developmental phenotype of *roco4*-null cells was used to determine essential structural elements in the protein. Remarkably, this phenotype can completely be rescued by expression of a chimeric Roco4 protein, in which its kinase domain has been replaced with the LRRK2 domain (Fig. 3, third panel) [115]. Furthermore, Roco4 kinase activity is inhibited by LRRK2 inhibitors (Fig. 3, right panel), and LRRK2 phosphorylates specific developed artificial substrates for LRRK2 *in vitro* [115, 117]. This shows that Roco4 has properties very much resembling those described for LRRK2, indicating that Roco4 protein thus can serve as a valid model to understand the complex structure and regulatory mechanism of LRRK2.

3.3. LRRK2 kinase activity

Protein kinases catalyze the transfer of γ-phosphate of ATP to the hydroxyl group of serine/ threonine/tyrosine in peptide substrates. Due to the simplicity, stability, and reversibility, protein phosphorylation is chosen by nature for modulating protein functions. Phosphorylation allows specific and dedicated control over enzymatic activities, regulation of protein localization and the transition between the ordered and disordered states of proteins [118]. Therefore, protein kinases are essential for many biological processes such as energy metabolism, cell cycle progression, transcription and cytoskeleton rearrangement. There are more than 500 protein kinases identified in the human genome, of which the majority are serine/ threonine kinases, a much smaller amount is tyrosine specific and a trace amount are atypical kinases [119].

LRRK2 kinase activity is extensively studied since its discovery, and it is found to be essential for neuronal toxicity induced by PD mutant of LRRK2 [120, 121]. LRRK2 and Roco proteins are serine/threonine specific kinases. Previously the structures of Roco4 kinase wild-type and the PD-related mutants G1179S and L1180T (G2019S and I2020T in LRRK2) were solved [115]. Like almost all kinases, Roco4 consists of a canonical, two-lobed kinase structure, with an adenine nucleotide located in the conventional nucleotide binding site [118, 122]. The N-terminal lobe is smaller, which is composed of an anti-parallel β-sheet and the large conserved αC-helix. It is followed by a linker connecting the larger C-terminal lobe, which is composed predominantly of α-helices and is containing the activation loop with the conserved DFG motif at the N-terminus [115]. The ATP binding pocket is located between the N- and C-terminal lobes and forms together with the activation segment and αC-helix the catalytic site of the kinase. In its inactive (dephosphorylated) form, the activation segment of Roco4 is disordered, and not visible in the crystal structure. In the active (phosphorylated) conformation, the αC-helix is ordered and packs against the N-terminal lobe. This conformational change between the active and inactive conformation is conserved between most kinases, and often dependent on autophosphorylation of the activation loop [118, 122-124]. *In vitro* kinase and *in vivo* rescue experiments showed that Roco4 S1187 and S1189 are essential for regulating Roco4 kinase activity. Autophosphorylation is well demonstrated in LRRK2 by numerous studies. LRRK2 contains with T2031/S2032/T2035 three potential phosphorylation sites in the activation loop. Studies using phosphospecific antibodies have shown that all three sites are phosphorylated, but like for Roco4, only the two later sites, S2032 and T2035, are important for LRRK2 activity *in vivo* [125]. Most other autophosphorylation sites are located in the Roc domain and kinase domain, such as S1292, T1348, T1349, T1357, T1503, T1967, T1969 [22, 126, 127]. Mutations of these residues significantly affect the enzymatic activities of LRRK2. Importantly, mutating S1292 to alanine [22] or inhibiting kinase activity with inhibitors, completely rescues neurite outgrowth in LRRK2 PD mutants. This suggests that LRRK2 kinase activity is important for both the intramolecular activation mechanism, as well, for downstream signalling. Several putative LRRK2 kinase substrates have been identified so far. LRRK2 phosphorylates 4E-BP [128] and FoxO and thereby modulates their translation and transcription activities. However, the relevance of 4E-BP phosphorylation by LRRK2 for the progression in PD is still under debate [129-131]. Phosphorylation of FoxO induces expression of the pro-apoptotic Bcl-2 protein, Bim, and the endogenous caspase-8 inhibitor, c-FLIP, leading to programmed cell death [132-134]. Therefore, FoxO may be one of the missing links between LRRK2 and cell death in neurons. [135]. Several LRRK2 substrates are linked to cytoskeleton remodelling; moesin promotes actin rearrangement in neurons [136, 137], and β-tubulin and tubulin-associated tau are important for neurite outgrowth and axonal transport [138-140].

3.4. Mechanism of increased kinase activity in LRRK2 PD mutants

The most prevalent PD mutation in the kinase domain is G2019S, which enhances kinase activity, while the PD-related mutation I2020T shows a slightly decreased activity [108, 109, 117, 121, 141]. Recently the molecular mechanism by which the G2019S mutation enhances LRRK2 was resolved using *Dictyostelium* Roco4. The LRRK2 G2019 and I2020 residues are conserved in *Dictyostelium* Roco4 and correspond to G1179 and L1180, respectively. Overlay of the solved Roco4 wild-type and the Roco4 G1179S structure didn't show large differences in the overall structure, however closer observation revealed that S1179 makes a new hydrogen bond with R1077, thereby presumably stabilizing the activation loop and the αC-helix in their active conformation. R1077 is conserved in almost all Roco proteins and corresponds to LRRK2 R1918. Kinase activity measurement with the Roco4 double mutant G1179S/R1077A and the homologous LRRK2 double mutant G2019S/R1918A, in which the new hydrogen bond is no longer possible, confirmed the proposed mechanism since it shows wild type kinase activity [115].

The structure of the PD-related mutant L1180T showed that the T1180 side-chain points into the solvent and revealed that it is most likely not directly involved in regulating kinase activity. Importantly, the data show that the PD-related effect of LRRK2 mutations result from different defects in the LRRK2 activation mechanism and suggest that different LRRK2 mutations such as S2019 and T2020 might require different ways of inhibition for the purpose of drug development [115, 142].

3.5. The RocCOR tandem

The Roc domain of LRRK2 belongs to the family of small G-proteins. G-proteins are GTP binding proteins which switch between an active GTP- and inactive GDP-bound state. The G-domain has an universal switch mechanism that carries out the basic function of nucleotide binding and hydrolysis [143]. The universal switch mechanism between the inactive GDP and active GTP form often consist of only small structural changes in the so called switch regions [144]. Although, the two nucleotide-bound states have only a slightly different conformation, only the GTP-bound conformation possesses high affinity for effector proteins [145]. In Roco family members the G-domain always occurs in tandem with the COR domain. Studies with both LRRK2 and *Dictyostelium* Roco4 revealed that a functional Roc domain is essential for kinase activity, the COR domain functions as the dimerization device and disruption of Roc or the kinase domain by a single point mutation leads to the complete inactivation of the protein. These suggest that the Roc-COR tandem is regulating kinase activity and/or that the kinase is regulating the activity of Roc by autophosphorylation [146]. The cycle of "classical" small G-protein is strictly controlled by GEFs (Guanine nucleotide Exchange Factors), which catalyze the exchange from GDP to GTP, and the intrinsic low GTP hydrolysis rate is increased by GAPs (GTPase Activating Proteins) [147]. It is well established that LRRK2 and other Roco proteins are active as a dimer ([148-150], see also below). The previously solved structure of the Roco protein from the bacteria *Chlorobium tepidum,* revealed that COR is the dimerization device and that Roco proteins, including LRRK2, belong to the GAD class of molecular switches (G proteins activated by nucleotide dependent dimerization) [149, 151]. This class also includes proteins such as signal recognition particle, dynamin and septins [151]. It is proposed that the juxtaposition of the G domains of two monomers in the complex across the GTP-binding sites activates the GTPase reaction and thereby regulates the biological function of these proteins (Fig. 4). Since GTPase activity is regulated within the dimer complex, GTP hydrolysis by Roco proteins is not regulated by GAP's. LRRK2 and Roco proteins have a much lower affinity (µM range) compared to other small G-proteins (nM range), and therefore most likely do not need GEFs for activation [149, 152]. The PD-related mutations, R1441C/G/H in the Roc domain and Y1699C in the COR domain, do not affect nucleotide binding, but significantly decrease GTPase activity [153, 154]. Importantly, the structure of the *Chlorobium tepidum* Roco protein showed that the PD-analogous mutations of the Roc and COR domain are in close proximity to each other at the dimer interface. Furthermore, these mutations are present in a region of the protein that is strongly conserved between bacteria, *Dictyostelium* and man. PD-mutations in the *Chlorobium tepidum* protein, like that of LRRK2, decrease the GTPase reaction, most likely due to altered interaction in the dimer between the Roc and COR domains [149].

3.6. Function of the N-terminus of LRRK2

The N- terminal part of LRRK2 consists of Armadillo repeats (ARM), Ankyrin repeats (ANK), and leucine-rich repeats (LRR) (Fig. 1). All these domains are commonly found in signalling proteins, in which they have a role in protein-protein interaction or assembly of large protein complexes [155]. The N-terminal segment of LRRK2 is most likely involved in regulating activity and/or localization. ARM are approximately 40 amino acid long tandem repeated sequences that form superhelix of helices. ANK consist of seven structural repeats, each repeat forms two anti-parallel helices ending with a loop or hairpin [156, 157]. LRR are defined by an 11 amino acid long consensus sequence LxxLxLxxNxL, where leucine can be replaced by isoleucine, valine or phenylalanine [155]. The LRRK2 LRR domain is composed of 13 repeats, allowing the formation of its characteristic horseshoe shaped structure due to parallel lining β- sheets with ending α- helices [139, 158, 159]. The LRR domain of LRRK2, and *Dictyostelium* Roco4, are not involved in Roc or kinase activation *in vitro*, but are absolutely essential for activity of the protein *in vivo* [160, 161]. Recent data suggest that the LRR are directly involved in determining input/output specificity of the Roco proteins, most likely by binding upstream proteins that activate specifically the Roco protein and/or by selectively binding of the substrate (AK unpublished data). Previously, it has been shown that 14-3-3 proteins bind to the N-terminus of LRRK2 [25]. 14-3-3 are highly conserved proteins that have been found in a variety of organisms, including mammals, plants, yeast, *Drosophila*, and *Dictyostelium* [162, 163]. In human, the 14-3-3 protein family consists of 7 structural similar yet distinct isoforms: α, β, γ, δ, ε, ζ, η [162]. The proteins exist as homo- or functional active heterodimers and are important for various signalling pathways, including neurotransmitter synthesis in mammalian brain tissue, via direct ligand binding [163, 164]. Interaction of 14-3-3 with LRRK2 is dependent on the phosphorylation of two conserved serine residues (S910, S935), situated at the N- terminal part of LRRK2 anterior to the LRR domain [158]. Since several LRRK2 specific kinase inhibitors abolish 14-3-3 binding, it is proposed that the binding is regulated by autophosphorylation [165, 166]. However, other studies suggest that LRRK2 interaction is dependent on a so far unidentified upstream kinase [167]. Disrupted phosphorylation of the serine residues results in strong defects in LRRK2 signalling; the protein is delocalized and accumulates in inclusion like bodies instead of being transported to the cell membrane [158, 166]. Interestingly, pathogenic PD mutants of LRRK2 display a similar dysfunctional phenotype, suggesting a direct link between LRRK2 and 14-3-3 signalling.

3.7. WD40 domain at the C-Terminus of LRRK2

LRRK2 contains a C-terminal WD40 domain. It comprises seven repeats each of which consists of antiparallel, four stranded β- sheets resulting in a circular propeller-like structure. WD40 repeats have a high positive net charge and several hydrophilic surfaces, and are therefore often involved in membrane binding and interaction with negatively charged proteins [157]. Two non-conserved mutations which are suggested to be involved in the onset of PD are found in the WD40 domain of LRRK2: G2385R and T2356I [157]. A yeast-two hybrid screen showed a direct interaction of WD40 repeats with the Roc domain [168]. In addition, LRRK2 lacking the WD40 domain has abolished abilities to form dimers, displays impaired activity and localization [169]. Together these results suggest an important role for the WD40 domain in the intramolecular regulation of LRRK2 activity.

3.8. LRRK2/Roco activation model

We have translated all biochemical, genetic and structural data into a model for the regulatory mechanism of LRRK2 (Fig. 4). LRRK2 is monomeric and inactive in the cytosol, but attains pre-

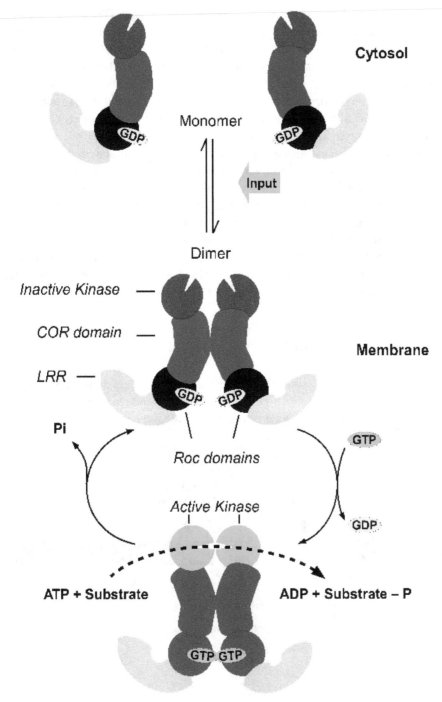

Figure 4. Proposed model for the function and activation mechanism of LRRK2.

dominantly dimeric and in the active state at the membrane [150]. These results suggest that LRRK2 cycles between a low activity monomeric state and high activity dimeric state. The previously solved structure of the Roco protein from *Chlorobium tepidum* revealed that COR is the dimerization device and that Roco proteins belong to the GAD class of molecular switches. In the GDP-bound inactive state the G-domains are flexible, but in the active form the G-domains come in close proximity to each other. This conformational change is transmitted to the kinase domains to allow the activation loops of the two kinase protomers to be autophosphorylated and activated. The GTPase reaction is also dependent on dimerization, because efficient catalytic machinery is formed by complementation of the active site of one protomer with that of the other protomer. In this way the GTPase reaction functions as a timing device for the activation of the kinase and the biological function of the protein. Consistently, PD-related mutations have reduced GTPase activity and enhanced kinase activity (MS in preparation, [16]). The N- and C- terminal segments are not important for kinase activity *in vitro*, but appear to be essential *in vivo* [114, 160, 161] and most likely determine the input and/or output specificity of the proteins. One of these upstream regulators might be 14-3-3, which binds in a phosphorylation dependent way to the N-terminal segment of LRRK2, thereby regulating its subcellular localization and secretion in exosomes [158, 170, 171].

4. Therapeutic targeting LRRK2

The multiple allosteric and enzymatic functions within one protein make LRRK2 an excellent therapeutic target (Fig. 5). Below we highlight the recent progress in identifying LRRK2 kinase inhibitors and discuss alternative ways of targeting LRRK2-mediated PD-disease.

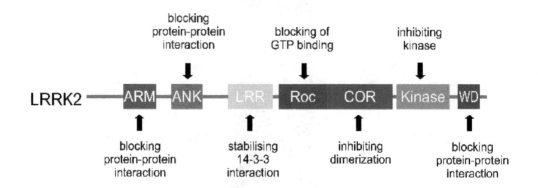

Figure 5. Strategies of LRRK2 inhibition.

4.1. LRRK2 kinase as a therapeutic target

Kinases are one of the most potent classes of drug targets and have been effectively used in the treatment of cancer, immunological, neurological and infectious diseases [172]. The majority of inhibitors directly target the ATP binding site. They are divided into three groups; most of the inhibitors reported are type I inhibitors, which target the active conformation and directly compete with ATP for the binding pocket. Type II inhibitors also bind in the ATP binding pocket resulting in a change from the active DFG-in into an inactive DFG-out conformation. Type III inhibitors directly target the DFG – out conformation. One of the approved kinase inhibitors for renal cell carcinoma treatment is Sunitinib (Sutent(®), Pfizer Inc.). It is a tyrosine kinase inhibitor which has several targets and inhibits tumor cell proliferation, and angiogenesis [173]. LRRK2 kinase activity is critically linked to clinical effects, and the most prevalent PD mutation, LRRK2 G2019S in the kinase domain, enhances kinase activity by 2-4 folds [108, 141]. Therefore LRRK2 kinase inhibitors are an intensively pursued class of drug targets. Several non selective inhibitors were found to inhibit LRRK2 with their IC50 values in nanomolar range, including staurosporin, K252A and Su-11248 (Sunitinib) [141, 174]. Several ROCK inhibitors have also been found to inhibit LRRK2 with similar efficiencies (low micromolar range), such as isoquinolinesulfonamides hydroxyfasudil and H1152, and the structurally unrelated Y-27632. Noteworthy, not all ROCK inhibitors inhibit LRRK2; isoquinolinesulfonamides do not inhibit LRRK2 as effective as ROCK and the aminofurazan ROCK inhibitor GSK269962A cannot inhibit LRRK2 [175]. Despite a high degree of conservation in the ATP binding site of kinases, it is possible to develop highly selective kinase inhibitors [172]. LRRK2-IN-1 is the first one discovered by compound-centric high throughput library screening [165]. It inhibits both wild-type (IC50 = 13 nM) and G2019S mutant (IC50 = 6 nM) of LRRK2, and shows high selectivity. Among a panel of 442 kinases, only 12 kinases were inhibited, with up to 10 μM of LRRK2-IN-1. LRRK2-IN-1 also inhibits LRRK2 activity in human cells, however dephosphorylation of LRRK2 can only be observed in the kidney and not in the brain of the mice received intraperitoneal injection of the inhibitor, suggesting that this potent and selective LRRK2 inhibitor is incapable of crossing the blood brain barrier [165].

The recently identified LRRK2 inhibitors, HG-10-102-01 [176] and GNE-7915 [177] are selective and brain penetrant [178]. However, long-term inhibition of LRRK2 with these inhibitors leads, similar to disrupting LRRK2 in mice, to kidney abnormality [179-181]. Developing kinase inhibitors specific to PD mutants of LRRK2, not affecting wild-type, might therefore be the most promising approach. The previous solved structure of the Roco4 kinase PD mutant and Roco4 kinase in complex with the LRRK2 inhibitor H1152 might be instrumental in this process [115]. Although current available LRRK2 kinase inhibitor can not be used for PD treatment yet [178], they provide an excellent tool to study PD *in vitro* and *in vivo* and form a good starting point to develop better PD drugs.

4.2. Alternative therapeutic approaches

Although most attention has concentrated on targeting LRRK2 kinase activity so far, only for the G2019S consistently an increased kinase activity has been reported. All other pathogenic mutations show inconsistent-, modest- or no effect on kinase activity. This suggests that different PD mutations in LRRK2 have a different defect in the activation mechanism and might require different ways of inhibition for the purpose of drug development (Fig. 5). The LRRK2 mutations in the Roc (R1441C/G/H), and COR (Y1699C) domain have a decreased

GTPase activity [153, 154], suggesting GTPase activity forms a good therapeutic target. Since Ras is the most common oncogene in human cancer, many studies have focussed on identifying Ras inhibitors. Targeting the G-domain could be done by using small compounds that bind to the nucleotide binding site and resemble the GDP bound off state or increase the GTPase reaction. Due to the high nucleotide affinity and the high cytosolic concentration, it has been very challenging to identify a therapeutic target of Ras. However, since LRRK2 has a much lower nucleotide affinity and the GTPase activity is regulated by dimerization, the LRRK2 G-domain may provide a better therapeutic target.

The N- and C-terminal segments of LRRK2 contain several protein-protein interaction domains which are involved in regulating kinase activity, oligomerization, and/or localization (Fig 5). As described above, LRRK2 cycles between a low active monomeric cytosolic state and high active dimeric membrane bound state. The regulation of LRRK2 membrane association is not well understood, but probably includes dimerization, post-translational modification and protein-protein interactions [158, 170, 182]. 14-3-3 proteins bind in a phosphorylation dependent manner to the N-terminus of LRRK2, which is important for LRRK2 localization and activity [25]. All purified or co-immunoprecipitated LRRK2 fragments are dimeric [148], and LRRK2 kinase activity seems to be dependent on dimerization [150, 170]. Active LRRK2 is a constitutive dimer by high affinity interaction of the COR domains, suggesting that in the cytosol the dimerization is most likely covered by regulatory proteins. Importantly, since LRRK2 activation is dependent on membrane localization and dimerization, inhibiting either of these properties may be a good therapeutic approach.

5. Conclusion

The multiple disease-linked mutations and enzyme functions within one protein make LRRK2 an excellent therapeutic target. Since several PD mutants result in an increase in LRRK2 kinase activity, the focus so far has been to develop kinase domain inhibitors as potential PD therapeutics. However, alternative approaches that target other domains of LRRK2, localization, dimerization, or allosteric modulation of the kinase domain may have significantly improved therapeutic benefits. To explore these potential therapeutic approaches, it will be essential to completely understand the molecular activation mechanism, identify upstream and downstream regulators, and characterize the cellular function of LRRK2. Work with model organism and biochemical and structural characterization of related Roco proteins from lower organisms might be important in this enterprise.

Acknowledgements

This work is supported by the Michael J. Fox foundation for Parkinson's research and a NWO-VIDI grant to AK. We want to thank Bernd Gilsbach for his input in this chapter.

Author details

F.Y. Ho[1], K.E. Rosenbusch[2] and A. Kortholt[2*]

*Address all correspondence to: a.kortholt@rug.nl

1 Department of Biochemistry, University of Groningen, Groningen, The Netherlands

2 Department of Cell Biochemistry, University of Groningen, Groningen, The Netherlands

References

[1] Lees A.J., Hardy J., and Revesz T. (2009). Parkinson's disease. Lancet 373: 2055-2066.

[2] Bekris L.M., Mata I.F., and Zabetian C.P. (2010). The genetics of Parkinson disease. J. Geriatr. Psychiatry Neurol. 23: 228-242.

[3] Satake W., Nakabayashi Y., Mizuta I., Hirota Y., Ito C., Kubo M., Kawaguchi T., Tsunoda T., Watanabe M., Takeda A. et al. (2009). Genome-wide association study identifies common variants at four loci as genetic risk factors for Parkinson's disease. Nat. Genet. 41: 1303-1307.

[4] Singleton A.B., Farrer M.J., and Bonifati V. (2013). The genetics of Parkinson's disease: progress and therapeutic implications. Mov Disord. 28: 14-23.

[5] Sundal C., Fujioka S., Uitti R.J., and Wszolek Z.K. (2012). Autosomal dominant Parkinson's disease. Parkinsonism. Relat Disord. 18 Suppl 1: S7-10.

[6] Paisan-Ruiz C., Jain S., Evans E.W., Gilks W.P., Simon J., van der B.M., Lopez d.M., Aparicio S., Gil A.M., Khan N. et al. (2004). Cloning of the gene containing mutations that cause PARK8-linked Parkinson's disease. Neuron 44: 595-600.

[7] Zimprich A., Biskup S., Leitner P., Lichtner P., Farrer M., Lincoln S., Kachergus J., Hulihan M., Uitti R.J., Calne D.B. et al. (2004). Mutations in LRRK2 cause autosomal-dominant parkinsonism with pleomorphic pathology. Neuron 44: 601-607.

[8] Gilks W.P., bou-Sleiman P.M., Gandhi S., Jain S., Singleton A., Lees A.J., Shaw K., Bhatia K.P., Bonifati V., Quinn N.P. et al. (2005). A common LRRK2 mutation in idiopathic Parkinson's disease. Lancet 365: 415-416.

[9] Farrer M.J. (2006). Genetics of Parkinson disease: paradigm shifts and future prospects. Nat. Rev. Genet. 7: 306-318.

[10] Healy D.G., Falchi M., O'Sullivan S.S., Bonifati V., Durr A., Bressman S., Brice A., Aasly J., Zabetian C.P., Goldwurm S. et al. (2008). Phenotype, genotype, and world-

wide genetic penetrance of LRRK2-associated Parkinson's disease: a case-control
study. Lancet Neurol. 7: 583-590.

[11] Marras C., Schule B., Munhoz R.P., Rogaeva E., Langston J.W., Kasten M., Meaney
C., Klein C., Wadia P.M., Lim S.Y. et al. (2011). Phenotype in parkinsonian and nonparkinsonian LRRK2 G2019S mutation carriers. Neurology 77: 325-333.

[12] Gaig C., Marti M.J., Ezquerra M., Rey M.J., Cardozo A., and Tolosa E. (2007). G2019S
LRRK2 mutation causing Parkinson's disease without Lewy bodies. J. Neurol. Neurosurg. Psychiatry 78: 626-628.

[13] Goldwurm S., Zini M., Di F.A., De G.D., Siri C., Simons E.J., van D.M., Tesei S., Antonini A., Canesi M. et al. (2006). LRRK2 G2019S mutation and Parkinson's disease: a
clinical, neuropsychological and neuropsychiatric study in a large Italian sample.
Parkinsonism. Relat Disord. 12: 410-419.

[14] Zhu X., Siedlak S.L., Smith M.A., Perry G., and Chen S.G. (2006). LRRK2 protein is a
component of Lewy bodies. Ann. Neurol. 60: 617-618.

[15] Bosgraaf L. and van Haastert P.J. (2003). Roc, a Ras/GTPase domain in complex proteins. Biochim. Biophys. Acta 1643: 5-10.

[16] Cookson M.R. and Bandmann O. (2010). Parkinson's disease: insights from pathways. Hum. Mol. Genet. 19: R21-R27.

[17] Cookson M.R. (2010). The role of leucine-rich repeat kinase 2 (LRRK2) in Parkinson's
disease. Nat. Rev. Neurosci. 11: 791-797.

[18] MacLeod D., Dowman J., Hammond R., Leete T., Inoue K., and Abeliovich A. (2006).
The familial Parkinsonism gene LRRK2 regulates neurite process morphology. Neuron 52: 587-593.

[19] Sepulveda B., Mesias R., Li X., Yue Z., and Benson D.L. (2013). Short- and long-term
effects of LRRK2 on axon and dendrite growth. PLoS. One. 8: e61986.

[20] Dachsel J.C., Behrouz B., Yue M., Beevers J.E., Melrose H.L., and Farrer M.J. (2010). A
comparative study of Lrrk2 function in primary neuronal cultures. Parkinsonism. Relat Disord. 16: 650-655.

[21] Winner B., Melrose H.L., Zhao C., Hinkle K.M., Yue M., Kent C., Braithwaite A.T.,
Ogholikhan S., Aigner R., Winkler J. et al. (2011). Adult neurogenesis and neurite
outgrowth are impaired in LRRK2 G2019S mice. Neurobiol. Dis. 41: 706-716.

[22] Sheng Z., Zhang S., Bustos D., Kleinheinz T., Le Pichon C.E., Dominguez S.L., Sola-
noy H.O., Drummond J., Zhang X., Ding X. et al. (2012). Ser1292 autophosphorylation is an indicator of LRRK2 kinase activity and contributes to the cellular effects of
PD mutations. Sci. Transl. Med. 4: 164ra161.

[23] Zechel S., Meinhardt A., Unsicker K., and von Bohlen Und H.O. (2010). Expression of leucine-rich-repeat-kinase 2 (LRRK2) during embryonic development. Int. J. Dev. Neurosci. 28: 391-399.

[24] varez-Buylla A. and Lim D.A. (2004). For the long run: maintaining germinal niches in the adult brain. Neuron 41: 683-686.

[25] Bahnassawy L., Nicklas S., Palm T., Menzl I., Birzele F., Gillardon F., and Schwamborn J.C. (2013). The Parkinson's Disease-Associated LRRK2 Mutation R1441G Inhibits Neuronal Differentiation of Neural Stem Cells. Stem Cells Dev. 22: 2487-2496.

[26] Liu G.H., Qu J., Suzuki K., Nivet E., Li M., Montserrat N., Yi F., Xu X., Ruiz S., Zhang W. et al. (2012). Progressive degeneration of human neural stem cells caused by pathogenic LRRK2. Nature 491: 603-607.

[27] Winner B., Melrose H.L., Zhao C., Hinkle K.M., Yue M., Kent C., Braithwaite A.T., Ogholikhan S., Aigner R., Winkler J. et al. (2011). Adult neurogenesis and neurite outgrowth are impaired in LRRK2 G2019S mice. Neurobiol. Dis. 41: 706-716.

[28] Schulz C., Paus M., Frey K., Schmid R., Kohl Z., Mennerich D., Winkler J., and Gillardon F. (2011). Leucine-rich repeat kinase 2 modulates retinoic acid-induced neuronal differentiation of murine embryonic stem cells. PLoS. One. 6: e20820.

[29] Paus M., Kohl Z., Ben Abdallah N.M., Galter D., Gillardon F., and Winkler J. (2013). Enhanced dendritogenesis and axogenesis in hippocampal neuroblasts of LRRK2 knockout mice. Brain Res. 1497: 85-100.

[30] Caesar M., Zach S., Carlson C.B., Brockmann K., Gasser T., and Gillardon F. (2013). Leucine-rich repeat kinase 2 functionally interacts with microtubules and kinase-dependently modulates cell migration. Neurobiol. Dis. 54: 280-288.

[31] Chan D., Citro A., Cordy J.M., Shen G.C., and Wolozin B. (2011). Rac1 protein rescues neurite retraction caused by G2019S leucine-rich repeat kinase 2 (LRRK2). J. Biol. Chem. 286: 16140-16149.

[32] Gandhi P.N., Wang X., Zhu X., Chen S.G., and Wilson-Delfosse A.L. (2008). The Roc domain of leucine-rich repeat kinase 2 is sufficient for interaction with microtubules. J. Neurosci. Res. 86: 1711-1720.

[33] Sancho R.M., Law B.M., and Harvey K. (2009). Mutations in the LRRK2 Roc-COR tandem domain link Parkinson's disease to Wnt signalling pathways. Hum. Mol. Genet. 18: 3955-3968.

[34] Stafa K., Trancikova A., Webber P.J., Glauser L., West A.B., and Moore D.J. (2012). GTPase activity and neuronal toxicity of Parkinson's disease-associated LRRK2 is regulated by ArfGAP1. PLoS. Genet. 8: e1002526.

[35] Ille F. and Sommer L. (2005). Wnt signaling: multiple functions in neural development. Cell Mol. Life Sci. 62: 1100-1108.

[36] Inestrosa N.C. and Arenas E. (2010). Emerging roles of Wnts in the adult nervous system. Nat. Rev. Neurosci. 11: 77-86.

[37] Ding S., Wu T.Y., Brinker A., Peters E.C., Hur W., Gray N.S., and Schultz P.G. (2003). Synthetic small molecules that control stem cell fate. Proc. Natl. Acad. Sci. U. S. A 100: 7632-7637.

[38] Hirabayashi Y., Itoh Y., Tabata H., Nakajima K., Akiyama T., Masuyama N., and Gotoh Y. (2004). The Wnt/beta-catenin pathway directs neuronal differentiation of cortical neural precursor cells. Development 131: 2791-2801.

[39] Berwick D.C. and Harvey K. (2013). LRRK2: an eminence grise of Wnt-mediated neurogenesis? Front Cell Neurosci. 7: 82.

[40] Kroemer G. and Levine B. (2008). Autophagic cell death: the story of a misnomer. Nat. Rev. Mol. Cell Biol. 9: 1004-1010.

[41] Janda E., Isidoro C., Carresi C., and Mollace V. (2012). Defective autophagy in Parkinson's disease: role of oxidative stress. Mol. Neurobiol. 46: 639-661.

[42] Rami A. (2009). Review: autophagy in neurodegeneration: firefighter and/or incendiarist? Neuropathol. Appl. Neurobiol. 35: 449-461.

[43] Sharon R., Bar-Joseph I., Frosch M.P., Walsh D.M., Hamilton J.A., and Selkoe D.J. (2003). The formation of highly soluble oligomers of alpha-synuclein is regulated by fatty acids and enhanced in Parkinson's disease. Neuron 37: 583-595.

[44] Walsh D.M., Klyubin I., Fadeeva J.V., Cullen W.K., Anwyl R., Wolfe M.S., Rowan M.J., and Selkoe D.J. (2002). Naturally secreted oligomers of amyloid beta protein potently inhibit hippocampal long-term potentiation in vivo. Nature 416: 535-539.

[45] Maeda S., Sahara N., Saito Y., Murayama S., Ikai A., and Takashima A. (2006). Increased levels of granular tau oligomers: an early sign of brain aging and Alzheimer's disease. Neurosci. Res. 54: 197-201.

[46] Webb A., Clark P., Skepper J., Compston A., and Wood A. (1995). Guidance of oligodendrocytes and their progenitors by substratum topography. J. Cell Sci. 108 (Pt 8): 2747-2760.

[47] Wang Y., Kruger U., Mandelkow E., and Mandelkow E.M. (2010). Generation of tau aggregates and clearance by autophagy in an inducible cell model of tauopathy. Neurodegener. Dis. 7: 103-107.

[48] Sarkar S. and Rubinsztein D.C. (2008). Huntington's disease: degradation of mutant huntingtin by autophagy. FEBS J. 275: 4263-4270.

[49] Hara T., Nakamura K., Matsui M., Yamamoto A., Nakahara Y., Suzuki-Migishima R., Yokoyama M., Mishima K., Saito I., Okano H. et al. (2006). Suppression of basal autophagy in neural cells causes neurodegenerative disease in mice. Nature 441: 885-889.

[50] Komatsu M., Wang Q.J., Holstein G.R., Friedrich V.L., Jr., Iwata J., Kominami E., Chait B.T., Tanaka K., and Yue Z. (2007). Essential role for autophagy protein Atg7 in the maintenance of axonal homeostasis and the prevention of axonal degeneration. Proc. Natl. Acad. Sci. U. S. A 104: 14489-14494.

[51] Komatsu M., Waguri S., Chiba T., Murata S., Iwata J., Tanida I., Ueno T., Koike M., Uchiyama Y., Kominami E. et al. (2006). Loss of autophagy in the central nervous system causes neurodegeneration in mice. Nature 441: 880-884.

[52] Nishiyama J., Miura E., Mizushima N., Watanabe M., and Yuzaki M. (2007). Aberrant membranes and double-membrane structures accumulate in the axons of Atg5-null Purkinje cells before neuronal death. Autophagy. 3: 591-596.

[53] Ahmed I., Liang Y., Schools S., Dawson V.L., Dawson T.M., and Savitt J.M. (2012). Development and characterization of a new Parkinson's disease model resulting from impaired autophagy. J. Neurosci. 32: 16503-16509.

[54] Plowey E.D., Cherra S.J., III, Liu Y.J., and Chu C.T. (2008). Role of autophagy in G2019S-LRRK2-associated neurite shortening in differentiated SH-SY5Y cells. J. Neurochem. 105: 1048-1056.

[55] egre-Abarrategui J., Christian H., Lufino M.M., Mutihac R., Venda L.L., Ansorge O., and Wade-Martins R. (2009). LRRK2 regulates autophagic activity and localizes to specific membrane microdomains in a novel human genomic reporter cellular model. Hum. Mol. Genet. 18: 4022-4034.

[56] Bravo-San Pedro J.M., Niso-Santano M., Gomez-Sanchez R., Pizarro-Estrella E., iastui-Pujana A., Gorostidi A., Climent V., Lopez de M.R., Sanchez-Pernaute R., Lopez de M.A. et al. (2013). The LRRK2 G2019S mutant exacerbates basal autophagy through activation of the MEK/ERK pathway. Cell Mol. Life Sci. 70: 121-136.

[57] Gomez-Suaga P., Luzon-Toro B., Churamani D., Zhang L., Bloor-Young D., Patel S., Woodman P.G., Churchill G.C., and Hilfiker S. (2012). Leucine-rich repeat kinase 2 regulates autophagy through a calcium-dependent pathway involving NAADP. Hum. Mol. Genet. 21: 511-525.

[58] Ramonet D., Daher J.P., Lin B.M., Stafa K., Kim J., Banerjee R., Westerlund M., Pletnikova O., Glauser L., Yang L. et al. (2011). Dopaminergic neuronal loss, reduced neurite complexity and autophagic abnormalities in transgenic mice expressing G2019S mutant LRRK2. PLoS. One. 6: e18568.

[59] Manzoni C., Mamais A., Dihanich S., Abeti R., Soutar M.P., Plun-Favreau H., Giunti P., Tooze S.A., Bandopadhyay R., and Lewis P.A. (2013). Inhibition of LRRK2 kinase activity stimulates macroautophagy. Biochim. Biophys. Acta 1833: 2900-2910.

[60] Orenstein S.J., Kuo S.H., Tasset I., Arias E., Koga H., Fernandez-Carasa I., Cortes E., Honig L.S., Dauer W., Consiglio A. et al. (2013). Interplay of LRRK2 with chaperone-mediated autophagy. Nat. Neurosci. 16: 394-406.

[61] Biskup S., Moore D.J., Celsi F., Higashi S., West A.B., Andrabi S.A., Kurkinen K., Yu S.W., Savitt J.M., Waldvogel H.J. et al. (2006). Localization of LRRK2 to membranous and vesicular structures in mammalian brain. Ann. Neurol. 60: 557-569.

[62] Papkovskaia T.D., Chau K.Y., Inesta-Vaquera F., Papkovsky D.B., Healy D.G., Nishio K., Staddon J., Duchen M.R., Hardy J., Schapira A.H. et al. (2012). G2019S leucine-rich repeat kinase 2 causes uncoupling protein-mediated mitochondrial depolarization. Hum. Mol. Genet. 21: 4201-4213.

[63] Mortiboys H., Johansen K.K., Aasly J.O., and Bandmann O. (2010). Mitochondrial impairment in patients with Parkinson disease with the G2019S mutation in LRRK2. Neurology 75: 2017-2020.

[64] Lin M.T. and Beal M.F. (2006). Mitochondrial dysfunction and oxidative stress in neurodegenerative diseases. Nature 443: 787-795.

[65] Valente E.M., bou-Sleiman P.M., Caputo V., Muqit M.M., Harvey K., Gispert S., Ali Z., Del T.D., Bentivoglio A.R., Healy D.G. et al. (2004). Hereditary early-onset Parkinson's disease caused by mutations in PINK1. Science 304: 1158-1160.

[66] Wang X., Yan M.H., Fujioka H., Liu J., Wilson-Delfosse A., Chen S.G., Perry G., Casadesus G., and Zhu X. (2012). LRRK2 regulates mitochondrial dynamics and function through direct interaction with DLP1. Hum. Mol. Genet. 21: 1931-1944.

[67] Perry G., Zhu X., Babar A.K., Siedlak S.L., Yang Q., Ito G., Iwatsubo T., Smith M.A., and Chen S.G. (2008). Leucine-rich repeat kinase 2 colocalizes with alpha-synuclein in Parkinson's disease, but not tau-containing deposits in tauopathies. Neurodegener. Dis. 5: 222-224.

[68] Guerreiro P.S., Huang Y., Gysbers A., Cheng D., Gai W.P., Outeiro T.F., and Halliday G.M. (2013). LRRK2 interactions with alpha-synuclein in Parkinson's disease brains and in cell models. J. Mol. Med. (Berl) 91: 513-522.

[69] Maroteaux L., Campanelli J.T., and Scheller R.H. (1988). Synuclein: a neuron-specific protein localized to the nucleus and presynaptic nerve terminal. J. Neurosci. 8: 2804-2815.

[70] Kahle P.J., Neumann M., Ozmen L., Muller V., Jacobsen H., Schindzielorz A., Okochi M., Leimer U., van Der P.H., Probst A. et al. (2000). Subcellular localization of wild-type and Parkinson's disease-associated mutant alpha -synuclein in human and transgenic mouse brain. J. Neurosci. 20: 6365-6373.

[71] Fortin D.L., Troyer M.D., Nakamura K., Kubo S., Anthony M.D., and Edwards R.H. (2004). Lipid rafts mediate the synaptic localization of alpha-synuclein. J. Neurosci. 24: 6715-6723.

[72] Burre J., Sharma M., Tsetsenis T., Buchman V., Etherton M.R., and Sudhof T.C. (2010). Alpha-synuclein promotes SNARE-complex assembly in vivo and in vitro. Science 329: 1663-1667.

[73] Diao J., Burre J., Vivona S., Cipriano D.J., Sharma M., Kyoung M., Sudhof T.C., and Brunger A.T. (2013). Native alpha-synuclein induces clustering of synaptic-vesicle mimics via binding to phospholipids and synaptobrevin-2/VAMP2. Elife. 2: e00592.

[74] Larsen K.E., Schmitz Y., Troyer M.D., Mosharov E., Dietrich P., Quazi A.Z., Savalle M., Nemani V., Chaudhry F.A., Edwards R.H. et al. (2006). Alpha-synuclein overexpression in PC12 and chromaffin cells impairs catecholamine release by interfering with a late step in exocytosis. J. Neurosci. 26: 11915-11922.

[75] Thayanidhi N., Helm J.R., Nycz D.C., Bentley M., Liang Y., and Hay J.C. (2010). Alpha-synuclein delays endoplasmic reticulum (ER)-to-Golgi transport in mammalian cells by antagonizing ER/Golgi SNAREs. Mol. Biol. Cell 21: 1850-1863.

[76] Sancenon V., Lee S.A., Patrick C., Griffith J., Paulino A., Outeiro T.F., Reggiori F., Masliah E., and Muchowski P.J. (2012). Suppression of alpha-synuclein toxicity and vesicle trafficking defects by phosphorylation at S129 in yeast depends on genetic context. Hum. Mol. Genet. 21: 2432-2449.

[77] Qing H., Wong W., McGeer E.G., and McGeer P.L. (2009). Lrrk2 phosphorylates alpha synuclein at serine 129: Parkinson disease implications. Biochem. Biophys. Res. Commun. 387: 149-152.

[78] Tong Y., Yamaguchi H., Giaime E., Boyle S., Kopan R., Kelleher R.J., III, and Shen J. (2010). Loss of leucine-rich repeat kinase 2 causes impairment of protein degradation pathways, accumulation of alpha-synuclein, and apoptotic cell death in aged mice. Proc. Natl. Acad. Sci. U. S. A 107: 9879-9884.

[79] Westerlund M., Ran C., Borgkvist A., Sterky F.H., Lindqvist E., Lundstromer K., Pernold K., Brene S., Kallunki P., Fisone G. et al. (2008). Lrrk2 and alpha-synuclein are co-regulated in rodent striatum. Mol. Cell Neurosci. 39: 586-591.

[80] Dalfo E., Barrachina M., Rosa J.L., Ambrosio S., and Ferrer I. (2004). Abnormal alpha-synuclein interactions with rab3a and rabphilin in diffuse Lewy body disease. Neurobiol. Dis. 16: 92-97.

[81] Shin N., Jeong H., Kwon J., Heo H.Y., Kwon J.J., Yun H.J., Kim C.H., Han B.S., Tong Y., Shen J. et al. (2008). LRRK2 regulates synaptic vesicle endocytosis. Exp. Cell Res. 314: 2055-2065.

[82] Klein C. and Lohmann-Hedrich K. (2007). Impact of recent genetic findings in Parkinson's disease. Curr. Opin. Neurol. 20: 453-464.

[83] Clark I.E., Dodson M.W., Jiang C., Cao J.H., Huh J.R., Seol J.H., Yoo S.J., Hay B.A., and Guo M. (2006). Drosophila pink1 is required for mitochondrial function and interacts genetically with parkin. Nature 441: 1162-1166.

[84] Gautier C.A., Kitada T., and Shen J. (2008). Loss of PINK1 causes mitochondrial functional defects and increased sensitivity to oxidative stress. Proc. Natl. Acad. Sci. U. S. A 105: 11364-11369.

[85] Matsuda S., Kitagishi Y., and Kobayashi M. (2013). Function and characteristics of PINK1 in mitochondria. Oxid. Med. Cell Longev. 2013: 601587.

[86] Ng C.H., Guan M.S., Koh C., Ouyang X., Yu F., Tan E.K., O'Neill S.P., Zhang X., Chung J., and Lim K.L. (2012). AMP kinase activation mitigates dopaminergic dysfunction and mitochondrial abnormalities in Drosophila models of Parkinson's disease. J. Neurosci. 32: 14311-14317.

[87] Venderova K., Kabbach G., bdel-Messih E., Zhang Y., Parks R.J., Imai Y., Gehrke S., Ngsee J., LaVoie M.J., Slack R.S. et al. (2009). Leucine-Rich Repeat Kinase 2 interacts with Parkin, DJ-1 and PINK-1 in a Drosophila melanogaster model of Parkinson's disease. Hum. Mol. Genet. 18: 4390-4404.

[88] Ariga H., Takahashi-Niki K., Kato I., Maita H., Niki T., and Iguchi-Ariga S.M. (2013). Neuroprotective function of DJ-1 in Parkinson's disease. Oxid. Med. Cell Longev. 2013: 683920.

[89] Bjorkblom B., Adilbayeva A., Maple-Grodem J., Piston D., Okvist M., Xu X.M., Brede C., Larsen J.P., and Moller S.G. (2013). Parkinson Disease Protein DJ-1 Binds Metals and Protects against Metal-induced Cytotoxicity. J. Biol. Chem. 288: 22809-22820.

[90] Kinumi T., Kimata J., Taira T., Ariga H., and Niki E. (2004). Cysteine-106 of DJ-1 is the most sensitive cysteine residue to hydrogen peroxide-mediated oxidation in vivo in human umbilical vein endothelial cells. Biochem. Biophys. Res. Commun. 317: 722-728.

[91] Betarbet R., Canet-Aviles R.M., Sherer T.B., Mastroberardino P.G., McLendon C., Kim J.H., Lund S., Na H.M., Taylor G., Bence N.F. et al. (2006). Intersecting pathways to neurodegeneration in Parkinson's disease: effects of the pesticide rotenone on DJ-1, alpha-synuclein, and the ubiquitin-proteasome system. Neurobiol. Dis. 22: 404-420.

[92] Irrcher I., Aleyasin H., Seifert E.L., Hewitt S.J., Chhabra S., Phillips M., Lutz A.K., Rousseaux M.W., Bevilacqua L., Jahani-Asl A. et al. (2010). Loss of the Parkinson's disease-linked gene DJ-1 perturbs mitochondrial dynamics. Hum. Mol. Genet. 19: 3734-3746.

[93] Thomas K.J., McCoy M.K., Blackinton J., Beilina A., van der B.M., Sandebring A., Miller D., Maric D., Cedazo-Minguez A., and Cookson M.R. (2011). DJ-1 acts in parallel to the PINK1/parkin pathway to control mitochondrial function and autophagy. Hum. Mol. Genet. 20: 40-50.

[94] Saunders-Pullman R., Barrett M.J., Stanley K.M., Luciano M.S., Shanker V., Severt L., Hunt A., Raymond D., Ozelius L.J., and Bressman S.B. (2010). LRRK2 G2019S mutations are associated with an increased cancer risk in Parkinson disease. Mov Disord. 25: 2536-2541.

[95] Inzelberg R., Cohen O.S., haron-Peretz J., Schlesinger I., Gershoni-Baruch R., Djaldetti R., Nitsan Z., Ephraty L., Tunkel O., Kozlova E. et al. (2012). The LRRK2 G2019S

mutation is associated with Parkinson disease and concomitant non-skin cancers. Neurology 78: 781-786.

[96] Pons B., Armengol G., Livingstone M., Lopez L., Coch L., Sonenberg N., and Cajal S. (2012). Association between LRRK2 and 4E-BP1 protein levels in normal and malignant cells. Oncol. Rep. 27: 225-231.

[97] Martin D., Nguyen Q., Molinolo A., and Gutkind J.S. (2013). Accumulation of dephosphorylated 4EBP after mTOR inhibition with rapamycin is sufficient to disrupt paracrine transformation by the KSHV vGPCR oncogene. Oncogene.

[98] Guertin D.A. and Sabatini D.M. (2005). An expanding role for mTOR in cancer. Trends Mol. Med. 11: 353-361.

[99] Barrett J.C., Hansoul S., Nicolae D.L., Cho J.H., Duerr R.H., Rioux J.D., Brant S.R., Silverberg M.S., Taylor K.D., Barmada M.M. et al. (2008). Genome-wide association defines more than 30 distinct susceptibility loci for Crohn's disease. Nat. Genet. 40: 955-962.

[100] Zhang F.R., Huang W., Chen S.M., Sun L.D., Liu H., Li Y., Cui Y., Yan X.X., Yang H.T., Yang R.D. et al. (2009). Genomewide association study of leprosy. N. Engl. J. Med. 361: 2609-2618.

[101] Marks D.J., Harbord M.W., MacAllister R., Rahman F.Z., Young J., Al-Lazikani B., Lees W., Novelli M., Bloom S., and Segal A.W. (2006). Defective acute inflammation in Crohn's disease: a clinical investigation. Lancet 367: 668-678.

[102] Actis G.C. and Rosina F. (2013). Inflammatory bowel disease: An archetype disorder of outer environment sensor systems. World J. Gastrointest. Pharmacol. Ther. 4: 41-46.

[103] Hakimi M., Selvanantham T., Swinton E., Padmore R.F., Tong Y., Kabbach G., Venderova K., Girardin S.E., Bulman D.E., Scherzer C.R. et al. (2011). Parkinson's disease-linked LRRK2 is expressed in circulating and tissue immune cells and upregulated following recognition of microbial structures. J. Neural Transm. 118: 795-808.

[104] Maekawa T., Kubo M., Yokoyama I., Ohta E., and Obata F. (2010). Age-dependent and cell-population-restricted LRRK2 expression in normal mouse spleen. Biochem. Biophys. Res. Commun. 392: 431-435.

[105] Gardet A., Benita Y., Li C., Sands B.E., Ballester I., Stevens C., Korzenik J.R., Rioux J.D., Daly M.J., Xavier R.J. et al. (2010). LRRK2 is involved in the IFN-gamma response and host response to pathogens. J. Immunol. 185: 5577-5585.

[106] Liu Z., Lee J., Krummey S., Lu W., Cai H., and Lenardo M.J. (2011). The kinase LRRK2 is a regulator of the transcription factor NFAT that modulates the severity of inflammatory bowel disease. Nat. Immunol. 12: 1063-1070.

[107] Greggio E. and Cookson M.R. (2009). Leucine-rich repeat kinase 2 mutations and Par-
       kinson's disease: three questions. ASN. Neuro. 1.

[108] Luzon-Toro B., Rubio d.l.T., Delgado A., Perez-Tur J., and Hilfiker S. (2007). Mecha-
       nistic insight into the dominant mode of the Parkinson's disease-associated G2019S
       LRRK2 mutation. Hum. Mol. Genet. 16: 2031-2039.

[109] West A.B., Moore D.J., Biskup S., Bugayenko A., Smith W.W., Ross C.A., Dawson
       V.L., and Dawson T.M. (2005). Parkinson's disease-associated mutations in leucine-
       rich repeat kinase 2 augment kinase activity. Proc. Natl. Acad. Sci. U. S A 102:
       16842-16847.

[110] Itoh N. and Nagata S. (1993). A novel protein domain required for apoptosis. Muta-
       tional analysis of human Fas antigen. J. Biol. Chem. 268: 10932-10937.

[111] Eichinger L., Pachebat J.A., Glockner G., Rajandream M.A., Sucgang R., Berriman M.,
       Song J., Olsen R., Szafranski K., Xu Q. et al. (2005). The genome of the social amoeba
       Dictyostelium discoideum. Nature 435: 43-57.

[112] Muller-Taubenberger A., Kortholt A., and Eichinger L. (2013). Simple system--sub-
       stantial share: the use of Dictyostelium in cell biology and molecular medicine. Eur. J.
       Cell Biol. 92: 45-53.

[113] Marin I. (2006). The Parkinson disease gene LRRK2: evolutionary and structural in-
       sights. Mol. Biol. Evol. 23: 2423-2433.

[114] van Egmond W.N. and van Haastert P.J. (2010). Characterization of the Roco protein
       family in Dictyostelium discoideum. Eukaryot. Cell 9: 751-761.

[115] Gilsbach B.K., Ho F.Y., Vetter I.R., van Haastert P.J., Wittinghofer A., and Kortholt A.
       (2012). Roco kinase structures give insights into the mechanism of Parkinson disease-
       related leucine-rich-repeat kinase 2 mutations. Proc. Natl. Acad. Sci. U. S. A.

[116] Bonner J.T. (1947). Evidence for the formation of cell aggregates by chemotaxis in the
       development of the slime mold Dictyostelium discoideum. J. Exp. Zool. 106: 1-26.

[117] Jaleel M., Nichols R.J., Deak M., Campbell D.G., Gillardon F., Knebel A., and Alessi
       D.R. (2007). LRRK2 phosphorylates moesin at threonine-558: characterization of how
       Parkinson's disease mutants affect kinase activity. Biochem. J. 405: 307-317.

[118] Taylor S.S. and Kornev A.P. (2011). Protein kinases: evolution of dynamic regulatory
       proteins. Trends Biochem. Sci. 36: 65-77.

[119] Endicott J.A., Noble M.E., and Johnson L.N. (2012). The structural basis for control of
       eukaryotic protein kinases. Annu. Rev. Biochem. 81: 587-613.

[120] Greggio E., Jain S., Kingsbury A., Bandopadhyay R., Lewis P., Kaganovich A., van
       der Brug M.P., Beilina A., Blackinton J., Thomas K.J. et al. (2006). Kinase activity is
       required for the toxic effects of mutant LRRK2/dardarin. Neurobiol. Dis. 23: 329-341.

[121] Smith W.W., Pei Z., Jiang H., Dawson V.L., Dawson T.M., and Ross C.A. (2006). Kinase activity of mutant LRRK2 mediates neuronal toxicity. Nat. Neurosci. 9: 1231-1233.

[122] Huse M. and Kuriyan J. (2002). The conformational plasticity of protein kinases. Cell 109: 275-282.

[123] Adams J.A. (2003). Activation loop phosphorylation and catalysis in protein kinases: is there functional evidence for the autoinhibitor model? Biochemistry 42: 601-607.

[124] Kornev A.P., Haste N.M., Taylor S.S., and Eyck L.F. (2006). Surface comparison of active and inactive protein kinases identifies a conserved activation mechanism. Proc. Natl. Acad. Sci. U. S. A 103: 17783-17788.

[125] Li X., Moore D.J., Xiong Y., Dawson T.M., and Dawson V.L. (2010). Reevaluation of phosphorylation sites in the Parkinson disease-associated leucine-rich repeat kinase 2. J. Biol. Chem. 285: 29569-29576.

[126] Kamikawaji S., Ito G., and Iwatsubo T. (2009). Identification of the autophosphorylation sites of LRRK2. Biochemistry 48: 10963-10975.

[127] Webber P.J., Smith A.D., Sen S., Renfrow M.B., Mobley J.A., and West A.B. (2011). Autophosphorylation in the leucine-rich repeat kinase 2 (LRRK2) GTPase domain modifies kinase and GTP-binding activities. J. Mol. Biol. 412: 94-110.

[128] Imai Y., Gehrke S., Wang H.Q., Takahashi R., Hasegawa K., Oota E., and Lu B. (2008). Phosphorylation of 4E-BP by LRRK2 affects the maintenance of dopaminergic neurons in Drosophila. EMBO J. 27: 2432-2443.

[129] Kumar A., Greggio E., Beilina A., Kaganovich A., Chan D., Taymans J.M., Wolozin B., and Cookson M.R. (2010). The Parkinson's disease associated LRRK2 exhibits weaker in vitro phosphorylation of 4E-BP compared to autophosphorylation. PLoS. One. 5: e8730.

[130] Lee S., Liu H.P., Lin W.Y., Guo H., and Lu B. (2010). LRRK2 kinase regulates synaptic morphology through distinct substrates at the presynaptic and postsynaptic compartments of the Drosophila neuromuscular junction. J. Neurosci. 30: 16959-16969.

[131] Trancikova A., Mamais A., Webber P.J., Stafa K., Tsika E., Glauser L., West A.B., Bandopadhyay R., and Moore D.J. (2012). Phosphorylation of 4E-BP1 in the mammalian brain is not altered by LRRK2 expression or pathogenic mutations. PLoS. One. 7: e47784.

[132] Kanao T., Venderova K., Park D.S., Unterman T., Lu B., and Imai Y. (2010). Activation of FoxO by LRRK2 induces expression of proapoptotic proteins and alters survival of postmitotic dopaminergic neuron in Drosophila. Hum. Mol. Genet. 19: 3747-3758.

[133] Gilley J., Coffer P.J., and Ham J. (2003). FOXO transcription factors directly activate bim gene expression and promote apoptosis in sympathetic neurons. J. Cell Biol. 162: 613-622.

[134] Park S.J., Sohn H.Y., Yoon J., and Park S.I. (2009). Down-regulation of FoxO-dependent c-FLIP expression mediates TRAIL-induced apoptosis in activated hepatic stellate cells. Cell Signal. 21: 1495-1503.

[135] Xu P., Das M., Reilly J., and Davis R.J. (2011). JNK regulates FoxO-dependent autophagy in neurons. Genes Dev. 25: 310-322.

[136] Parisiadou L., Xie C., Cho H.J., Lin X., Gu X.L., Long C.X., Lobbestael E., Baekelandt V., Taymans J.M., Sun L. et al. (2009). Phosphorylation of ezrin/radixin/moesin proteins by LRRK2 promotes the rearrangement of actin cytoskeleton in neuronal morphogenesis. J. Neurosci. 29: 13971-13980.

[137] Parisiadou L. and Cai H. (2010). LRRK2 function on actin and microtubule dynamics in Parkinson disease. Commun. Integr. Biol. 3: 396-400.

[138] Gillardon F. (2009). Leucine-rich repeat kinase 2 phosphorylates brain tubulin-beta isoforms and modulates microtubule stability--a point of convergence in parkinsonian neurodegeneration? J. Neurochem. 110: 1514-1522.

[139] Kawakami F., Yabata T., Ohta E., Maekawa T., Shimada N., Suzuki M., Maruyama H., Ichikawa T., and Obata F. (2012). LRRK2 phosphorylates tubulin-associated tau but not the free molecule: LRRK2-mediated regulation of the tau-tubulin association and neurite outgrowth. PLoS. One. 7: e30834.

[140] Lin C.H., Tsai P.I., Wu R.M., and Chien C.T. (2010). LRRK2 G2019S mutation induces dendrite degeneration through mislocalization and phosphorylation of tau by recruiting autoactivated GSK3ss. J. Neurosci. 30: 13138-13149.

[141] Anand V.S., Reichling L.J., Lipinski K., Stochaj W., Duan W., Kelleher K., Pungaliya P., Brown E.L., Reinhart P.H., Somberg R. et al. (2009). Investigation of leucine-rich repeat kinase 2 : enzymological properties and novel assays. FEBS J. 276: 466-478.

[142] Reichling L.J. and Riddle S.M. (2009). Leucine-rich repeat kinase 2 mutants I2020T and G2019S exhibit altered kinase inhibitor sensitivity. Biochem. Biophys. Res. Commun. 384: 255-258.

[143] Vetter I.R. and Wittinghofer A. (2001). The guanine nucleotide-binding switch in three dimensions. Science 294: 1299-1304.

[144] Milburn M.V., Tong L., deVos A.M., Brunger A., Yamaizumi Z., Nishimura S., and Kim S.H. (1990). Molecular switch for signal transduction: structural differences between active and inactive forms of protooncogenic ras proteins. Science 247: 939-945.

[145] Repasky G.A., Chenette E.J., and Der C.J. (2004). Renewing the conspiracy theory debate: does Raf function alone to mediate Ras oncogenesis? Trends in Cell Biology 14: 639-647.

[146] Biosa A., Trancikova A., Civiero L., Glauser L., Bubacco L., Greggio E., and Moore D.J. (2013). GTPase activity regulates kinase activity and cellular phenotypes of Parkinson's disease-associated LRRK2. Hum. Mol. Genet. 22: 1140-1156.

[147] Bourne H.R., Sanders D.A., and Mccormick F. (1991). The Gtpase Superfamily - Conserved Structure and Molecular Mechanism. Nature 349: 117-127.

[148] Civiero L., Vancraenenbroeck R., Belluzzi E., Beilina A., Lobbestael E., Reyniers L., Gao F., Micetic I., De M.M., Bubacco L. et al. (2012). Biochemical characterization of highly purified leucine-rich repeat kinases 1 and 2 demonstrates formation of homodimers. PLoS. One. 7: e43472.

[149] Gotthardt K., Weyand M., Kortholt A., van Haastert P.J., and Wittinghofer A. (2008). Structure of the Roc-COR domain tandem of C. tepidum, a prokaryotic homologue of the human LRRK2 Parkinson kinase. EMBO J. 27: 2239-2249.

[150] James N.G., Digman M.A., Gratton E., Barylko B., Ding X., Albanesi J.P., Goldberg M.S., and Jameson D.M. (2012). Number and Brightness Analysis of LRRK2 Oligomerization in Live Cells. Biophys. J. 102: L41-L43.

[151] Gasper R., Meyer S., Gotthardt K., Sirajuddin M., and Wittinghofer A. (2009). It takes two to tango: regulation of G proteins by dimerization. Nat. Rev. Mol. Cell Biol. 10: 423-429.

[152] Ito G., Okai T., Fujino G., Takeda K., Ichijo H., Katada T., and Iwatsubo T. (2007). GTP binding is essential to the protein kinase activity of LRRK2, a causative gene product for familial Parkinson's disease. Biochemistry 46: 1380-1388.

[153] Guo L., Gandhi P.N., Wang W., Petersen R.B., Wilson-Delfosse A.L., and Chen S.G. (2007). The Parkinson's disease-associated protein, leucine-rich repeat kinase 2 (LRRK2), is an authentic GTPase that stimulates kinase activity. Exp. Cell Res. 313: 3658-3670.

[154] Lewis P.A., Greggio E., Beilina A., Jain S., Baker A., and Cookson M.R. (2007). The R1441C mutation of LRRK2 disrupts GTP hydrolysis. Biochem. Biophys. Res. Commun. 357: 668-671.

[155] Kobe B. and Kajava A.V. (2001). The leucine-rich repeat as a protein recognition motif. Curr. Opin. Struct. Biol. 11: 725-732.

[156] Marin I. (2006). The Parkinson disease gene LRRK2: evolutionary and structural insights. Mol. Biol. Evol. 23: 2423-2433.

[157] Mata I.F., Wedemeyer W.J., Farrer M.J., Taylor J.P., and Gallo K.A. (2006). LRRK2 in Parkinson's disease: protein domains and functional insights. Trends Neurosci. 29: 286-293.

[158] Nichols R.J., Dzamko N., Morrice N.A., Campbell D.G., Deak M., Ordureau A., Macartney T., Tong Y., Shen J., Prescott A.R. et al. (2010). 14-3-3 binding to LRRK2 is disrupted by multiple Parkinson's disease-associated mutations and regulates cytoplasmic localization. Biochem. J. 430: 393-404.

[159] Greggio E., Taymans J.M., Zhen E.Y., Ryder J., Vancraenenbroeck R., Beilina A., Sun P., Deng J., Jaffe H., Baekelandt V. et al. (2009). The Parkinson's disease kinase LRRK2 autophosphorylates its GTPase domain at multiple sites. Biochem. Biophys. Res. Commun. 389: 449-454.

[160] Iaccarino C., Crosio C., Vitale C., Sanna G., Carri M.T., and Barone P. (2007). Apoptotic mechanisms in mutant LRRK2-mediated cell death. Hum. Mol. Genet. 16: 1319-1326.

[161] van Egmond W.N., Kortholt A., Plak K., Bosgraaf L., Bosgraaf S., Keizer-Gunnink I., and van Haastert P.J. (2008). Intramolecular activation mechanism of the Dictyostelium LRRK2 homolog Roco protein GbpC. J. Biol. Chem. 283: 30412-30420.

[162] Aitken A., Jones D., Soneji Y., and Howell S. (1995). 14-3-3 proteins: biological function and domain structure. Biochem. Soc. Trans. 23: 605-611.

[163] Fu H., Subramanian R.R., and Masters S.C. (2000). 14-3-3 proteins: structure, function, and regulation. Annu. Rev. Pharmacol. Toxicol. 40: 617-647.

[164] Xiao B., Smerdon S.J., Jones D.H., Dodson G.G., Soneji Y., Aitken A., and Gamblin S.J. (1995). Structure of a 14-3-3 protein and implications for coordination of multiple signalling pathways. Nature 376: 188-191.

[165] Deng X., Dzamko N., Prescott A., Davies P., Liu Q., Yang Q., Lee J.D., Patricelli M.P., Nomanbhoy T.K., Alessi D.R. et al. (2011). Characterization of a selective inhibitor of the Parkinson's disease kinase LRRK2. Nat. Chem. Biol. 7: 203-205.

[166] Dzamko N., Deak M., Hentati F., Reith A.D., Prescott A.R., Alessi D.R., and Nichols R.J. (2010). Inhibition of LRRK2 kinase activity leads to dephosphorylation of Ser(910)/Ser(935), disruption of 14-3-3 binding and altered cytoplasmic localization. Biochem. J. 430: 405-413.

[167] Li X., Wang Q.J., Pan N., Lee S., Zhao Y., Chait B.T., and Yue Z. (2011). Phosphorylation-dependent 14-3-3 binding to LRRK2 is impaired by common mutations of familial Parkinson's disease. PLoS. One. 6: e17153.

[168] Greggio E., Zambrano I., Kaganovich A., Beilina A., Taymans J.M., Daniels V., Lewis P., Jain S., Ding J., Syed A. et al. (2008). The Parkinson disease-associated leucine-rich repeat kinase 2 (LRRK2) is a dimer that undergoes intramolecular autophosphorylation. J. Biol. Chem. 283: 16906-16914.

[169] Jorgensen N.D., Peng Y., Ho C.C., Rideout H.J., Petrey D., Liu P., and Dauer W.T. (2009). The WD40 domain is required for LRRK2 neurotoxicity. PLoS. One. 4: e8463.

[170] Sen S., Webber P.J., and West A.B. (2009). Dependence of leucine-rich repeat kinase 2 (LRRK2) kinase activity on dimerization. J. Biol. Chem. 284: 36346-36356.

[171] Fraser K.B., Moehle M.S., Daher J.P., Webber P.J., Williams J.Y., Stewart C.A., Yacoubian T.A., Cowell R.M., Dokland T., Ye T. et al. (2013). LRRK2 secretion in exosomes is regulated by 14-3-3. Hum. Mol. Genet.

[172] Zhang J., Yang P.L., and Gray N.S. (2009). Targeting cancer with small molecule kinase inhibitors. Nat. Rev. Cancer 9: 28-39.

[173] Mihaly Z., Sztupinszki Z., Surowiak P., and Gyorffy B. (2012). A comprehensive overview of targeted therapy in metastatic renal cell carcinoma. Curr. Cancer Drug Targets. 12: 857-872.

[174] Covy J.P. and Giasson B.I. (2009). Identification of compounds that inhibit the kinase activity of leucine-rich repeat kinase 2. Biochem. Biophys. Res. Commun. 378: 473-477.

[175] Nichols R.J., Dzamko N., Hutti J.E., Cantley L.C., Deak M., Moran J., Bamborough P., Reith A.D., and Alessi D.R. (2009). Substrate specificity and inhibitors of LRRK2, a protein kinase mutated in Parkinson's disease. Biochem. J. 424: 47-60.

[176] Choi H.G., Zhang J., Deng X., Hatcher J.M., Patricelli M.P., Zhao Z., Alessi D.R., and Gray N.S. (2012). Brain Penetrant LRRK2 Inhibitor. ACS Med. Chem. Lett. 3: 658-662.

[177] Estrada A.A., Liu X., Baker-Glenn C., Beresford A., Burdick D.J., Chambers M., Chan B.K., Chen H., Ding X., DiPasquale A.G. et al. (2012). Discovery of highly potent, selective, and brain-penetrable leucine-rich repeat kinase 2 (LRRK2) small molecule inhibitors. J. Med. Chem. 55: 9416-9433.

[178] Chen H., Chan B.K., Drummond J., Estrada A.A., Gunzner-Toste J., Liu X., Liu Y., Moffat J., Shore D., Sweeney Z.K. et al. (2012). Discovery of selective LRRK2 inhibitors guided by computational analysis and molecular modeling. J. Med. Chem. 55: 5536-5545.

[179] Herzig M.C., Kolly C., Persohn E., Theil D., Schweizer T., Hafner T., Stemmelen C., Troxler T.J., Schmid P., Danner S. et al. (2011). LRRK2 protein levels are determined by kinase function and are crucial for kidney and lung homeostasis in mice. Hum. Mol. Genet. 20: 4209-4223.

[180] Ness D., Ren Z., Gardai S., Sharpnack D., Johnson V.J., Brennan R.J., Brigham E.F., and Olaharski A.J. (2013). Leucine-rich repeat kinase 2 (LRRK2)-deficient rats exhibit renal tubule injury and perturbations in metabolic and immunological homeostasis. PLoS. One. 8: e66164.

[181] Tong Y., Giaime E., Yamaguchi H., Ichimura T., Liu Y., Si H., Cai H., Bonventre J.V., and Shen J. (2012). Loss of leucine-rich repeat kinase 2 causes age-dependent bi-phasic alterations of the autophagy pathway. Mol. Neurodegener. 7: 2.

[182] Berger Z., Smith K.A., and LaVoie M.J. (2010). Membrane localization of LRRK2 is associated with increased formation of the highly active LRRK2 dimer and changes in its phosphorylation. Biochemistry 49: 5511-5523.

3

Parkinson's Disease and Peripheral Neuropathy

Peter Podgorny and Cory Toth

1. Introduction

Idiopathic Parkinson's disease (IPD), an age-dependent neurodegenerative disorder without known cause, is well known to manifest with rest tremor, rigidity, bradykinesia and gait instability on examination [1, 2]. However, other ancillary manifestations have become accepted over the years, including cognitive decline, depression, and autonomic dysfunction [3]. All of these clinically presenting features have long been known to result from disease within the central nervous system, where IPD is pathologically associated with degeneration of the substantia nigra [4].

The possibility of peripheral nervous system functional or pathological involvement in IPD has only recently been considered. One form of peripheral nervous system disease is a peripheral neuropathy, a distal-predominant process affecting the feet and legs, and in more severe cases, the hands and torso [5]. Peripheral neuropathy can manifest as a disease of the axons or the myelin, or both, within nerve fibers. In addition, sensory nerve fibers carrying information for touch, pain and temperature sensations (small nerve fibers termed Aδ and C fibers) as well as for vibration detection and proprioception (large nerve fibers termed Aα and Aβ fibers) can be selectively affected. In most cases, sensory dysfunction appears first, followed by further disease of large nerve fibers leading to loss of reflexes and the possible development of weakness. Symptoms of a peripheral neuropathy may include the early onset of numbness, tingling or prickling sensations, followed by the later onset of incoordination, weakness and pain [6]. The presence of such symptoms in patients should lead to a detailed neurological examination of the peripheral nervous system. Physical examination findings in a patient with peripheral neuropathy will often include abnormal responses to touch, pinprick, temperature, vibration and proprioception, as well as abnormal reflexes, weakness and ataxia. These features will typically display a stocking-glove pattern of distribution due to the distal predominance of peripheral neuropathy with the feet being implicated first.

Recently, an association of peripheral neuropathy with IPD has been demonstrated [7-10]. The importance of this finding has been the new appreciation of peripheral nervous system presentations in patients with IPD. However, for patients with IPD already suffering mobility issues [11], a concurrent peripheral neuropathy may contribute to immobility, risk of falling and autonomic dysfunction. In addition, a peripheral neuropathy may contribute to development of new symptoms including sensory phenomena, distal limb weakness, and pain. This chapter will examine the occurrence of peripheral neuropathy and IPD, its potential causes, progression, and its management.

2. Peripheral neuropathy

2.1. General assessment of peripheral neuropathy

Peripheral neuropathy, as compared with IPD, can be due to hundreds of different etiologies [12], and is associated with a variety of pathological changes within a peripheral nerve. The most common causes of peripheral neuropathy are metabolic or endocrine disorders such as with diabetes mellitus, uremia, or thyroid disease, infections such as with human immuno-deficiency virus or leprosy, toxic effects as with chemotherapy or alcohol excess, genetic disorders such as with Charcot-Marie-Tooth disease, amongst other causes. Another poten-tially underdiagnosed cause of peripheral neuropathy is a nutritional deficiency such as with insufficient vitamin B1, vitamin B6, vitamin B12, folate or thiamine [13, 14]. Many other causes of peripheral neuropathy occur, but between 40-50% of patients with peripheral neuropathy have no determined cause for their peripheral neuropathy, leading to its designation as an idiopathic peripheral neuropathy [15]. Typically, idiopathic peripheral neuropathy occurs in older patients and has a slow progression over many years, but its overall clinical presentation and course of progression is similar when compared with other forms of peripheral neuropa-thy. There are likely a number of causes of idiopathic peripheral neuropathy, many of which may be due to neurodegenerative conditions which have not yet been determined.

The diagnosis of peripheral neuropathy, unlike that of IPD, does not depend upon clinical criteria. Instead, the diagnosis can be supported by electrophysiological testing of peripheral nerves using nerve conduction studies and electromyography. Pathological investigations include nerve biopsy and skin biopsies for the identification of epidermal nerve fibers [16, 17]. Peripheral neuropathy will often develop from an asymptomatic (mild signs, no symp-toms) or subclinical (no signs or symptoms) peripheral neuropathy [18] in which neurological changes have already begun but can only be detected electrophysiologically, pathologically or through quantitative sensory testing. Because peripheral nerves have some regenerative capacity, early recognition of the peripheral neuropathy could reduce morbidity. Although there is no gold standard diagnostic test for peripheral neuropathy, nerve conduction studies are considered a well established method of diagnosis, classification and quantification of peripheral neuropathy [19]. However, nerve conduction studies and electromyography cannot detect all forms of peripheral neuropathy, such as with a small fiber dominant neuropathy [20], where clinical assessment and skin biopsy findings may be abnormal. In other forms of peripheral neuropathy, such as with remitted immune-mediated peripheral neuropathies, only electrophysiological testing may be abnormal. Therefore, the diagnosis of peripheral neuropathy is subject to the overall impression of the assessing neurologist. In order to assist the clinician, clinical scoring systems have been validated for the assessment of peripheral neuropathy, particularly with diabetic polyneuropathy. The Toronto Clinical Scoring System [21] and the Utah Early Neuropathy Scale [22] have been developed to assist with quantification of peripheral neuropathy, specifically for clinical trials. Overall, the clinician must examine a number of aspects when assessing for a peripheral neuropathy, including clinical presentation and examination findings, electrophysiological results, and pathological investigations. In some cases, a subclinical peripheral neuropathy may only be captured by a combination of physical examination, electrophysiology and pathological investigations.

2.2. Peripheral neuropathy in idiopathic Parkinson's disease

A number of non-motor features have been reported to occur in IPD (Table 1). These may range from cognitive dysfunction and neuropsychiatric presentations to dysautonomia and sleep disorders. Sensory manifestations, such as may occur with a peripheral neuropathy were first recognized in 1976 [23]. Nearly half of IPD patients were described to have sensory manifestations with normal clinical examination; less than 10% of these patients had sensory manifestations initiate before motor symptoms onset. Due to patient reports of sensory manifestations being more likely to be present when IPD patients were in an "off" medication state rather than in the "on" medication state, the possibility of sensory symptoms emanating from the central nervous system arose [24-26]. Furthermore, earlier electrophysiological studies for peripheral and central-peripheral sensory conduction failed to determine any abnormalities, leading to a belief that all sensory manifestations occurring in IPD patients occur without the involvement of the somatosensory pathways [27]. The possibility of sensory manifestations in IPD patients occurring due to an "off" medication state previously led to beliefs of a dopamine-mediated origin for all sensory phenomena in IPD patients. Furthermore, hypotheses had arisen regarding the dysfunction of the basal ganglia and pathways involving the striatum in particular [28]. Some older papers have reported sensory symptoms to occur in 40-70% of IPD patients, often consisting of pain, paresthesias, itching and burning sensations [29]; many of these symptoms are often unreported [30]. In particular, it was felt that pain was most often related to the presence of concurrent dystonia [31]. The beliefs that sensory features in IPD patients were only related to medication (dopamine) and the "off" state and/or abnormalities in the basal ganglia likely contributed to decades of a relative absence of studies to better determine the nature of sensory symptoms in IPD patients. However, work in the most recent years has re-examined the potential for peripheral nervous system involvement in patients with IPD.

Any consideraton for involvement of the peripheral nervous system in IPD patients must first begin with consideration of concurrent conditions in the same patient. The most well established estimation for the prevalence of peripheral neuropathy in the general population is 2.4% overall, but this may rise to as high as 8% in older populations, with diabetic and idiopathic forms being the most common cause [32]. Certainly, this high prevalence needs to be consid-

Cognitive dysfunction
Executive impairment
Inattention
Impaired visuomotor processing
Mild Cognitive Impairment
Dementia

Neuropsychiatric manifestations
Mood and anxiety disorders
Anhedonia and apathy
Psychosis and hallucinosis

Autonomic dysfunction
Arrhythmias and other cardiovascular manifestations
Orthostatic hypotension
Urinary urgency, incontinence or nocturia
Gastrointestinal manifestations including constipation
Thermoregulatory dysfunction including change in sweating function

Sleep disorders
REM behavioral disorder (RBD)
Periodic limb movements/restless legs syndrome
Excessive daytime somnolence
Insomnia

Sensory symptoms
Numbness, tingling, pain

Other
Fatigue
Dysphagia
Olfactory dysfunction
Visual disturbances including lack of accommodation
Seborrhoeic dermatitis

Table 1. Non-motor manifestations in Idiopathic Parkinson's Disease

ered in any population, particular an older population of IPD patients. The estimated preva-
lance of IPD is 0.1-0.2% of the general population, but this also rises to 1% of those above 60
years of age [33]. Thus, a small percentage of the general population may have concurrent and
unrelated Parkinsonism and peripheral neuropathy which may be estimated to be less than
0.01% of those above 60 years of age if based upon chance alone.

Genetic considerations have been considered as well for the concurrence of IPD and peripheral
neuropathy. In one study of IPD patients with a parkin gene mutation, a genetic mutation
related to younger onset of IPD, one out of 24 patients had a sensory and autonomic peripheral

neuropathy based upon nerve conduction studies and nerve biopsy [34]. Another single case report identified a patient with IPD and peripheral neuropathy using similar methods [35]. In both of these cases, the peripheral neuropathy appeared axonal in nature. The potential role of parkin is interesting, as parkin mRNA is present within human peripheral nerve [36]. In IPD patients with parkin mutations and presence of a sensory dominant axonal peripheral neuropathy [37], two fragments of the parkin gene product could be identified [36]. In addition, abnormal electrophysiological findings in patients with PARK2 mutations suggest there are pre-symptomatic neurodegenerative processes occuring in the periphery [38] and may be indicative of a sensory neuropathy [39].

Concurrent peripheral neuropathy may occur in conditions related to Parkinson's Disease, such as multiple system atrophy (MSA). Patients with MSA may have peripheral neuropathy present in as many as 40% of cases when the peripheral nervous system is specifically examined [40-42]. Another clue may be the co-occurrence of peripheral neuropathy and Parkinsonism in patients with mitochondrial disorders while Parkinsonism may be seen with mitochondrial disorders [43, 44]. However, these disorders have important differences from Parkinson's disease, including the presence of peripheral nervous system pathology. For example, patients with MSA have pathological changes within autonomic ganglia, where α-synuclein accumulation occurs within neurons of the sympathetic ganglia. Many forms of mitochondrial diseases have axonal atrophy and loss in the peripheral nerves along with concurrent development of ragged red fibers and myopathic changes. Finally, even patients with IPD can have presence of α-synuclein accumulation in sympathetic ganglia and in the enteric nervous system [45] as well as in some sensory nerves innervating the pharynx [46]. Despite this knowledge, there has been no literature reports investigating the prevalence of peripheral neuropathy within a large population of IPD patients until recently.

Our group began to identify patients with IPD and concurrent peripheral neuropathy beginning in 2002 [7]. Patients identified in a tertiary care Movement Disorders Clinic were assessed prospectively for presence of peripheral neuropathy and potential causative relationships. All patients with IPD and potential peripheral neuropathy were assessed for other potential causes of peripheral neuropathy and had documentation for other comorbid conditions, treatment for IPD, and the nature of peripheral neuropathy present. Each patient was assessed clinically with a Toronto Clinical Scoring System (TCSS) calculated for each patient and electrophysiological assessment using nerve conduction studies of the upper and lower limbs. Following assessment of routine blood work investigations obtained for determination for other related causes of peripheral neuropathy, patients were reassessed for causation of identified peripheral neuropathies. Studies included assessment of fasting methylmalonic acid, which is recommended for investigation of undetermined peripheral neuropathy [47].

Interestingly, and somewhat unexpectedly, we identified a total of 40 IPD patients with both clinical and electrophysiological evidence of a concurrent peripheral neuropathy [7]. Of these 40 patients, 30% had another etiology for peripheral neuropathy – diabetes mellitus was determined in 13% of patients, a monoclonal gammopathy of uncertain significance with possible relationship to peripheral neuropathy was determined in 10% of patients, and possible or probable chronic inflammatory demyelinating peripheral neuropathy was discovered in 7% of patients. However, the remaining 70% of IPD patients had no defined cause for peripheral neuropathy, a much higher anticipated prevalence than would be anticipated in the general population (up to 40%). Clinical and electrophysiological abnormalities of peripheral neuropathy in the remaining population suggested an axonal form of peripheral neuropathy. In this remaining population, fasting methylmalonic acid elevation was seen in 93% of patients, considerably higher than in patients with IPD without peripheral neuropathy and than in patients without IPD with otherwise idiopathic peripheral neuropathy. The reasons for the elevated fasting methylmalonic acid were not immediately understood, nor the importance. The levels of cobalamin, or vitamin B12, were not significantly abnormal in the majority of patients; cobalamin deficiency is the most well reported cause of methylmalonic acid elevations. However, examination of the severity of peripheral neuropathy using the Toronto Clinical Scoring System revealed a strong positive association with lifetime consumption of levodopa, the mainstay of therapy for IPD. The daily levodopa equivalence dose, particularly when administered as an intestinal gel infusion, also appeared to correlate with neuropathic impairment [48]. Although this could be explained by longer duration and worse severity of illness in IPD patients with concurrent peripheral neuropathy, another relationship also emerged. Severity of peripheral neuropathy also correlated positively with the degree of elevation of fasting methylmalonic acid.

Although cobalamin deficiency is most classically associated with subacute combined degeneration manifesting as a myelopathy in combination with peripheral neuropathy, an exclusive presentation with peripheral neuropathy can also occur [49] as an axonal form of peripheral neuropathy [50]. Typically, cobalamin deficiency has been identified as a cause of peripheral neuropathy in 8% of patients with cryptogenic peripheral neuropathy [51]. Making the diagnosis of cobalamin deficiency-associated peripheral neuropathy can be problematic, since a significant proportion of up to 50% of cobalamin deficient patients will have normal serum cobalamin levels [13, 52]. However, measurement of the serum metabolite methylmalonic acid improves diagnostic specificity and sensitivity [53] and is now recommended [5].

A mainstay of PD therapy for several decades has been levodopa [54]. Although arguably the most effective long-term therapeutic option in IPD patients, several long-term complications have emerged from the use of long-term levodopa. These have included dyskinesias, dopamine dysregulation syndrome, addiction, impulse control disorders, punding, and compulsive medication use [55, 56, 57]. In addition to these adverse effects, levodopa's catabolism is associated with elevation of serum homocysteine and methylmalonic acid [58]. This occurs via levodopa exerting its influence upon methyltetrahydrofolate (methyl-THF) pathways during folate metabolism (Figure 1). One-carbon fragments are stepwise reduced to methyl groups in cobalamin-dependent reactions from methyl-THF to homocysteine, forming methionine. Adenosylation of methionine then follows, leading to S-adenosylmethionine (SAM) formation - this serves as the methyl group donor in several transmethylation reactions, some of which are catalyzed by catechol-O-methyltransferase (COMT). Whereas demethylation of SAM leads to formation of S-adenosylhomocysteine (SAH), this is immediately cleaved to form homocysteine. During these transmethylations, homocysteine may be remethylated by methyl-THF and cobalamin to form methionine and SAM. Upon introduction of levodopa, the process of its methylation likely leads to the depletion of SAM and subsequently leads to elevated plasma homocysteine. Cobalamin is an essential cofactor in the conversion of homocysteine to methionine and SAM, and is likely depleted as SAM levels return to normal. Further downstream in the pathway, cobalamin serves as a cofactor for the isomerisation of succinyl-CoA; hence, a cobalamin deficiency may lead to methylmalonic acid accumulation [59]. Systemic aromatic L-amino acid decarboxylase inhibitors (such as carbidopa) given to IPD patients also direct the systemic metabolism of levodopa to occur through COMT to 3-O-methyldopa (3-OMD); this reaction also involves methylation by SAM, further contributing to increasing homocysteine and methylmalonic acid formation. The methylation potential within an individual can be measured by the SAM/SAH ratio and appeared to be an important factor for neurodegeneration, in one study [60]. The B complex vitamins including cobalamin are important in the control of one-carbon metabolism (Figure 1), it is possible for plasma concentrations of cobalamin to decline in IPD patients due to increasing methylation demands of daily levodopa consumption. As a result of these biochemical implications, it can be speculated that levodopa's interaction with these methylation pathways precipitates elevations in both homocysteine and methylmalonic acid in IPD patients.

It was previously shown that homocysteine was elevated amongst IPD patients when compared to control subjects [61-63], with greatest elevation noted in those with levodopa usage [64-66]. In IPD patients initiating levodopa therapy, homocysteine levels elevate and cobalamin levels fall at about 3 months after levodopa initiation. Similar elevations in homocysteine and depression in cobalamin occur in IPD patients who double their daily levodopa intake [67]. As well, IPD patients treated with levodopa for at least a year have significantly lower cobalamin levels than matched controls [68]. Although it could be speculated that the use of a COMT inhibitor could prevent these changes, this may or may not be the case [67, 69, 70]. Patients with IPD and concurrent homocysteine elevation may also be subject to a genetic alteration – approximately 1/3 of IPD patients with homocysteine elevation have a more inefficient (thermolabile) form of methylenetetrahydrofolate reductase (MTHFR), the key enzyme for the remethylation of homocysteine to methionine [71]. This may indicate that specific IPD patients are genetically susceptible to the development of homocysteine and methylmalonic acid elevation due to levodopa therapy. However, it is not known if IPD individuals are more susceptible to MTHFR polymorphisms, as they occur in healthy individuals as well [72]. This may also explain why only a proportion of patients we have studied with IPD and levodopa use were identified to have peripheral neuropathy.

The identification of a series of patients with IPD, levodopa usage, and elevations in homocysteine and methylmalonic acid led to a further prospective cohort investigation to attempt to identify if the association with IPD and peripheral neuropathy was more than chance [8]. We selected IPD patients randomly from a comprehensive database at a tertiary clinic and compared these patients to control subjects without IPD or levodopa usage. This study format was used to determine the relationship of levodopa use with serum levels of cobalamin, methylmalonic acid and homocysteine. We also explored the association between presence and severity of peripheral neuropathy and age, duration of IPD, cumulative levodopa dosing,

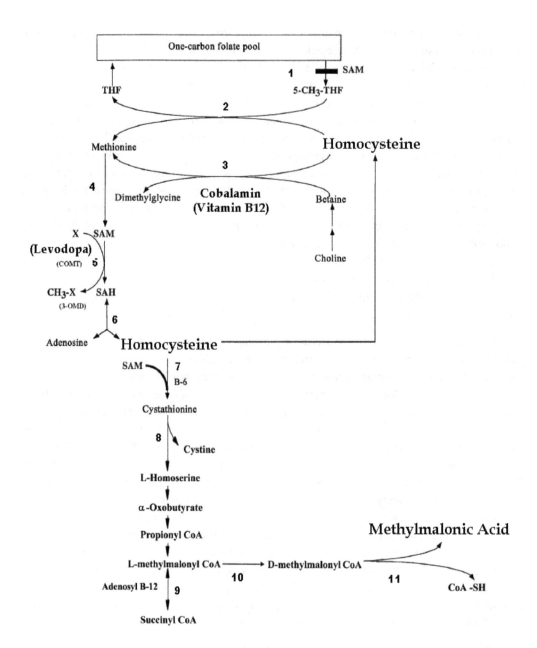

Figure 1. Folate and methyl group metabolism related to levodopa, methylmalonic acid and homocysteine. The numbers refer to the enzymes as listed: 1, methylenetetrahydrofolate (THF) reductase; 2, 5-methyltetrahydrofolate–homocysteine S-methyltransferase; 3, methionine synthase; 4, methionine adenosyltransferase; 5, a variety of methyltransferase reactions including catechol-O-methyltransferase (COMT); 6, adenosylhomocysteinase; 7, cystathionine-ß-synthase; 8, cystathionine lyase; 9, L-methylmalonyl CoA mutase; 10, D,L-methylmalonyl CoA racemase; 11, D-methylmalonyl CoA hydrolase. The heavy bar in reaction 1 denotes an allosteric inhibition by S-adenosylmethionine (SAM). The heavy arrow in reaction 7 denotes activation by SAM. SAH is S-adenosylhomocysteine. Note that levodopa acts in the methylation of SAH in enzymatic reaction 6, while cobalamin is an important factor in enzymatic reaction 3.

cobalamin, methylmalonic acid, and homocysteine levels. The majority (86%) of the 58 IPD patients assessed were taking levodopa at time of assessment. A blinded and unblinded Neurologist assessed the clinical and electrophysiological presentations for all patients and control subjects. A total of 58% of IPD patients assessed had clinical and electrophysiological features of peripheral neuropathy - 75% of these patients had symptomatic peripheral neuropathy, while 25% of these IPD patients had subclinical neuropathy. This was contrasted by only 9% of age- and sex-matched control subjects receiving a diagnosis of peripheral neuropathy.

Although the duration of IPD was similar between IPD patients with or without peripheral neuropathy, the severity of IPD, based upon the Unified Parkinson's Disease Rating Scale, was greater in IPD patients with peripheral neuropathy. This indicated that peripheral neuropathy was not likely to be present near the time of diagnosis of IPD, but appeared to occur later. Likewise, greater severities of disease would tend to indicate higher cumulative intakes of levodopa for disease management, which was the case for IPD patients with peripheral neuropathy. Interestingly, cobalamin levels were similar between IPD patients with and without peripheral neuropathy; however, both fasting homocysteine and methylmalonic acid levels were higher in those IPD patients with peripheral neuropathy than in IPD patients without peripheral neuropathy. An odds ratio of 12.4 emerged for levodopa exposure contributing to peripheral neuropathy. Cumulative levodopa exposure was significantly and positively associated with the severity of peripheral neuropathy using the Toronto Clinical Scoring System for all IPD patients studied. In addition, fasting methylmalonic acid levels were also positively associated with severity of peripheral neuropathy amongst all IPD patients. Finally, cumulative levodopa exposure was also directly associated with fasting methylmalonic acid levels in all IPD patients.

Although this may appear as though methylmalonic acid elevations are clearly responsible, it must be considered that a higher severity and longer duration of disease with IPD will lead to greater cumulative use of levodopa. Indeed, greater severity of disease in IPD was also positively associated with greater severity of peripheral neuropathy. At this time, it is not possible to separate the prospect of peripheral neuropathy developing based upon the severity of central nervous system disease occurring in IPD patients. There were no associations of peripheral neuropathy severity with advancing age such as is expected in the general population. Despite the association with levodopa usage that appeared, there was also no relationship to the use of COMT-inhibitors, dopamine agonists, anticholinergic agents, amantidine, or surgical interventions used for IPD. In particular, the use of a COMT-inhibitor did not appear to be protective against the occurrence of homocysteine or methylmalonic acid elevation in IPD patients.

These studies have been followed by case series, including two patients with IPD being treated with high dose levodopa (duodopa) developing subacute axonal peripheral neuropathy with associated cobalamin and vitamin B6 deficiency [73]; another case series suggests there may be an additional demyelinating component in some patients [74]. Another small case series identified clinical and electrophysiological changes of peripheral neuropathy in patients with IPD; these patients had concurrent cobalamin deficiencies in most cases, but also identified other potential causes for peripheral neuropathy as well [75]. Similar observations were made in another population treated with duodopa [76].

2.3. Potential pathogenic mechanisms of peripheral neuropathy in idiopathic Parkinson's disease patients

The studies to date have been descriptive and associative in nature only. The precise pathogenic mechanisms for the development of peripheral neuropathy in IPD patients remain speculative. Before considering the mechanisms by which methylmalonic acid and/or homocysteine may be pathogenic, other considerations require discussion.

As mentioned, considerations for genetic influences are important. The potential implications of parkin mutations given the expression of parkin mRNA in peripheral nerve [36] may be of importance, but only a small percentage of IPD patients with parkin mutations appear to have an axonal form of peripheral neuropathy [34, 35]. The relationship of concurrent peripheral neuropathy to the so called Parkinson's Plus forms of disease, such as with multiple system atrophy must also be considered; patients with multiple system atrophy frequently (40%) have an axonal peripheral neuropathy present [40-42]. Associations such as this may suggest a neurodegenerative pathogenesis for peripheral neuropathy rather than a deficiency. Indeed, patients with greater severity and longer duration of IPD were more susceptible to development of peripheral neuropathy in our studies as well [8]. Further studies will be required to determine if the peripheral neuropathy present in IPD patients develops in an analagous fashion to the central nervous system neurodegeneration in IPD.

It is possible that alpha-synuclein protein deposits in IPD may exhibit neurotoxic properties in peripheral nerves leading to a neuropathy [77]. This is consistent with recent studies demonstrating the presence of alpha-synuclein deposits in the periphery, but in autonomic nerves, not somatic sensory nerves [78]. One study has also demonstrated impaired CNS axonal transport, especially where alpha-synuclein deposits were present, leading to neuronal degeneration in both experimental and human forms of IPD; whether this may also be the case in peripheral neurons has yet to be investigated [79].

The mechanisms by which homocysteine and/or methylmalonic acid may contribute to development of peripheral neuropathy are not as clear. Homocysteine may increase susceptibility to mitochondrial toxins, contribute to free radical formation, exert glutaminergic-associated neurotoxicity, and impair DNA repair mechanisms [62, 80]. Elevated levels of homocyteine may also increase systemic oxidative stress [81]. Thus, homocysteine may exert toxic effects in multiple ways, although which of these may be relevant at the level of the peripheral nerve is not established as of yet. Another nutritional deficiency was detected in a separate population of patients with peripheral neuropathy and IPD: pyridoxine (vitamin B6) [82]; relevance of this finding remains uncertain.

Methylmalonic acid elevations can be detected within both tissues and blood. *In vitro*, methylmalonic acid plays a role in lipid and protein oxidative damage and affects the production of reactive species in cerebral synaptosomes [83]. *In vivo*, MMA can induce preventable or modifiable lipid peroxidation and protein oxidative damage, as well as inhibition of glutathione peroxidase, suggesting that reactive oxygen species generation may be a main product of methylmalonic acid excess [84]. Further work is needed to determine the susceptibility of the dorsal root ganglia sensory neurons to excessive levels of methylmalonic acid and subsequent mechanisms of toxicity.

In IPD patients that we have assessed, it is probable that methylmalonic acid accumulation or relative cobalamin deficiency is the cause of peripheral neuropathy for a number of reasons. In all cases in our prospective cohort study, symptoms of a peripheral neuropathy started years after the onset of IPD and the initiation of levodopa therapy. Second, higher severity levels of peripheral neuropathy were positively correlated with levodopa cumulative use over time, suggesting a treatment-related effect. Third, no other reason could be identified in the majority of cases of peripheral neuropathy identified in a randomly selected IPD population. Finally, treatment of the peripheral neuropathy, described below, appeared to stabilize progression of peripheral neuropathy.

2.4. Treatment options for peripheral neuropathy in idiopathic Parkinson's disease patients

In our initial case series with IPD patients identified to have peripheral neuropathy [7], all patients identified to have one of cobalamin deficiency, methylmalonic acid elevation, or elevated homocystine levels were prescribed monthly intramuscular injections of 1000 μg of cobalamin (vitamin B12). This was provided via intramuscular injections and not oral therapy due to concerns of potential inadequate absorption from the gastrointestinal tract. All patients initialized on therapy were subjected to repeated clinical examinations using the Toronto Clinical Scoring System and electrophysiological evaluations at 6, 12, and 24 months after diagnosis of the peripheral neuropathy when cobalamin therapy was initiated. Repeated blood tests for cobalamin, fasting methylmalonic acid and fasting homocysteine were concurrently performed.

Beginning at 6 months after monthly cobalamin injections were initiated, significant improvements in each of cobalamin, fasting methylmalonic acid and fasting homocysteine were noted all measurements were noted, with cobalamin returning to normal levels in all patients and with fasting homocysteine and fasting methylmalonic acid levels improving to normal levels in approximately 2/3 of cases. Interestingly, clinical assessments and electrophysiological measurements essentially stabilized over follow-up at 12 and 24 months after initiation of intramuscular cobalamin treatment. When compared to a cohort of patients without IPD but with idiopathic peripheral neuropathy identified to have isolated methylmalonic acid elevation, differences in clinical course could be identified; this patient population continued to exhibit mild clinical and electrophysiological decline over the 12 and 24 months follow-up as compared to the IPD patient population receiving cobalamin injections. This initial data is supportive of management of the identified elevated methylmalonic academia, but further studies are required before definitive suggestions can be applied.

3. Conclusion

Peripheral neuropathy developing concurrently in patients with established IPD can be problematic and should be investigated. A further contribution to disability and mobility may certainly develop in an already compromised patient population. Fortunately, we are starting to learn some of the relationships and the potential iatrogenic effect of levodopa therapy. Future studies should examine the potential mechanisms by which methylmalonic acid may exert its toxic effects, and the prospective options for management of concurrent peripheral neuropathy in IPD patients. Therapeutic intervention studies are required to establish whether cobalamin replacement may be viable. Further genetic susceptibility testing may determine the heterogenous development of peripheral neuropathy in IPD patients. Finally, the possibility of prophylactic interventions at the time of diagnosis of IPD or at the time of levodopa initiation for the prevention of peripheral neuropathy may be a future endeavour. We do not yet know the role of dopamine antagonists and COMT inhibitors, amongst other IPD interventions, but future studies may assist in our understanding. Our knowledge of the development of peripheral neuropathy in IPD patients has developed over a short duration of time, but is certain to expand over the coming generations.

Acknowledgements

We would like to thank the Alberta Heritage Foundation for salary and research support during the time of studies performed in the IPD population. We would also like to thank the Movement Disorders Clinic at the University of Calgary and Dr. O. Suchowersky for their support of the clinical studies performed to date. Finally, we would like to thank all of the IPD patients and control subjects who assisted in the prospective cohort study to help identify this important clinical problem.

Author details

Peter Podgorny and Cory Toth

University of Calgary, Canada

References

[1] Lang, A. E. & Lozano, A. M. Parkinson's disease. First of two parts. *New England Journal of Medicine* 339, 1044-1053 (1998).

[2]   Lang, A. E. & Lozano, A. M. Parkinson's disease. Second of two parts. *New England Journal of Medicine* 339, 1130-1143 (1998).

[3]   Mendis, T., Suchowersky, O., Lang, A. & Gauthier, S. Management of parkinson's disease: a review of current and new therapies. *Canadian Journal of Neurological Sciences* 26, 89-103 (1999).

[4]   Lang, A. E. & Obeso, J. A. Time to move beyond nigrostriatal dopamine deficiency in Parkinson's disease. *Annals of Neurology* 55, 761-765 (2004).

[5]   England, J. D. *et al.* Evaluation of distal symmetric polyneuropathy: the role of laboratory and genetic testing (an evidence-based review). *Muscle Nerve* 39, 116-125, doi: 10.1002/mus.21226 (2009).

[6]   Wolfe, G. I. *et al.* Chronic cryptogenic sensory polyneuropathy: clinical and laboratory characteristics. *Archives of Neurology* 56(5), 540-547 (1999).

[7]   Toth, C., Brown, M. S., Furtado, S., Suchowersky, O. & Zochodne, D. Neuropathy as a potential complication of levodopa use in Parkinson's disease. *Mov Disord* 23, 1850-1859, doi:10.1002/mds.22137 (2008).

[8]   Toth, C. *et al.* Levodopa, methylmalonic acid, and neuropathy in idiopathic Parkinson disease. *Ann Neurol* 68, 28-36, doi:10.1002/ana.22021 (2010).

[9]   Rajabally, Y. A. & Martey, J. Neuropathy in Parkinson disease: prevalence and determinants. *Neurology* 77, 1947-1950, doi:WNL.0b013e31823a0ee4 [pii] 10.1212/WNL. 0b013e31823a0ee4 (2011).

[10] Streitova, H., Bursova, S., Minks, E., Bednarik, J. & Bares, M. High incidence of small fiber neuropathy in patients with Parkinson's disease: Electrophysiological and histopathological study [abstract]. *Movement Disorders* 27, 659 (2012).

[11] Wallace, M. *et al.* Once-daily OROS hydromorphone for the management of chronic nonmalignant pain: a dose-conversion and titration study. *Int J Clin Pract* 61, 1671-1676, doi:IJCP1500 [pii] 10.1111/j.1742-1241.2007.01500.x (2007).

[12] Dyck, P. J. & Thomas, P. K. *Peripheral Neuropathy.* (Elsevier Saunders, 2005).

[13] Nations, S. P. & et.al. Clinical profile of vitamin B12 neuropathy. *Neurology* 50, A208-A209 (1998).

[14] Skelton, W. P. d. & Skelton, N. K. Thiamine deficiency neuropathy. It's still common today. *Postgraduate Medical Journal* 85, 301-306 (1989).

[15] Notermans, N. C. *et al.* Chronic idiopathic axonal polyneuropathy: a five year follow up. *Journal of Neurology, Neurosurgery & Psychiatry* 57, 1525-1527 (1994).

[16] Lauria, G. *et al.* EFNS guidelines on the use of skin biopsy in the diagnosis of peripheral neuropathy. *European Journal of Neurology* 12, 747-758 (2005).

[17] Malik, R. A. *et al.* Sural nerve pathology in diabetic patients with minimal but progressive neuropathy. *Diabetologia* 48, 578-585 (2005).

[18] Albers, J. W. & Berent, S. in *Neurobehavioral Toxicology: The peripheral nervous system* Vol. 2 Ch. 14, 661-662 (Taylor & Francis, 2005).

[19] Perkins, B. A., Ngo, M. & Bril, V. Symmetry of nerve conduction studies in different stages of diabetic polyneuropathy. *Muscle & Nerve* 25, 212-217 (2002).

[20] Lacomis, D. Small-fiber neuropathy. *Muscle and Nerve* 26, 173-188 (2002).

[21] Bril, V. & Perkins, B. A. Validation of the Toronto Clinical Scoring System for diabetic polyneuropathy. *Diabetes Care* 25, 2048-2052 (2002).

[22] Hadi, I., Morley-Forster, P. K., Dain, S., Horrill, K. & Moulin, D. E. Brief review: Perioperative management of the patient with chronic non-cancer pain: [Article de synthese court : Prise en charge perioperatoire des patients souffrant de douleur chronique non cancereuse]. *Can J Anaesth* 53, 1190-1199, doi:53/12/1190 [pii] (2006).

[23] Snider, S. R., Fahn, S., Isgreen, W. P. & Cote, L. J. Primary sensory symptoms in parkinsonism. *Neurology* 26, 423-429 (1976).

[24] Turk, D. C. *et al.* Developing patient-reported outcome measures for pain clinical trials: IMMPACT recommendations. *Pain* 125, 208-215, doi:S0304-3959(06)00501-X [pii] 10.1016/j.pain.2006.09.028 (2006).

[25] Moulin, D. Does acute pain associated with herpes zoster respond to treatment with gabapentin? *Nat Clin Pract Neurol* 2, 298-299, doi:ncpneuro0195 [pii] 10.1038/ncpneuro0195 (2006).

[26] Gilron, I., Watson, C. P., Cahill, C. M. & Moulin, D. E. Neuropathic pain: a practical guide for the clinician. *CMAJ* 175, 265-275, doi:175/3/265 [pii] 10.1503/cmaj.060146 (2006).

[27] Jovey, R. D. *et al.* Use of opioid analgesics for the treatment of chronic noncancer pain--a consensus statement and guidelines from the Canadian Pain Society, 2002. *Pain Res Manag* 8 Suppl A, 3A-28A (2003).

[28] Russell, A. *et al.* Evaluation of dosing guidelines for use of controlled-release codeine in chronic noncancer pain. *Pain Res Manag* 8, 143-148 (2003).

[29] Koller, W. C. Sensory symptoms in Parkinson's disease. *Neurology* 34, 957-959 (1984).

[30] Moulin, D. Use of methadone for neuropathic pain. *Pain Res Manag* 8, 131-132 (2003).

[31] Watson, C. P., Moulin, D., Watt-Watson, J., Gordon, A. & Eisenhoffer, J. Controlled-release oxycodone relieves neuropathic pain: a randomized controlled trial in painful diabetic neuropathy. *Pain* 105, 71-78, doi:S030439590300160X [pii] (2003).

[32] Dyck, P. J. The causes, classification and treatment of peripheral neuropathy. *New England Journal of Medicine* 307, 283-286 (1982).

[33] Sumpton, J. E. & Moulin, D. E. Treatment of neuropathic pain with venlafaxine. *Ann Pharmacother* 35, 557-559 (2001).

[34] Khan, N. L. *et al.* Parkin disease: a phenotypic study of a large case series. *Brain* 126, 1279-1292 (2003).

[35] Roy, M. K. Familial parkinsonism with peripheral neuropathy. *J Assoc.Physicians India* 49, 944 (2001).

[36] Abbruzzese, G. *et al.* Does parkin play a role in the peripheral nervous system? A family report. *Mov Disord.* 19, 978-981 (2004).

[37] Okuma, Y., Hattori, N. & Mizuno, Y. Sensory neuropathy in autosomal recessive juvenile parkinsonism (PARK2). *Parkinsonism.Relat Disord.* 9, 313-314 (2003).

[38] Ohsawa, Y. *et al.* Reduced amplitude of the sural nerve sensory action potential in PARK2 patients. *Neurology* 65, 459-462, doi:65/3/459 [pii] 10.1212/01.wnl. 0000171859.85078.3d (2005).

[39] Okuma, Y., Hattori, N. & Mizuno, Y. Sensory neuropathy in autosomal recessive juvenile parkinsonism (PARK2). *Parkinsonism Relat Disord* 9, 313-314, doi:S1353802002001141 [pii] (2003).

[40] Chand, R. P., Tharakan, J. K., Koul, R. L. & Kumar, S. D. Clinical and radiological features of juvenile onset olivopontocerebellar atrophy. *Clin.Neurol Neurosurg.* 98, 152-156 (1996).

[41] Rodolico, C. *et al.* Peripheral neuropathy as the presenting feature of multiple system atrophy. *Clinical Autonomic Research* 11, 119-121 (2001).

[42] Rossi, A., Ciacci, G., Federico, A., Mondelli, M. & Rizzuto, N. Sensory and motor peripheral neuropathy in olivopontocerebellar atrophy. *Acta Neurol Scand* 73, 363-371 (1986).

[43] Luoma, P. *et al.* Parkinsonism, premature menopause, and mitochondrial DNA polymerase gamma mutations: clinical and molecular genetic study. *Lancet* 364, 875-882 (2004).

[44] Liu, S. *et al.* Parkinson's disease-associated kinase PINK1 regulates Miro protein level and axonal transport of mitochondria. *PLoS Genet* 8, e1002537, doi:10.1371/journal.pgen.1002537 PGENETICS-D-11-02331 [pii] (2012).

[45] Zaza, C., Reyno, L. & Moulin, D. E. The multidimensional pain inventory profiles in patients with chronic cancer-related pain: an examination of generalizability. *Pain* 87, 75-82, doi:S0304-3959(00)00274-8 [pii] (2000).

[46] Mu, L. *et al.* Parkinson Disease Affects Peripheral Sensory Nerves in the Pharynx. *J Neuropathol Exp Neurol* 72, 614-623, doi:10.1097/NEN.0b013e3182965886 (2013).

[47] England, J. D. *et al.* Practice Parameter: evaluation of distal symmetric polyneuropathy: role of laboratory and genetic testing (an evidence-based review). Report of the

American Academy of Neurology, American Association of Neuromuscular and Electrodiagnostic Medicine, and American Academy of Physical Medicine and Rehabilitation. *Neurology* 72, 185-192, doi:01.wnl.0000336370.51010.a1 [pii] 10.1212/01.wnl. 0000336370.51010.a1 (2009).

[48] Jugel, C. *et al.* Neuropathy in Parkinson's Disease Patients with Intestinal Levodopa Infusion versus Oral Drugs. *PLoS One* 8, e66639, doi:10.1371/journal.pone.0066639 PONE-D-13-08087 [pii] (2013).

[49] Saperstein, D. S. & Barohn, R. J. Peripheral neuropathy due to cobalamin deficiency. *Curr.Treat.Options.Neurol* 4, 197-201 (2002).

[50] Fine, E. J., Soria, E., Paroski, M. W., Petryk, D. & Thomasula, L. The neurophysiological profile of vitamin B12 deficiency. *Muscle and Nerve* 13, 158-164 (1990).

[51] Saperstein, D. S. *et al.* Challenges in the identification of cobalamin-deficiency polyneuropathy. *Arch.Neurol* 60, 1296-1301 (2003).

[52] Savage, D. G., Lindenbaum, J., Stabler, S. P. & Allen, R. H. Sensitivity of serum methylmalonic acid and total homocysteine determinations for diagnosing cobalamin and folate deficiencies. *Am J Med* 96, 239-246 (1994).

[53] Lindenbaum, J., Savage, D. G., Stabler, S. P. & Allen, R. H. Diagnosis of cobalamin deficiency: II. Relative sensitivities of serum cobalamin, methylmalonic acid, and total homocysteine concentrations. *Am J Hematol.* 34, 99-107 (1990).

[54] Fahn, S. *et al.* Levodopa and the progression of Parkinson's disease. *New England Journal of Medicine* 351, 2498-2508 (2004).

[55] Sloan, P. A., Moulin, D. E. & Hays, H. A clinical evaluation of transdermal therapeutic system fentanyl for the treatment of cancer pain. *J Pain Symptom Manage* 16, 102-111, doi:S088539249800044X [pii] (1998).

[56] Babul, N., Provencher, L., Laberge, F., Harsanyi, Z. & Moulin, D. Comparative efficacy and safety of controlled-release morphine suppositories and tablets in cancer pain. *J Clin Pharmacol* 38, 74-81 (1998).

[57] Moulin, D. E., Hagen, N., Feasby, T. E., Amireh, R. & Hahn, A. Pain in Guillain-Barre syndrome. *Neurology* 48, 328-331 (1997).

[58] Postuma, R. B. *et al.* Vitamins and entacapone in levodopa-induced hyperhomocysteinemia: a randomized controlled study. *Neurology.* 66(12), 1941-1943 (2006).

[59] Postuma, R. B. & Lang, A. Homocysteine and levodopa;should Parkin disease patients recieve preventative therapy? *Arch Neurol*, 1296 - 1301 (2004).

[60] Obeid, R. *et al.* Methylation status and neurodegenerative markers in Parkinson disease. *Clin Chem* 55, 1852-1860, doi:10.1373/clinchem.2009.125021 clinchem. 2009.125021 [pii] (2009).

[61] Blandini, F. *et al.* Plasma homocysteine and l-dopa metabolism in patients with Par-kinson disease. *Clinical Chemistry* 47, 1102-1104 (2001).

[62] Kuhn, W., Roebroek, R., Blom, H., van, O. D. & Muller, T. Hyperhomocysteinaemia in Parkinson's disease. *J Neurol* 245, 811-812 (1998).

[63] Kuhn, W. *et al.* Elevated plasma levels of homocysteine in Parkinson's disease. *Eur.Neurol* 40, 225-227 (1998).

[64] Muller, T., Werne, B., Fowler, B. & Kuhn, W. Nigral endothelial dysfunction, homo-cysteine, and Parkinson's disease. *Lancet* 354, 126-127 (1999).

[65] Rogers, J. D., Sanchez-Saffon, A., Frol, A. B. & Diaz-Arrastia, R. Elevated plasma ho-mocysteine levels in patients treated with levodopa: association with vascular dis-ease. *Arch Neurol* 60, 59-64, doi:noc20099 [pii] (2003).

[66] Miller, J. W. *et al.* Effect of L-dopa on plasma homocysteine in PD patients: relation-ship to B-vitamin status. *Neurology* 60, 1125-1129 (2003).

[67] O'Suilleabhain, P. E., Bottiglieri, T., Dewey, R. B., Jr., Sharma, S. & az-Arrastia, R. Modest increase in plasma homocysteine follows levodopa initiation in Parkinson's disease. *Mov Disord.* 19, 1403-1408 (2004).

[68] Triantafyllou, N. I. *et al.* Folate and vitamin B12 levels in levodopa-treated Parkin-son's disease patients: their relationship to clinical manifestations, mood and cogni-tion. *Parkinsonism Relat Disord* 14, 321-325, doi:S1353-8020(07)00214-3 [pii] 10.1016/j.parkreldis.2007.10.002 (2008).

[69] Valkovic, P. *et al.* Reduced plasma homocysteine levels in levodopa/entacapone treat-ed Parkinson patients. *Parkinsonism.Relat Disord.* 11, 253-256 (2005).

[70] Zoccolella, S. *et al.* Plasma homocysteine levels in Parkinson's disease: role of antipar-kinsonian medications. *Parkinsonism.Relat Disord.* 11, 131-133 (2005).

[71] Yasui, K., Kowa, H., Nakaso, K., Takeshima, T. & Nakashima, K. Plasma homocys-teine and MTHFR C677T genotype in levodopa-treated patients with PD. *Neurology* 55, 437-440 (2000).

[72] Bialecka, M. *et al.* Association of COMT, MTHFR, and SLC19A1(RFC-1) polymor-phisms with homocysteine blood levels and cognitive impairment in Parkinson's dis-ease. *Pharmacogenet Genomics* 22, 716-724, doi:10.1097/FPC.0b013e32835693f7 (2012).

[73] Urban, P. P. *et al.* Subacute axonal neuropathy in Parkinson's disease with cobalamin and vitamin B6 deficiency under duodopa therapy. *Mov Disord* 25, 1748-1752, doi:10.1002/mds.23342 (2010).

[74] Kobylecki, C., Marshall, A. G., Gosal, D., Silverdale, M. A. & Kellett, M. W. 114 Suba-cute axonal and demyelinating peripheral neuropathy complicating Duodopa thera-py for Parkinson's disease. *Journal of Neurology, Neurosurgery & Psychiatry* 83, e1, doi:10.1136/jnnp-2011-301993.156 (2012).

[75] Gilron, I. Gabapentin and pregabalin for chronic neuropathic and early postsurgical pain: current evidence and future directions. *Curr Opin Anaesthesiol* 20, 456-472, doi: 10.1097/ACO.0b013e3282effaa7 00001503-200710000-00010 [pii] (2007).

[76] Merola, A. *et al.* Prospective assessment of peripheral neuropathy in Duodopa-treated parkinsonian patients. *Acta Neurol Scand*, doi:10.1111/ane.12164 (2013).

[77] Siebert, H. *et al.* Over-expression of alpha-synuclein in the nervous system enhances axonal degeneration after peripheral nerve lesion in a transgenic mouse strain. *J Neurochem* 114, 1007-1018, doi:10.1111/j.1471-4159.2010.06832.x JNC6832 [pii] (2010).

[78] Wang, N., Freeman, R. & Gibbons, C. Cutaneous α-Synuclein Is a Biomarker of Parkinson Disease Severity (S37.002) *Neurology* 80, S37.002 (2013).

[79] Chu, Y. *et al.* Alterations in axonal transport motor proteins in sporadic and experimental Parkinson's disease. *Brain* 135, 2058-2073, doi:10.1093/brain/aws133 aws133 [pii] (2012).

[80] Lipton, S. A. *et al.* Neurotoxicity associated with dual actions of homocysteine at the N-methyl-D-aspartate receptor. *Proc.Natl.Acad.Sci U.S.A* 94, 5923-5928 (1997).

[81] Gorgone, G. *et al.* Coenzyme Q10, hyperhomocysteinemia and MTHFR C677T polymorphism in levodopa-treated Parkinson's disease patients. *Neuromolecular Med* 14, 84-90, doi:10.1007/s12017-012-8174-1 (2012).

[82] DopplerK, Ebert S, ÜçeylerN, Volkmann J & CL, S. in *Peripheral Nerve Society.*

[83] Shinnar, S. & Singer, H. Cobalamin C mutation (methylmalonic aciduria and homocystinuria) in adolescence. *New England Journal of Medicine* 311, 451-451 (1984).

[84] Boscariol, R., Gilron, I. & Orr, E. Chronobiological characteristics of postoperative pain: diurnal variation of both static and dynamic pain and effects of analgesic therapy. *Can J Anaesth* 54, 696-704, doi:54/9/696 [pii] (2007).

4

Long-Term Multimodal Exercise Program Improves Motor and Non-Motor Parameters of People with Parkinson's Disease

L.T.B. Gobbi, F.A. Barbieri, R. Vitório, M.P. Pereira,
C. Teixeira-Arroyo, P.C.R. Santos, L.C. Morais,
P.H.S. Pelicioni, L. Simieli, D. Orcioli-Silva, J. Lahr,
A.Y.Y. Hamanaka, A.C. Salles, A.P.T. Alves,
C.B. Takaki, E. Lirani-Silva, F.A. Cezar, F. Stella,
M.D.T.O. Ferreira, M.J.D. Caetano, N.M. Rinaldi,
P.M. Formaggio, R.A. Batistela and V. Raile

1. Introduction

Parkinson's disease (PD) is a neurodegenerative pathology characterized by progressive death of the dopamine-containing neurons in the *substantia nigra pars compacta*. Although motor symptoms (i.e. resting tremor, postural instability, rigidity and gait impairment) are more commonly described in the literature, people with PD can also show cognitive symptoms (i.e. deficits in executive function, depression and dementia). Furthermore, these clinical characteristics of PD negatively impact functional capacity (Barbieri et al., 2012) and tend to get worse progressively (Karlsen et al., 2000).

Physical exercise has been described to benefit both clinical symptoms (motor and cognitive symptoms) and functional capacity of people with PD. In this concern, our research group has published a couple of studies demonstrating the benefits offered by a long-term multimodal exercise program on executive functions (Tanaka et al., 2009), balance (Gobbi et al., 2009), gait parameters (Vitório et al., 2011), and mobility (Pereira et al., 2012).

The aim of current chapter is to discuss the effects of long-term multimodal exercise program on motor and cognitive symptoms, as well as on function capacity in people with PD. To reach this objective, this chapter is going to revisit the findings of our research group.

2. Intervention

Although promising, studies of exercise in PD have been limited in scope (program duration and specificity). Most have addressed the effects of short-term (over 4 to 12 weeks) specific exercise programs. The benefits of longer and nonspecific exercise intervention remain poorly understood. The cardinal clinical manifestations of PD are resting tremor, rigidity, bradyki-nesia, and gait dysfunction (Damier, Hirsch, Agid & Graybiel, 1999; Olanow; Stern & Sethi, 2009). However, it is known that PD is also associated with many non-motor features, including autonomic dysfunction, pain and sensory disturbances, mood disorders and sleep and cognitive impairment (Olanow; Stern & Sethi, 2009). In this way, a specific physical activity program may not be efficient in achieving many of these symptoms, and consequently to improve the quality of life of these patients. Furthermore, studies have shown that the annual rate of clinical decline in people with PD is between 3.5% (Alves, Wentzel-Larsen, Aarsland & Larsen, 2005) and 11.2% (García-Ruiz, Meseguer, Del Val & Vazquez, 2004), indicating the importance of knowing the effects of exercise are opposed to the advancement of the disease in the long term.

In this context, all the studies reviewed and included in this chapter used the same training protocol, characterized by a long duration multimodal program. Our multimodal exercise program aimed to develop the patients' functional capacities and to improve their quality of life. In contrast to specific programs, this one targeted a holistic improvement of PD patients.

The multimodal program took place over a 6-month period (72 sessions, 3 times a week and 60 minutes per session). Each session consisted of five parts (warm-up, pre-exercise stretching, exercise session, cool down and post-exercise stretching). The main exercise session lasted 40 minutes. The program was structured into six phases; each phase was composed of 12 sessions, each lasting approximately one month. At the end of each phase there was a progressive load increment. In each session, exercise intensity (remained between 60% and 80% of maximum heart rate, 220 minus the participant's age in years) was controlled by a heart rate monitor (Polar®).

The exercise program execution was supervised by at least three physical education profes-sionals and one physiotherapist each time. The multimodal program was composed of a variety of activities that simultaneously focus on the components of functional capacity, such as muscular resistance (specific exercises for gastrocnemius, quadriceps femoralis, hamstrings, rectus abdominalis, and trunk dorsal muscles), motor coordination (rhythmic activities), and balance (recreational motor activities on different surfaces and obstacles) (Table 1).

Phases	Coordination	Muscular Resistance	Balance
1	Movements of upper, and lower limbs	Exercises without weights	Recreational activities stimulating the vestibular system
2	Movements of trunk, upper, and lower limbs	Exercises with hoops, ropes, and batons	Recreational activities stimulating the vestibular system
3	Head movements instead of trunk	Exercises with barbells, ankle, weights, and medicine balls	Stimulation of visual and somatosensory systems
4	Head, trunk, upper, and lower limb movements	Increase in intensity or repetitions (volume increment)	Integration of visual, somatosensory, and vestibular systems
5	Four different movement sequences: two with same movements for upper and lower limbs and two alternating movements	Gym exercises: leg press, pulley, seated cable rows, peck deck, and bench press. Two series with 15 repetitions	Activities including static balance, and half-turn and complete turn (all with visual cues)
6	Four different movement sequences: two alternate movements for upper and lower limbs and two with different movements	Increase in load and volume: addition of series of 15 repetitions	Addition of tactile cues

Table 1. Phases of the multimodal exercise protocol with progressive increments in volume, intensity and complexity.

2.1. Evaluations

Participants were tested before commencing the multimodal program (pretest) and upon completion (posttest). All assessments were carried out in the morning, in the "on-medication" state, 1 hour after participants' first morning dose of medication. The assessments included clinical, cognitive and motor standard instruments.

2.2. Clinical evaluations

Unified Parkinson's Disease Rating Scale (UPDRS; Fahn & Elton, 1987) was used to follow the longitudinal course of Parkinson's disease and assessed the impairments in psychological, functional and motor functions. This scale ranges from 0 to 176 points (I- psychological: 16 points, II-functional: 52 points, III-motor: 108 points).

Hoehn and Yahr Scale (Hoehn & Yahr, 1967; Goetz et al., 2004) was used for describing how the stages of Parkinson's disease progress. This scale ranges from 1 to 5 stages: stage 1 - Unilateral involvement only; stage 1.5 - Unilateral and axial involvement; stage 2 - Bilateral involvement without impairment of balance; stage 2.5 - Mild bilateral disease with recovery on pull test; stage 3 - Mild to moderate bilateral disease; some postural instability; physically independent; stage 4 - Severe disability; still able to walk or stand unassisted; and stage 5 - Wheelchair bound or bedridden unless aided.

2.3. Cognitive evaluations

Mini-Mental State Examination (MMSE) (Folstein, Folstein, & Mchugh, 1975; Brucki et al., 2003), a brief 30-point questionnaire test was used to screening cognitive impairment. This test evaluates orientation, memory, arithmetic and visuo-constructive praxis. For Brazilian population the cutoff score for cognitive impairment considers the educational level (illiterate people - 19 points; from 1 to 4 years of schooling - 24 points; from 5 to 8 years of schooling - 26 points; from 9 to 11 years of schooling - 28 points and educational level $\geq$ 12 years - 29 points).

Wisconsin Card Sorting Test (WCST; Heaton, Chelune, Talley, Kay, & Curtiss, 1993; Paolo, Troster, Axelrod, & Koller, 1995) specifically assessed abstraction, mental flexibility and attention respectively by the subtests "Categories Completed", "Perseverative Errors" and "Failure to Maintain Set".

Wechsler Memory Scale – Revised (WMS-R; Wechsler, 1997), a neuropsychological test designed to measure different memory functions. Subtests used in reviewed studies were logical memory, for short-term memory (logical memory I) and episodic declarative memory (logical memory I I), and Symbol Search, for attention capacity.

State-Trait Anxiety Inventory (STAI; Spielberger, Gorsuch, & Lushene, 1979; Gorenstein & Andrade, 1996), a psychological inventory based on a 4-point Likert scale and consisted in 2 self-report questionnaires that measured two types of anxiety: state anxiety (anxiety about an event) and trait anxiety (anxiety level as a personal characteristic). Higher scores represent higher levels of anxiety.

2.4. Motor evaluations

Functional capacity was assessed by means of AAHPERD tests (flexibility, muscle strength, agility, coordination and aerobic endurance; Osness et al., 1990). Flexibility test: a standard sit-and-reach test in which participants were seated, with their heels 12-in apart and over a line that runs perpendicular to a measuring tape. They were asked to reach with both hands as far along the measuring tape as they comfortably can while keeping both knees straight. The score was their highest tape measure mark in three attempts.

Muscular strength: requires female participants to lift a 4-lb object, and male participants to lift an 8-lb object, using a biceps curl motion, as many times as possible in 30-s.

Agility: patients started from a seated position and were asked to rise from a chair, walk to the right around a cone, and return to the seat and sit down, stand again, walk to the left around a cone, return to their seat and sit down, and then repeat the entire procedure. Two attempts were given to the participants, and the raw score represented the faster of the two.

Coordination: involved the movement of three 12-oz soda cans, using the dominant hand. The cans are placed on a table, topside-up and on a line indicated by a 30-in length of masking tape. The cans are located at 10-in intervals. The participants were seated at the table with the line of cans well within their grasp and they were then asked to place each can top-side-down in a space adjacent to its original position. Then they returned the cans to their original top-side-up position. Each attempt consisted of performing these movements twice, and the raw score reflected the faster of two attempts.

Aerobic resistance: an 880-yd walk, at the participant's maximum speed.

Modified Timed "Up and Go" test (TUG; Schilling et al., 2009; Gobbi et al., 2009) consisted of the participant stand up from a sitting position in an armless chair with a seat height of 46.5 cm, walk a 3-m distance, pass around a cone, return, and sit back down in the chair. Each participant was instructed to perform the task as quickly as possible, but without running. At least one practice attempt was offered to the participants at the beginning of the procedure so that they could become familiar with it. Three attempts were performed for testing purposes, and the time to perform the task was measured in seconds. Time was recorded from the instant the person's buttocks left the chair until the next contact with the chair. The mean value of the three attempts was considered for statistical analysis.

Berg's Functional Balance Scale (FBS; Scalzo et al., 2009), measured the static and dynamic balance abilities by 14 simple balance related tasks, ranging from standing up from a sitting position, to standing on one foot. For each task this test ranged from 0 (unable) to 4 (independent). The better score is 56 points with the increased risk of falls below a score of 45 and a significant increase below 40 points.

Postural-Locomotor-Manual Test (PLM; Hong & Steen, 2007) was designed to assess movement patterns. The test movement is a compound movement involving a postural phase (rising up), a locomotion phase (walking), and a manual phase (pendulous arm movement and positioning of a test object on a pedestal). The PLM test consisted of a complex motion during which the patients moved an object from the floor 1.5-m forward and positioned it on a stand at their chin height, as fast as possible. The time to complete the test was record.

Kinematic gait parameters: the walking task required participants to walk, at a self speed, on an 8m long pathway. Three attempts were performed. For the kinematic data recording, two passive markers (reflective, adhesive Styrofoam) were attached to the following anatomic landmarks: lateral face of the right calcaneus and medial face of the left calcaneus. The images of the right sagittal plane of one stride at center of the pathway were recorded with a frequency of 60Hz by one digital camcorder (JVC, GR-DVL 9800), generating 2D kinematic data. Markers were digitized automatically on Digital Video for Windows (DVIDEOW) software.

3. Results

The multimodal exercise program improved several aspects related to quality of life of patients with PD. First, we showed the benefits of six months of the exercise program on clinical parameters. Exercise program improved the UPDRS-II (functional aspects) score. After exercise program patients with PD decreased the score (Table 2). The exercise program seems be able to improve clinical parameters, agreeing with the benefits to functional capacity components, mobility and locomotion, which are aspects relate to functional activities. Therefore, the improvement in the clinical parameters is important for quality of life for this population.

DEMOGRAPHIC CHARACTERISTICS			
Age (years)	67.77 ± 7.28		
Body height (cm)	161.00 ± 8.74		
Body mass (kg)	70.70 ± 15.87		
CLINICAL PARAMETERS			
Dependent Variables	Pre exercise	Post exercise	p values
H&Y (stage)	1.47 ± 0.72	1.53 ± 0.72	0.15
UPDRS - Functional (score)	11.07 ± 6.36	9.73 ± 6.04	0.02
UPDRS - Motor (score)	20.13 ± 12.26	21.00 ± 14.53	0.72
UPDRS – Total (score)	34.87 ± 18.89	34.07 ± 20.71	0.45
MMSE (score)	26.20 ± 3.47	25.90 ± 4.35	0.77

H&Y: Hoehn & Yahr Stage; UPDRS: Unified Parkinson's Disease Rating Scale; MMSE: Mini-Mental State Examination.

Table 2. Means and standard deviations for the demographic characteristics and clinical dependent variables at before (pre) and after (post) the multimodal exercise program.

Second, the exercise program affected motor aspects. The multimodal exercise program was efficient to improve the functional parameters, such as functional capacity (some components), mobility and locomotion. For functional capacity components, the coordination and muscle strength (Table 3) improved after the multimodal exercise program, which indicates a control of the motor symptoms effects. Moreover, the exercise program maintained the other components, which was an important finding since PD and ageing decreases progressively the functional capacity. For functional mobility, patients with PD were faster in TUG and PLM (Table 3) after the enrolment in the multimodal exercise program. The exercise seems to act on bradykinesia symptom revealing that patients PD were able to perform functional tasks faster. In addition, our results for locomotion corroborated with functional mobility. Patients with PD increased gait velocity after exercise program (Table 3). Still, the multimodal exercise program improved stride length (Table 3), indicating a positive change for hypometria symptom. Therefore, the exercise program seems to be an important aspect for PD patients, improving the quality of life and decreasing the dependency.

FUNCTIONAL CAPACITY			
Dependent Variables	**Pre exercise**	**Post exercise**	**p values**
balance (score)	52.86 ± 4.15	53.57 ± 2.71	0.19
flexibility (cm)	47.56 ± 12.10	50.14 ± 10.53	0.17
coordination (s)	18.50 ± 7.58	15.89 ± 6.84	0.01
agility (s)	28.82 ± 12.37	30.74 ± 11.54	0.64
strength (rep)	19.79 ± 6.57	23.50 ± 5.33	0.01
aerobic resistance (min)	10.08 ± 2.45	10.13 ± 2.90	0.83
TUG (s)	10.10 ± 4.32	8.46 ± 2.16	0.01
PLM (s)	4.03 ± 1.42	3.58 ± 0.76	0.01
GAIT PARAMETERS			
Dependent Variables	**Pre exercise**	**Post exercise**	**p values**
Stride Length (cm)	95.1 ± 14.8	102.4 ± 15.5	0.01
Stride duration (s)	1.06 ± 0.17	0.97 ± 0.11	0.06
Stride velocity (cm/s)	92.7 ± 21.1	105.7 ± 15.5	0.01
Cadence (strides/s)	0.97 ± 0.13	1.04 ± 0.12	0.07
Swing phase (%)	36.5 ± 4.1	37.2 ± 2.3	0.93
Single support (%)	37.5 ± 3.7	38.3 ± 2.3	0.83
Double support (%)	26.0 ± 7.3	24.5 ± 4.0	0.86

TUG: Timed Up and Go Test; PLM: Posture-Locomotor-Manual Test.

Table 3. Means and standard deviations for each functional capacity component and gait dependent variables at before (pre) and after (post) the multimodal exercise program.

Third, even though it was not the purpose of the multimodal exercise program, the individuals with PD improved the non-motor symptoms (Table 4). Patients with PD improved short-term memory (logical memory I), episodic declarative memory (logic memory II), abstraction capacities (categories completed) and mental flexibility (perseverative errors) after the enrolment in the multimodal exercise program. Again, these findings indicated an improvement of quality of life for patients with PD. So, the multimodal exercise program seems to improve cognitive function.

COGNITIVE FUNCTIONS			
Dependent Variables	Pre exercise	Post exercise	p values
STAI - Trait	50.40 ± 8.01	48.70 ± 5.39	0.58
STAI - State	49.20 ± 6.95	48.50 ± 6.67	0.27
HAD	5.40 ± 2.59	5.40 ± 3.13	0.35
Logic memory I (score)	15.50 ± 3.60	19.50 ± 5.00	0.04
Logic memory II (score)	8.6 ± 5.95	13.8 ± 6.38	0.01
Symbol Search	22.50 ± 7.73	24.20 ± 9.12	0.60
Categories Completed (WCST)	2.80 ± 1.68	4.10 ± 1.37	0.04
Perserverative Errors (WCST)	4.00 ± 3.49	0.30 ± 0.94	0.04
Failure to Maintain Set (WCST)	6.00 ± 2.40	5.20 ± 2.34	0.64

WCST: Wisconsin Card Sorting Test; STAI: State-Trait Anxiety Inventory; HAD: Hospital Anxiety and Depression Scale.

Table 4. Means and standard deviations for the cognitive functions at before (pre) and after (post) the multimodal exercise program.

In summary, a multimodal exercise program of six months seems to improve motor and non-motor symptoms of PD. Aspects related to functional activity, mobility and cognition showed benefits with exercise program, which is a relevant finding for functionality and quality of life of PD patients.

4. Final considerations

The aim of this chapter was to discuss the effects of long-term multimodal exercise program on motor and cognitive symptoms, as well as on functional capacity in people with PD. To reach this aim, we reviewed the published data of our group and as main results we found improvements in four different domains: clinical aspects, gait parameters, functional capacity and cognitive status. All these improvements certainly increased patients' independency, mobility, functional aspects and quality of life. For functional aspects, this is clear according to the improvement of UPDRS II score. Since the UPRDS II is a self-related scale, this is also important to the patients' quality of life: patients self-perceived their own functional aspects as better after the enrolment in our program. This certainly increases patients' quality of life. However, the benefits did not only rely on PD clinical aspects, but also on peripheral gains (as strength) and improvements in brain functions, as memory and executive function. We show during this section that there is not a main cause as responsible for our results. In another way, we demonstrate that enrolling into our exercise program allowed the patients to improve different aspects of their life.

Considering functional capacity, PD patients showed improvements on muscular strength, motor coordination, dynamic balance and functional mobility (Orcioli-Silva et al., 2013, submitted for publication). Muscular strength is a function of length and velocity (Winter, 1990), where its gain can leads to an improvement of both stride velocity and length. Motor coordination is a motor act that requires the control of body segments in an integrated way, with the aim to create a successful movement pattern. In this way, both improvements of strength and coordination could drive patients to increase their gait velocity and stride length. This is reinforced by the results of some studies which demonstrated that gait is highly influenced by coordination in PD patients (Plotnik, Giladi & Hausdorff, 2008). Due to the improvement of these both motor capacities, a more stable level was acquired, thus reflecting on functional mobility, measured through TUG and PLM tests.

Lower limbs muscular strength decrease, a reduction of stride length and velocity, and poor levels of balance and functionality can lead to higher risk of falling in PD patients (Cole et al., 2010; Kerr et al., 2010; Latt et al., 2009; Vitório, Lirani-Silva & Pelicioni, 2013). In this way, even without assessing the number of falls during our exercise program, we can suggest that the enrolment on our multimodal exercise program leads to a reduction of patients' risk of falls. Also, since patients increased their self-judgment about their functionality (increase in UPDRS II scores), this could also result in a falling risk reduction. This is based on the study of Vellas et al. (1997), which indicates that fear of falling (and therefore a reduction of own judgment about functional capacity) is direct related to the number of falling episodes.

Beyond the benefits in patients' quality of life, we cannot forget to mention another important aspect of our motor results. The improvement of both strength and coordination after a 6-month multimodal exercise program show us that peripheral benefits observed in healthy elderly, from exercise enrolment, can be transferred, at least in part, to PD patients. Also, the improvement on coordination leaves an open window to discuss the maintenance of learning capacity in PD patients.

Finally, about the motor benefits of our multimodal exercise program, we need to discuss the maintenance of UPRDS III score. Someone can argue that our program did not reduced motor impairments and therefore, is not so attractive. However, since a decrease of 3.2% in HY stage score per year is expected (Alves et al., 2005), the maintenance of UPRDS III score is an important result. We must remember that our program has a long lasting period and the maintenance of motor impairments after 6 months has important effects on patients' quality of life.

However, the most exciting results are those related to cognitive aspects. The improvement in executive functions (responsible to successfully plan, select and execute motor plans) could also be responsible to higher performance of gait. This is based on the study of Yogev et al. (2005), which relates the gait performance to cognitive status in PD patients. Furthermore, a higher cognitive performance can also leads to a better self-perception of functional state, increasing the UPDRS II score.

These are exciting results since they demonstrate that exercise cannot benefits only healthy adult brain, but also mental function of PD patients. Some studies had demonstrated that the practice of moderate and intense physical exercise can result in compensatory changes on the dopaminergic neurotransmission (Petzinger et al., 2007). In addition, some studies had shown that exercise could also be responsible to neural adaptations as the increase of blood flow (Hirsch & Farley, 2009) and to an increase of metabolic and neurochemical function in the brain (Petzinger et al., 2010). Other results point to an increase of neuroprotection and even to an increase of neural growth factors (Zigmond et al., 2009) in the brain after exercise programs. These results were seen mainly on animal models and at this time, we cannot assure that our exercise program promoted these adaptations. However, even without assessing these morphological and physiological aspects of physical exercise (and this is not the objective of our group), the improvement in memory and executive function point to some adaptations in brain levels. The PD brain also shows a high capacity to redesign itself in response to physical activity, providing a plausible argument related to the neuroplasticity mechanism in PD patients after physical exercises (Hirsch & Farley, 2009).

It is believed that these adaptations are due to our program design and to the exercises intensity level. High intensity exercises have shown more positive effects in PD patients when compared to low intensity exercises (Burini et al., 2006; Fisher et al., 2008). Also, physical activity programs lasting longer than 10 weeks, with a frequency more than 3 days a week and with 45-60minutes of duration per session can lead to higher benefits to PD patients (Barbieri et al., 2013). Also, it is indicated that activities with intensity between moderate to high (Barbieri et al., 2013). Our multimodal exercise program fully respected all these statements as well as it had a continuous progression during each phase, whereas the intensity of physical exercises was kept between moderate to high. It is believed that this exercise design is better for PD patients than others since it results in compensatory changes in the dopaminergic neurotransmission (Petzinger et al., 2007; Petzinger et al., 2010).

It is also important to consider that patients enrolled in our multimodal exercise program were in between the mild to moderate stages of disease. Since these patients have a better physical condition than those on severe stages, possibly these last could not be able to execute the exercises properly. Also, patients in mild to moderate disease stages are still able to learn new motor skills (Canning, Ada & Woodhouse, 2008).

In resume, the results of our group clearly show that a 6-months multimodal exercise program was feasible and improved patients' physical and cognitive status (Gobbi et al., 2011). After 6 months, patients enrolled in our exercise program maintained their motor impairments and, moreover, improved their independency and functionality. We can state that our exercise program increased patient's mobility, with the reduction of two main symptoms: bradikynesia and hypometria. At this time is not possible to state if the positive results found after our program are mainly due to a reduction in the physiological aging process, to neural adaptations or to a combination of both. However, these improvements are not only result of motor aspects but they are also related to improvement on cognitive domain. Finally, after reviewing our results we can properly affirm that our 6-months multimodal exercise program increased patients' independency, which certainly, improved their quality of life.

Author details

L.T.B. Gobbi[1], F.A. Barbieri[1], R. Vitório[1], M.P. Pereira[1], C. Teixeira-Arroyo[1], P.C.R. Santos[1], L.C. Morais[1], P.H.S. Pelicioni[1], L. Simieli[1], D. Orcioli-Silva[1], J. Lahr[1], A.Y.Y. Hamanaka[2], A.C. Salles[2], A.P.T. Alves[2], C.B. Takaki[2], E. Lirani-Silva[2], F.A. Cezar[2], F. Stella[1], M.D.T.O. Ferreira[2], M.J.D. Caetano[1], N.M. Rinaldi[2], P.M. Formaggio[1], R.A. Batistela[2] and V. Raile[2]

1 UNESP Univ Estadual Paulista, Rio Claro, Brazil

2 The PROPARKI Group, Brazil

References

[1] Alves, G.; Wentzel-Larsen, T.; Aarsland, D. & Larsen, J. P. (2005) Progression of motor impairment and disability in Parkinson disease: a population-based study. *Neurology*, 65, 1436-1441.

[2] Barbieri, F. A.; Simieli, L.; Orcioli-Silva, D. & Gobbi, L. T. B. (2013). Benefícios do exercício físico para pacientes com doença de Parkinson. In. Coelho, F. G. M.; Gobbi, S.; Costa, J. L. R. & Gobbi, L. T. B. *Exercício físico no envelhecimento saudável e patológico: da teoria à prática*. Curitiba, PR: CRV, 325-339.

[3] Barbieri, F.A.; Rinaldi, N.M.; Santos, P.C.R.; Lirani-Silva, E; Vitório, R.; Teixeira-Arroyo, C.; Stella, F.; Gobbi, L.T.B. (2012) "Functional capacity of Brazilian patients with Parkinson's disease (PD): Relationship between clinical characteristics and disease severity." *Archives of Gerontology and Geriatrics*, 54, e83-e88.

[4] Brucki, S. M. D., Nitrini, R., Caramelli, P., Bertolucci, P. H. F., & Okamoto, I. H. (2003) Suggestions for utilization of the mini-mental state examination in Brazil. *Arquivos de Neuro-Psiquiatria*, 61(3B), 777-781.

[5] Burini, D.; Farabollini, B.; Iacucci, S.; Rimatori, C.; Riccardi, G.; Capecci, M.; Provinciali, L. & Ceravolo, M. G. (2006). A randomized controlled cross-over trial of aerobic training versus qigong in advanced Parkinson's disease. *Europa Medicophysica*, 42(3), 231-238.

[6] Canning, C. G; Ada, L; Woodhouse, E. (2008). Multiple-task walking training in people with mild to moderate Parkinson's disease: a pilot study. *Clinical Rehabilitation*, 22(3), 226-233.

[7] Cole, M. H.; Silburn, P.A.; Wood, J.M.; Worringham, C. J. & Kerr, G.K. (2010). Falls in Parkinson's disease: kinematic evidence for impaired head and trunk control. *Movement Disorders*, 5(14), 2369 – 2378.

[8]   Damier, P., Hirsch, E. C., Agid, Y., Graybiel, A. M. (1999) The substantia nigra of the human brain II. Patterns of loss of dopamine-containing neurons in Parkinson's disease. *Brain*, 122, 1437-1448.

[9]   Fahn, S., & Elton, R. Members of the UPDRS Development Committee. (1987) The Unified Parkinson's disease rating scale. In: Fahn, S., Marsden, C. D., Calne, D. B., & Goldstein, M. (Eds). *Recent Developments in Parkinson's Disease*. Florham Park NJ: McMellam Health Care Information, v. 2, 153-164.

[10] Fisher, B. E.; Wu, A. D.; Salem, G. J.; Song, J.; Lin, C. H.; Yip, J.; Cen, S.; Gordon, J.; Jakowec, M. & Petzinger, G. (2008). The effect of exercise training in improving motor performance and corticomotor excitability in people with early Parkinson's disease. *Archives of Physical Medicine and Rehabilitation*, 89(7), 1221-1229.

[11] Folstein, M. F., Folstein, S. E., & Mchug, P. R. (1975) Minimental state: a practical method for grading the cognitive state of patients for the clinician. *Journal of Psychiatry Research*, 12, 189-198.

[12] García-Ruiz, P. J., Meseguer, E., Del Val, J., & Vazquez, A. (2004) Motor complications in Parkinson's disease: A prospective follow-up study. *Clinical Neuropharmacology*, 27, 49-52.

[13] Gobbi, L. T. B., Barbieri, F. A., Vitório, R., Pereira, M. P., & Teixeira-Arroyo, C. (2011). Effects of a multimodal exercise program on clinical, functional mobility and cognitive parameters of idiopathic Parkinson's disease patients. In: Dushanova, J. (Org.). Diagnostics and Rehabilitation of Parkinson's Disease. Rijeka-Croacia: Intech, 339-352.

[14] Gobbi, L.T.B.; Oliveira-Ferreira, M.D.T.; Caetano, M.J.D.; Lirani-Silva, E.; Barbieri, F.A.; Stella, F.; Gobbi, S. "Exercise programs improve mobility and balance in people with Parkinson's disease. *Parkinsonism and Related Disorders*, 15S3, S49-S52, 2009.

[15] Goetz, C. G., Poewe, W., Rascol. O., Sampaio, C. Stebbins, G. T., Counsell, C., ... Seidl, L. (2004) Movement Disorder Society Task Force report on the Hoehn and Yahr staging scale: status and recommendations. *Movement Disorders*, 19, 1020-1028.

[16] Gorenstein, C., & Andrade, L. (1996) Validation of a Portuguese version of the Beck Depression Inventory and the State-Trait Anxiety Inventory in Brazilian subjects. *Brazilian Journal of Medical and Biological Research*, 29, 453–457.

[17] Heaton, R. K., Chelune, G. J., Talley, J. L., Kay, G. C., & Curtiss, G. (1993) *Wisconsin card sorting test manual*. USA: Psychological Assessment Resources.

[18] Hirsch, M. A., & Farley, B. G. (2009). Exercise and neuroplasticity in persons living with Parkinson's disease. *European Journal of Physical and Rehabilitation Medicine*, 45(2), 215-229.

[19] Hoehn, M. M., & Yahr, M. D. (1967) Parkinsonism: onset, progression and mortality. *Neurology*, 17, 573-581.

[20] Hong, S. & Steen, B. (2007) A population-based study on motor performance in elderly men. *Korean Journal of Clinical Geriatric*, 8(4).

[21] Karlsen, K.H.; Tandberg, E.; Arsland, D.; Larse, J.P. (2000) Health related quality of life in Parkinson's disease: a prospective longitudinal study. *Journal of Neurology Neurosurgery and Psychiatry*, 69(5), 584–589.

[22] Kerr, G. K.; Worringham, C. J.; Cole, M. H.; Lacherez, P. F.; Wood, J. M. & Silburn, P.A. (2010). Predictors of future falls in Parkinson's disease. *Neurology*, 75(2), 116-124.

[23] Latt, M. D.; Lord, S. R.; Morris, J. G. & Fung, V. S. (2009). Clinical and physiological assessment for elucidating falls risk in Parkinson's disease. *Movement Disorders*, 24, 1280-1289.

[24] Olanow, C. W., Stern, M. B., & Sethi, K. (2009) The scientific and clinical basis for the treatment of Parkinson disease. *Neurology*, 72, Suppl. 4, S1-S136.

[25] Orcioli-Silva, D., Simieli, L., Barbieri, F., Rinaldi, N. M., & Gobbi, L. (2013, submitted for publication). Effects of a multimodal exercise program on the functional capacity of Parkinson's disease patients considering disease severity and gender. *Motriz*.

[26] Osness, W. H., Adrian, M., Clark, B., Hoeger, W., Raab, D., & Wiswell, R. (1990) *Functional fitness assessment for adults over 60 years* (a field based assessment). Reston: American Alliance for Health, Physical Education, Recreation and Dance.

[27] Paolo, A. M., Troster, A. I., Axelrod, B. N., & Koller, W. C. (1995) Construct validity of the WCST in normal elderly and persons with Parkinson's disease. *Archives of Clinical Neuropsychology*, 10(5), 463–473.

[28] Pereira, M.P.; Oliveira-Ferreira, M.D.T.; Caetano, M.J.D.; Vitório, R.; Lirani-Silva, E.; Barbieri, F.A.; Stella, F.; Gobbi, L.T.B. (2012) Long-term multimodal exercise program enhances mobility of patients with Parkinson's disease. *ISRN Rehabilitation*, pp. 1-7.

[29] Petzinger, G. M., Fisher, B. E., Van Leeuwen, J. E., Vukovic, M., Akopian, G., Meshul, C. K., . . . Jakowec, M. W. (2010). Enhancing neuroplasticity in the basal ganglia: the role of exercise in Parkinson's disease. *Movement Disorders*, 25(Suppl 1), S141-145.

[30] Petzinger, G. M.; Walsh, J. P.; Akopian, G.; Hogg, E.; Abernathy, A.; Arevalo, P.; Turnquist, P.; Vucković, M.; Fisher, B. E.; Togasaki, D. M. & Jakowec, M.W. (2007). Effects of treadmill exercise on dopaminergic transmission in the 1-methyl-4-phenyl-1, 2, 3, 6-tetrahydropydrine-lesioned mouse model of basal ganglia injury. *Journal of Neuroscience*, 27(20), 5291-5300.

[31] Plotnik, M.; Giladi, N. & Hausdorff, J. M. (2008). Bilateral coordination of walking and freezing of gait in Parkinson's disease. *European Journal of Neuroscience*, 27, 1999-2006.

[32] Scalzo, P. L., Nova, I. C., Perracini, M. R., Sacramento, D. R. C., Cardoso, F., ... Teix-eira, A. L. (2009) Validation of the Brazilian version of the Berg balance scale for pa-tients with Parkinson's disease. *Arquivos de Neuro Psiquiatria*, 67(3), 831–835.

[33] Schilling, B. K., Karlage, R. E., LeDoux, M. S., Pfeiffer, R. F., Weiss, L. W., & Falvo, M. J. (2009) Impaired leg extensor strength in individuals with Parkinson's disease and relatedness to functional mobility. *Parkinsonism and Related Disorders*, 15(10), 776–780.

[34] Spielberger, C. D., Gorsuch, R. L., Lushene, R. E. (1979). *Inventário de ansiedade traço – estado*: IDATE (State-Trait Anxiety Inventory – STAI). Rio de Janeiro: Centro de Estu-dos de Psicologia Aplicada (CEPA).

[35] Tanaka, K.; Quadros Jr., A.C.; Santos, R.F.; Stella, F.; Gobbi, L.T.B.; Gobbi, S. (2009). Benefits of physical exercise on executive function in older people with Parkinson's disease. *Brain and Cognition*, 69, 435-441.

[36] Vellas B.J., Wayne S.J., Romero LJ., Baumgartner R.N. & Garry P.J. (1997) Fear of fall-ing and restriction of mobility in elderly fallers. *Age Ageing*, 26, 189-93.

[37] Vitório, R.; Lirani-Silva, E. & Pelicioni, P. H.S. (2013). Controle motor, ocorrência de quedas e doença de Parkinson. In. Coelho, F. G. M.; Gobbi, S.; Costa, J. L. R. & Gobbi, L. T. B. *Exercício físico no envelhecimento saudável e patológico: da teoria à prática*. Curiti-ba, PR: CRV, pp. 311-323.

[38] Vitório, R.; Teixeira-Arroyo, C.; Lirani-Silva, E.; Barbieri, F.A.; Caetano, M.J.D.; Gob-bi, S.; Stella, F.; Gobbi, L.T.B. (2011) Effects of 6-month multimodal exercise program on clinical and gait paremeters of patients with idiopathic Parkinson's disease: a pilot study. *ISRN Neurology*, pp. 1-7. (doi:10.5402/2011/714947)

[39] Wechsler, D. *The Wechsler Memory Scale – III Revised* (Manual). (1997). Santo Antonio Texas: Psychological Corporation.

[40] Winter, D. A. (1990). *Biomechanics and motor control of human movement*. 2 Ed. Water-loo: Wiley-Interscience Publication.

[41] Yogev, G., Giladi, N., Peretz, C., Springer, S., Simon, E. S., & Hausdorff, J. M. (2005). Dual tasking, gait rhythmicity and Parkinson's disease: which aspects of gait are at-tention demanding? *Eur J Neurosci*, 22, 1248-1256.

[42] Zigmond, M. J., Cameron, J. L., Leak, R. K., Mirnics, K., Russell, V. A., Smeyne, R. J., & Smith, A. D. (2009). Triggering endogenous neuroprotective processes through ex-ercise in models of dopamine deficiency. *Parkinsonism Relat Disord*, 15 Suppl 3, S42-45

5

Sleep Disturbances in Patients with Parkinson's Disease

Keisuke Suzuki, Tomoyuki Miyamoto,
Masayuki Miyamoto, Ayaka Numao, Hideki Sakuta,
Hiroaki Fujita, Yuji Watanabe,
Masaoki Iwanami and Koichi Hirata

1. Introduction

Parkinson's disease (PD) is clinically characterized by motor symptoms such as rigidity, bradykinesia, resting tremor, and postural instability, which are caused by the degeneration of striatonigral dopaminergic neurons [1]. Reflecting recent advances in therapeutic options and management in motor disabilities in PD, non-motor symptoms have received considerable attention due to substantial evidence that shows their significant impact on quality of life. Although some non-motor symptoms can be effectively treated by dopaminergic agents, their management and treatment remain clinically challenging [2]. Non-motor symptoms include sleep disturbances, cognitive impairment, mood disorders, hyposmia, pain, and dysautonomia, among which sleep disturbances are the central issue when considering their impact on disease course and clinical correlation. The presence of sleep disorders in PD was first described by James Parkinson in his "An Essay on the Shaking Palsy" published in 1817 [3].

– "In this stage, the sleep becomes much disturbed. The tremulous motion of the limbs occur during sleep, and augment until they awaken the patient, and frequently with much agitation and alarm" –

Sleep disturbances in PD are common and multifactorial problems with a reported incidence ranging from approximately 40% to 90% [4-7]. Disease-related intrinsic causes include impairment in thalamocortical arousal and degeneration of the brainstem regulatory centers for sleep/wakefulness maintenance and REM sleep [8]. Other causes include nocturnal motor symptoms, psychiatric symptoms, dementia, medication use, circadian rhythm sleep disorders, and comorbidities involving sleep apnea syndrome (SAS), restless legs syndrome (RLS), and rapid eye movement sleep behavior disorder (RBD). Table 1 shows the various causes of sleep problems in PD; when patients complain of or are likely to suffer from sleep problems such as difficulty initiating or maintaining sleep, early awakening, or daytime sleepiness, all of the possibilities should be considered in clinical practice, but they are often underestimated. In this chapter, we review the current understanding of sleep problems in PD and the methods used to evaluate these problems, focusing on the PD sleep scale (PDSS) and PDSS-2.

2. Evaluation of sleep disturbance

2.1. Polysomnography

Polysomnography is the gold standard in the assessment of sleep disorders because it provides sleep status information, including sleep efficiency, sleep latency, and sleep architecture. However, the cost, special equipment required, and limited availability may hamper its routine application. Sleep structure may be altered, reflecting disease-related changes in the brainstem in patients with PD: the degeneration of cholinergic neurons in the basal forebrain and brainstem, including the pedunculopontine nucleus and noradrenergic neurons in the locus coeruleus, results in disorders of REM sleep. A loss of serotoninergic neurons in the raphe nucleus is associated with a decreased percentage of slow-wave sleep [9] (Table 2). However, reported PSG findings on sleep architecture vary [10]. Reduced total sleep time and sleep efficiency were observed in PD patients compared with controls [11-13], although other studies did not find a difference. Reduced total sleep time was associated with increased age and increased levodopa dose [13], whereas the other study showed a weak positive correlation between the mean sleep latency and the daily dose of levodopa [14]. Sleep stages 1 and 2 appear to be unchanged in PD patients [15, 16]. Slow-wave sleep was reported to be unchanged, decreased, or increased [11, 17, 18]. REM sleep was also shorter or unchanged [11, 13, 19, 20].

These discrepancies may reflect individual night-to-night variation, medication effects, and differences in patient selection in the studies. PSG may detect abnormal REM sleep in PD, namely, REM sleep without atonia, excessive sustained or intermittent elevation of submental tone, or excessive phasic submental or limb twitching, which are required for a diagnosis of RBD. A recent review of case-control PSG studies provides a higher prevalence of RBD in PD than in controls (0-47% vs. 0-1.8%), but no significant increase of obstructive sleep apnea (27-60% vs. 13-65%) or periodic limb movements of sleep compared with controls [10]. In contrast, slightly but significantly increased periodic limb movements during sleep were described in patients with PD [21]. The clinical significance of sleep apnea in PD will be discussed later.

Regarding the effect of dopaminergic medication on the sleep architecture in PD, relative to controls, Wailke et al [18] reported that a significantly decreased total sleep time, REM sleep,

1. PD-related pathological changes
Impairment of the sleep-wake cycle, circadian rhythm sleep disorder, sundown syndrome
Impairment of sleep architecture (REM and non-REM sleep)
Impairment of the arousal system (orexin, serotonin, noradrenaline, acetylcholine)
2. Nocturnal motor symptoms
Wearing-off phenomenon, rigidity, akinesia, tremor, medication-related dyskinesia, dystonia
3. Nocturnal non-motor symptoms
Neuropsychiatric symptoms (depression, psychosis, cognitive impairment)
Sensory symptoms (pain, dysesthesia, restlessness of the arms or legs)
Hallucinations, nightmares and vivid dreams, nocturia
4. Medication use
Dopaminergic drugs, anti-psychotics
5. Comorbid primary sleep disorders
Sleep apnea syndrome
REM sleep behavior disorder
Restless legs syndrome, periodic limb movement disorder

Table 1. The cause of sleep-related problems in PD

Nucleus/area	Main transmitter	Function	Consequence of dysfunction
Pedunculopontine nucleus	Acetylcholine	Regulation of REM sleep	Disorders of REM sleep
Locus coeruleus	Noradrenaline	Regulation of REM sleep	Reduction/absence of REM sleep
Area peri-locus coeruleus	GABA, glutamate?	Inhibition of spinal motoneurons	Loss of muscle atonia during REM sleep
Raphe nuclei	Serotonin	Regulation of slow-wave sleep	Reduction of slow-wave sleep

Table 2. Impaired sleep architecture in PD [9].

and slow-wave sleep and an increased amount of time spent awake were found in PD patients whose usual dopaminergic treatments were discontinued after noon and that the administration of levodopa had no impact on any of these PSG parameters. In a study evaluating sleep status in de novo patients with PD, the sleep continuity, sleep architecture, and periodic limb movements index were similar between patients and controls, but an increased alpha activity in REM sleep was observed in de novo PD patients [16]. In another case control study including 15 de novo PD patients and 15 controls, compared with controls, the total sleep time and sleep efficiency in the de novo PD group decreased, the stage 1 sleep and the time spent awake increased, and REM sleep was reduced. A higher percentage of REM sleep without atonia in patients compared with controls was observed, whereas only one patient clinically manifested RBD [22]. Because RBD precedes the onset of PD and can manifest during the early phase of PD, abnormalities in REM sleep in the early phase of PD are supported by PSG findings.

2.2. Multiple sleep latency test

The multiple sleep latency test (MSLT) records the initial sleep latency of four or five sequential naps to evaluate objective daytime sleepiness. In 54 levodopa-treated PD patients who were referred for sleepiness, pathological sleepiness (mean SL < 5 min) was observed in 50% of the 54 patients [14], and a narcolepsy-like phenotype (2≥ sleep-onset REM periods) was found in 39% of the patients. Additionally, Rye et al [23] found that although the mean SL was similar between patients with PD and controls, abnormal sleepiness (mean SL≤5 min) was common (40 of 134 nap opportunities), and sleep-onset REM periods were also observed (13 of 134 nap opportunities) in PD patients. In contrast, Yong et al [13] reported that mean SL did not differ between PD and controls. No differences in mean SL between the levodopa-alone group and the levodopa and dopamine agonist group were reported [20]. In untreated PD patients, the mean SL on MSLT was not different compared with controls (11.7±4 vs. 12.5±2 min) [22]. The mean SL was in the pathological range (<8 min) in three PD patients and in none of the controls, and one patient with PD had a single sleep onset REM on MSLT. This observation suggests that some but not all patients exhibit pathological daytime sleepiness as measured by MSLT, irrespective of the quality and amount of nighttime sleep. However, one should note that sleepiness measured by MSLT does not always reflect subjective sleepiness.

2.3. Questionnaire-based assessment

2.3.1. Parkinson's disease sleep scale

To comprehensively and clinically address PD's common, disease-specific sleep problems, Chaudhuri et al [24] have developed the Parkinson's disease sleep scale (PDSS), a visual analogue scale, including 15 PD-related nocturnal symptoms for assessing nocturnal disability in PD. The subitems of the PDSS address the follows: item 1, overall quality of the night's sleep; items 2/3, sleep onset and maintenance insomnia; items 4/5, nocturnal restlessness; items 6/7, nocturnal psychosis; items 8/9, nocturia; items 10-13, nocturnal motor symptoms; item 14, sleep refreshment; and item 15, daytime dozing. This scale measures the patient's subjective evaluation of sleep and does not address the frequency of sleep problems. Scores for a given individual item range from 0 to 10; 10 represents the best and 0 represents the worst score. The maximum total score for PDSS is 150 (patient is free of symptoms associated with sleep disorders).

In the original study [24], PD patients showed a significantly impaired (lower) total PDSS score compared with controls (101.1±21.7 vs. 120.7±21.0), and advanced PD patients (Hoehn and Yahr (HY) stage 4-5) had a lower total PDSS score than early/moderate PD patients (HY stage 1-3) and controls. This scale is now regarded as a recommended and reliable scale for screening and assessing sleep disturbance in PD [25]. The PDSS has been validated and used extensively in a number of countries, with a high reliability [26-30]. Our multicenter study also showed an impaired total PDSS score in patients with PD compared with controls (112.8±25.4 vs. 126.6±17.8) and revealed more severe nocturnal disturbances measured by PDSS in advanced-stage PD patients (HY stage 4) compared with those with early/moderate stages (HY stage 1-3) (Figure 1). With regard to the subitems in PDSS, compared with controls, almost all the subitems were significantly impaired in PD patients except for item 2 (sleep onset insomnia), item 11 (painful muscle cramp), and item 14 (refreshment after sleep), and both groups had the most severe ratings in item 3 (sleep maintenance insomnia) and item 8 (nocturia) (Figure 2). Patients with HY 4 had significantly worse scores on item 1 (quality of sleep), item 3 (sleep maintenance insomnia), item 6 (distressing dream), item 11 (painful muscle cramps), and item 15 (daytime dozing) than those with HY 1-3 (Figure 3). In addition, sleep disturbances as measured by the total PDSS score were associated with a longer disease duration, depressive symptoms, and complications in the dopaminergic treatment (dyskinesia and wearing off) [29]. When dividing the PD patients into patients with and without depressive symptoms, we found that patients with depressive symptoms (Zung Self-Rating Depression Scale, SDS score ≥ 40) had significantly impaired scores in almost all PDSS items except item 2 (difficulty in initiating sleep) and item 11 (painful muscle cramps) compared with patients without depressive symptoms and controls [31]. The lack of significant differences between controls and nondepressed patients in PDSS subitems suggests that depressive symptoms play an important role in nocturnal disturbances in PD (Figure 4). From a detailed evaluation of nocturnal symptoms, it was determined that early morning tremor (item 13) and nocturnal dystonia (item 12) were closely associated with depressive symptoms.

In contrast, untreated PD patients can manifest various nocturnal symptoms as assessed by PDSS, such as nocturia, nighttime cramps, dystonia, and tremor [32], emphasizing that nocturnal disturbances should be recognized and managed early even in the early stage of PD.

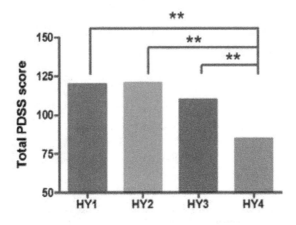

*p<0.05, ** p<0.01. Bonferroni test after adjustment for age. PD patients with HY stage 4 had a lower score compared with those with HY stages 1 to 3.

Figure 1. Total PDSS score classified by H&Y stage in patients with PD [29].

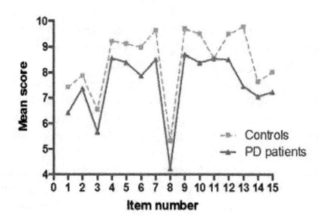

PD patients had a lower score on almost all PDSS scores compared with controls except for items 2 (sleep onset insomnia), 11 (painful muscle cramps), and 14 (tired and sleepy after waking).

Figure 2. PDSS subitems in patients with PD and controls [29].

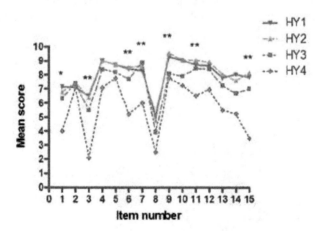

* $p<0.05$, ** $p<0.01$. One-way ANOVA followed by a Bonferroni test. Compared with patients with HY stages 1-3, PDSS subitems in patients with HY stage 4 were lower for difficulty staying asleep (item 3), nightmares (item 6), painful muscle cramps (item 11), and daytime sleepiness (item 15).

Figure 3. PDSS subitems classified by HY stage in patients with PD [29].

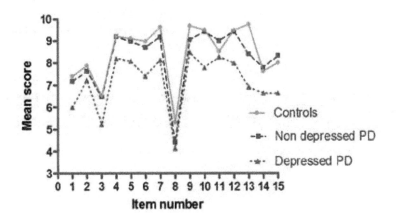

Significant differences in PDSS subitems, except items 2 (sleep onset insomnia) and 11 (painful muscle cramps), are observed among depressed patients, nondepressed patients, and controls.

Figure 4. PDSS subitems in depressed PD, nondepressed PD, and controls [31].

2.3.2. Parkinson's disease sleep scale-2

Trenkwalder et al have recently published the PDSS-2, a revised version of the PDSS, to address the frequency of nocturnal symptoms observed in PD patients [33]. A visual analog scale used in the original version of PDSS was transformed into a frequency measure in the PDSS-2. A question regarding daytime sleepiness (item 15 in PDSS) was removed because it reflects complex regulation in PD, and a screening question for SAS was added instead. The PDSS-2 consists of 15 questions about various sleep and nocturnal disturbances rated by the patients using one of five categories, from 0 (never) to 4 (very frequent). Unlike the PDSS, in which a lower score represents worse conditions in sleep, the PDSS-2 total score ranges from 0 (no disturbance) to 60 (maximum nocturnal disturbance) (Figure 5). The study showed satisfactory internal consistency, stability, construct validity, and precision for the PDSS-2 [33]. Nocturnal problems assessed by the PDSS-2 total score were correlated with impaired quality of life and motor impairment. The factor analysis of PDSS resulted in three domain scales: 1) motor problems at night; 2) PD symptoms at night, representing disease-specific symptoms; and 3) disturbed sleep, representing sleep-specific disturbances (Table 3). We have performed a validation study and confirmed the usefulness of the Japanese version of the PDSS-2 [34]. PD patients had significantly impaired scores for the PDSS-2 total score compared with control subjects (15.0 ± 9.7 vs. 9.1 ± 6.6, $p<0.001$) (Figure 6). Significant differences were found between PD patients and controls in three PDSS-2 domain scores and subscores (Figure 7). The PDSS-2 total score was correlated with the Pittsburgh Sleep Quality Index (PSQI), Epworth Sleepiness Scale (ESS), Beck Depression Inventory-II (BDI-II), Parkinson Fatigue Scale (PFS), Parkinson's Disease Questionnaire (PDQ-39) summary index, all of the PDQ-39 domains, and the Unified Parkinson's Disease Rating Scale part III (motor function). The PDSS-2 is simple and easy to use at the outpatient clinic or bedside and is suitable for assessing not only the current status on sleep but also evaluating treatment response [35]. For further improvement in the PDSS-2, subitems for the screening for RLS (items 4 and 5) and RBD (item 6) may not be sufficient to differentiate those conditions from RLS mimics, psychosis, and delirium. Adding a subjective evaluation of severity for each item may be useful.

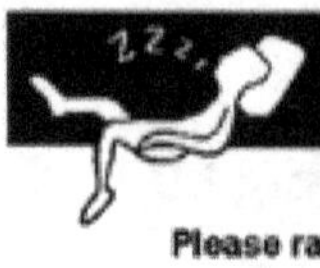

Parkinson's Disease Sleep Scale (PDSS-2)

Please rate the severity of the following based on your experiences during the past week (7 days). Please make a cross in the answer box

	Very often (This means 6 to 7 days a week)	Often (This means 4 to 5 days a week)	Sometimes (This means 2 to 3 days a week)	Occasionally (This means 1 day a week)	Never
1) Overall, did you sleep well during the last week?	0	1	2	3	4
2) Did you have difficulty falling asleep each night?	4	3	2	1	0
3) Did you have difficulty staying asleep?	4	3	2	1	0
4) Did you have restlessness of legs or arms at nights causing disruption of sleep?	4	3	2	1	0
5) Was your sleep disturbed due to an urge to move your legs or arms?	4	3	2	1	0
6) Did you suffer from distressing dreams at night?	4	3	2	1	0
7) Did you suffer from distressing hallucinations at night (seeing or hearing things that you are told do not exist)?	4	3	2	1	0
8) Did you get up at night to pass urine?	4	3	2	1	0
9) Did you feel uncomfortable at night because you were unable to turn around in bed or move due to immobility?	4	3	2	1	0
10) Did you feel pain in your arms or legs which woke you up from sleep at night?	4	3	2	1	0
11) Did you have muscle cramps in your arms or legs which woke you up whilst sleeping at night?	4	3	2	1	0
12) Did you wake early in the morning with painful posturing of arms and legs?	4	3	2	1	0
13) On waking, did you experience tremor?	4	3	2	1	0
14) Did you feel tired and sleepy after waking in the morning?	4	3	2	1	0
15) Did you wake up at night due to snoring or difficulties with breathing?	4	3	2	1	0

Total score ranges from 0 (no disturbance) to 60 (maximum nocturnal disturbance).

Figure 5. PDSS-2 (reproduced with permission from [33]).

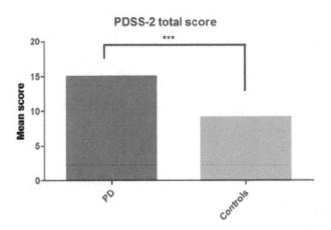

*p<0.001, Mann–Whitney U-test

Figure 6. PDSS-2 total score in PD patients and controls

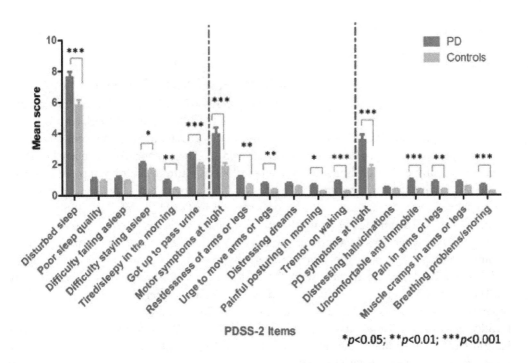

Figure 7. The mean PDSS-2 scores in the three domains between PD patients and controls

PDSS-2	Item
Disturbed sleep	
Poor sleep quality	1
Difficulty falling asleep	2
Difficulty staying asleep	3
Tired/sleepy in the morning	14
Get up to pass urine	8
Motor symptoms at night	
Restlessness of arms or legs	4
Urge to move arms or legs	5
Distressing dreams	6
Painful posturing in morning	12
Tremor on waking	13
PD symptoms at night	
Distressing hallucinations	7
Uncomfortable and immobile	9
Pain in arms or legs	10
Muscle cramps in arms or legs	11
Breathing problems/snoring	15

Table 3. PDSS-2 domain scale

3. Nocturnal problems in PD

The significant impact of nocturnal problems in PD patients has been emphasized by the study by Lees et al [4], which found that among 220 patients with PD, 215 (98%) reported sleep problems, and 29% took hypnotics or sedatives, but only 6% took any anti-parkinsonian drug during the night (Table 4). In the study using continuous activity monitoring, compared with the healthy elderly subjects, patients with PD showed an elevated nocturnal activity level and an increased proportion of time with movement [36]. Nocturnal motor symptoms such as worsened rigidity, tremor, dystonia, and akinesia can lead to nocturnal awakening and sleep maintenance insomnia, a common form of insomnia in PD [4, 7, 24, 29, 37]. Sleep-onset insomnia does not seem to account for the majority of insomnia cases in PD when compared with age-matched controls. In a community-based sleep study by Tandberg et al, sleep-onset insomnia, sleep-maintenance insomnia, and early awakening were observed in 31.8%, 38.9%, and 23.4% of PD patients compared with 22%, 12%, and 11% of healthy controls, respectively [7]. The frequency of sleep onset insomnia did not significantly differ between the groups. Self-reported sleep problems occurred significantly more often in patients with PD (60%) than in healthy controls (33%) and patients with diabetes mellitus (45%). Our cross-sectional studies have also found sleep-maintenance insomnia, but not sleep-onset insomnia, to be significantly more prevalent in patients with PD than in controls [29, 34]. Sleep disturbances correlate with motor impairment in PD patients [6]. However, even in untreated patients with PD, in addition to the changes in sleep architecture, motor symptoms may predominately occur at night rather than during the day [32]. Therefore, nocturnal motor symptoms can interfere with sleep and are not always parallel with daytime motor symptoms, which is supported by several studies showing a weak or nonexistent correlation between sleep disturbances and daytime motor symptoms (UPDRS motor score) [7, 38] and no correlation between nocturnal motor symptoms obtained by PDSS-2 and UPDRS motor scores [33]. In patients with an early to moderate stage of PD, a substantial number of patients may suffer from nocturnal problems; however, this may be missed in clinical practice unless physicians screen for it.

An international cross-sectional study comprising 242 patients with PD (HY 2 (n=121) being most frequent) revealed that a significant number of sleep-related symptoms were undeclared by patients before the administration of the non-motor questionnaire: nocturia, 43.9%; daytime sleepiness, 52.4%; insomnia, 43.9%; vivid dreams, 52.4%; acting out during dreams, 44.1%; and restless legs, 36.4% [39]. Patients in the advanced stages of the disease have motor dysfunction throughout the day; therefore, its impact on the nighttime period should always be considered.

Symptoms	Experienced by (%)	Most troublesome (%)
Need to visit lavatory	79	29
Inability to turn over in bed	65	39
Painful leg cramps	55	15
Vivid dreams / nightmares	48	9
Inability to get out of bed unaided	35	15
Limb or facial dystonia	34	10
Back pain	34	9
Jerks of legs	33	5
Visual hallucinations	16	3
None	4	

Table 4. Nocturnal problems in PD patients (adapted from Lees et al [4])

Although nocturia is associated with normal aging, 80% of PD patients show two or more episodes of nocturia per night resulting from overflow incontinence and a spastic bladder [4].Urinary bladder–related symptoms, such as frequency, urgency, and urge incontinence, are common in PD, resulting in frequent nocturnal awakenings. In animal studies, the stimulation of D1 receptors inhibits the micturition reflex, whereas the stimulation of D2 receptors facilitates the micturition reflex. D2 depletion of dopaminergic neurons induces an overactive bladder, and D1 receptor agonists produce a dose-dependent inhibition of the micturition reflex [40]. For the treatment of nocturia, first, a urologic examination is recommended to rule out underlying urologic diseases. Switching from bromocriptine to pergolide improved nocturia, thereby improving sleep status in patients with PD [41]. Anticholinergic drugs, such as oxybutynin and tolterodine, are commonly used for detrusor hyperreflexia. Subthalamic deep brain stimulation improved detrusor hyperreflexia [42]. When nocturia is related to wearing-off symptoms, adding a long-acting dopamine agonist before bedtime should be considered.

Pain has been reported in approximately 60% of PD patients [43] in association with sleep disturbances and depressive symptoms [44, 45], in addition to tremor, rigidity, akinesia, dystonia, and akathisia. Pain is classified into the following categories: musculoskeletal pain, radicular or neuropathic pain, dystonia-related pain, akathitic discomfort, and primary central parkinsonian pain [46]. Nocturnal pain is related to nocturnal awakening. To evaluate whether pain is related to wearing off is important because it can worsen during wearing-off periods. Primary central parkinsonian, akathitic, and dystonia-related pain may respond to dopaminergic treatment.

Increased severity in nocturnal motor symptoms such as rigidity, bradykinesia, and resting tremor may benefit from increasing the bedtime dose of dopaminergic treatment. A double-blinded, placebo-controlled trial demonstrated the efficacy of 24-h rotigotine on daytime motor function (UPDRS part III) and nocturnal disabilities, as evaluated by the PDSS-2 [35]. Subcutaneous overnight apomorphine infusion markedly reduced nocturnal awakenings, nocturnal off periods, pain, dystonia, and nocturia [47]. High-frequency subthalamic nucleus stimulation in 10 PD patients with insomnia reduced nighttime akinesia by 60% and completely suppressed axial and early-morning dystonia [48]. Furthermore, a 24-week, double-blind study showed that once-daily ropinirole prolonged release improved nocturnal symptoms (as assessed by PDSS) in patients with advanced PD who were not optimally controlled with levodopa and suffered troublesome nocturnal disturbances [49]. In contrast, some studies indicate that dopaminergic drugs can have alerting effects, possibly interfering with sleep continuity in patients with PD [14, 36, 50].

Hallucinations and psychosis affect 30 to 45% of PD patients who have been treated with levodopa for a long period [51]. Among a wide spectrum of hallucinations, visual hallucinations are commonly observed. Sleep disturbances, daily levodopa doses, older age, depression, and cognitive impairment are associated with an increased risk for hallucinations in PD patients [52, 53]. In contrast to nocturnal motor symptoms, nocturnal psychiatric symptoms including hallucination and psychosis can be effectively treated by reducing the bedtime dose of dopaminergic treatment or adding antipsychotics.

The prevalence of depression in PD patients varies, ranging from 2.7% to 89% [54]. Depression is associated with sleep disturbances and impaired quality of life in patients with PD [55, 56]. Nortripryline, desipramine, and selective serotonin reuptake inhibitors (venlafaxine and paroxetine) are more effective than placebo in treating depression in PD [57]. Additionally, it should be noted that depressive symptoms worsen during wearing-off periods and also contribute to worsened motor symptoms [58]. In this regard, antiparkinsonian drugs show beneficial effects not only on motor symptoms but also on a patient's mood. Pramipexole improved depressive symptoms in patients with PD mainly through a direct antidepressant effect rather than through improved motor symptoms [59].

Untreated nocturnal disturbances contribute not only to sleep fragmentation but also to daytime sleepiness and thus daytime motor dysfunction. The primary sleep disorders include RBD, RLS, and SAS, all of which should be properly managed because of their clinical significance in disease. RBD is a REM parasomnia characterized by loss of muscle atonia during

REM sleep and complex motor behavior in association with dream content [60]. Table 5 summarizes the management of sleep problems in PD.

Type of insomnia	Cause	Treatment
Difficulty initiating sleep	Unknown cause	Hypnotics (short-acting type; zolpidem, zopiclone, eszopiclone, brotizolam)
	Drug related (alerting effect)	Remove or reduce dose of causative drug
Difficulty maintaining sleep / early morning awakening	Unknown cause	Hypnotics (intermediate type; flunitrazepam)
	Wearing off, resting tremor, rigidity, akinesia,	Increase frequency of levodopa administration, add dopamine agonist, or switch to a different type of dopamine agonist
	Drug-induced dyskinesia	Increase frequency of levodopa and reduce dose of levodopa administration, add dopamine agonist
	Depression, anxiety	Antidepressant (SSRI, SNRI, tricyclic antidepressant) Anti-anxiety drug Dopamine agonist (D3 R)
	Nocturia	Oxybutynin, flavoxate Dopamine agonist (D1 R)
Excessive daytime sleepiness	Unknown cause	Daytime rehabilitation
	Drug related (sedative effect)	Remove or reduce dose of causative drug (including dopamine agonist)
	Refractory	Modafinil, caffeine
Hallucination, delusion, delirium		Reduce dopaminergic drugs, consider Yi-Gan San and atypical antipsychotics
REM sleep behavior disorder		Hazard avoidance (remove potentially dangerous objects from the bedroom and place a mattress on the floor), consider clonazepam and Yi-Gan San
Sleep apnea syndrome		Continuous positive airway pressure therapy (severe case)
Restless legs syndrome, periodic limb movement disorder		Adjustment of dopaminergic treatment, use dopamine agonist before bedtime, consider iron supplement (if serum ferritin are below 50 µg/L) and clonazepam

Table 5. Management of sleep problems in PD

4. Excessive daytime sleepiness and sudden-onset sleep episodes

Excessive daytime sleepiness (EDS) occurs in approximately 15%-50% of PD patients [61-63]. A high Epworth sleepiness scale (ESS) score, male gender status, longer disease duration, and high disease severity and dopaminergic medication have been associated with EDS [61, 62, 64]. Multifactorial nocturnal problems (Table 1) are the causes of sleep disturbances in PD and also lead to EDS, reflecting poor sleep quality and duration. In addition to nocturnal problems, PD-related pathological changes play a role in sleepiness: an impaired arousal system has been suggested in PD (Table 6; Figure 8). A subset of patients with PD exhibit EDS and a sudden onset of sleep episodes with a short sleep latency and a short sleep-onset REM period, independent of the nighttime sleep conditions. This finding suggests a narcolepsy phenotype in PD patients. Narcolepsy is a sleep disorder characterized by severe daytime sleepiness, cataplexy, hypnagogic hallucination, and sleep paralysis caused by loss of orexin neurons. However, cataplexy is lacking in patients with PD [65], and orexin levels in the cerebrospinal fluid in PD patients with EDS remains controversial [66-68]. Decreased orexin levels in the hypothalamus and a loss of orexin neurons have been observed in PD patients in correlation with clinical disease progression; however, no description was provided for EDS [69, 70].

Dopaminergic medication, i.e., taking dopamine agonists or levodopa, is associated with increased daytime sleepiness in patients with PD [61, 62, 64, 71, 72]. Although a higher levodopa equivalent dose is correlated with increased daytime sleepiness in PD [62, 64, 71], the association between the specific type of dopamine agonist and EDS is unclear [61, 62, 72, 73] (Figure 9). Untreated PD patients do not seem to have EDS compared with controls [22, 74]. However, the study consisting of 3078 men aged 71 to 93 years showed that there was more than a threefold excess (odds ratio 3.3) in the risk of PD in men with EDS versus men without EDS [75]. In a prospective study, of the 232 patients included at baseline, 138 were available for reevaluation after 4 years, and 89 patients were available after 8 years. The EDS frequency increased from 5.6% at the baseline to 22.5% at the 4-year follow up and 40.8% at the 8-year follow up. EDS was related to age, gender, and use of dopamine agonists in the logistic regression model, whereas in patients never having used dopamine agonists, hyper-somnia was associated with the HY stage only, suggesting that age- and disease-related disturbances of the sleep-wake regulation contribute to hypersomnia in PD and that treatment with dopamine agonists also contribute to EDS [76]. Regarding the interaction between dopamine and sleep [77], the D1 receptor agonist promotes wakefulness and decreases slow-wave sleep and REM sleep. In contrast, the D2 receptor agonist has a biphasic action: a lower dose reduces wakefulness and increases slow-wave sleep and REM sleep via the pre-synaptic auto D2 receptor, whereas a higher dose stimulates wakefulness via the post-synaptic D2 receptor. D3 receptor stimulation increases slow-wave sleep and promotes sleep. This result for D2 receptor stimulation differs from that observed in patients with PD: a higher dose of dopaminergic drugs is associated with EDS. Bliwise et al reported that increasing dosages of dopamine agonists were associated with less daytime alertness, whereas higher levels of levodopa were associated with higher levels of alertness [78].

Sudden-onset sleep episodes while driving have been reported in 3.8%-22.8% of PD patients and are associated with a high score on the ESS [61, 64, 73], although sleepiness is sometimes unrecognized by patients. However, similar to the findings by Tan et al, which showed that ESS scores ≥10 had a 71.4% sensitivity and 88.4% specificity for predicting a sleep attack [64], our study showed that an ESS score of ≥10 had a 75% sensitivity and 82.4% specificity for predicting sleep episodes [62]. This evidence suggests that PDS patients with EDS have a significant increased risk for sudden-onset sleep episodes.

Nucleus	Main neurotransmitter	Neuronal loss in Parkinsonian brain (%)
Locus coeruleus	Noradrenaline	40-50
Median raphe	Serotonin	20-40
Ventral periaqueductal gray matter	Dopamine	9
Pedunculopontine nucleus	Acetylcholine	57
Tuberomammillary nucleus	Histamine	Unchanged enzymatic activity
Lateral hypothalamus	Orexin (hypocretin)	23-62
Basal forebrain	Acetylcholine	32-93

Table 6. Neuronal loss in arousal systems in the brains of patients with PD (adapted from [79]).

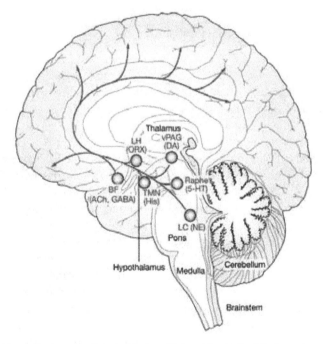

5-HT, 5-hydroxytryptamine (serotonin);ACh, acetylcholine; BF, basal forebrain; DA, dopamine; GABA, γ-aminobutyric acid; His, histamine; LC, locus ceruleus; LH, lateral hypothalamus; NE, norepinephrine; ORX, orexin; Raphe, median raphe nucleus; TMN, tuberomamillary nucleus; vPAG, ventral periaqueductal gray matter.

Figure 8. The ascending arousal systems in the human brain (reproduced with permission from [80]).

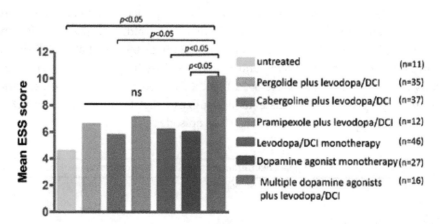

The ESS score is significantly higher in the group with multiple dopamine agonists plus levodopa/DCI; however, no differences in EDS among different types of dopamine agonist groups are shown.

Figure 9. Excessive daytime sleepiness and dopamine agonists in patients with PD (created based on the data from [62]).

5. Primary sleep disorders

5.1. Rapid eye movement sleep behavior disorder

REM sleep behavior disorder (RBD) is characterized by a loss of muscle atonia during REM sleep, resulting in dream-enacting behavior, leading to injury to the individual or bed partner [81]. The important implication is that idiopathic RBD patients are found to be at high risk of later developing neurodegenerative diseases in the synucleinopathies, such as PD, multiple system atrophy, and dementia with Lewy bodies [82]. Schenck and colleagues first reported that 3.7 ± 1.4 years after an initial diagnosis of idiopathic RBD, 38% of patients developed a parkinsonian syndrome [83]. In a prospective study of idiopathic RBD patients, the estimated 5-year risk of neurodegenerative disease was 17.7%, the 10-year risk was 40.6%, and the 12-year risk was 52.4% [84]. A recent clinicopathological study of 172 cases of RBD with or without coexisting neurological diseases revealed that among the neurodegenerative disorders associated with RBD (n=170), 160 (94%) were synucleinopathies [85]. The association between RBD and synucleinopathy was particularly high when RBD preceded the onset of other neurodegenerative syndrome features. Before the onset of motor symptoms, idiopathic RBD subjects already possess characteristics, such as olfactory impairment, impaired color vision, autonomic dysfunction, mild cognitive impairment, a decreased uptake of cardiac (123) I-metaiodobenzylguanidine (MIBG), and hyperechogenicity in the substantia nigra [86-90], that are similar to PD. These may be potential predictive markers for future development of PD. In the subjects with idiopathic RBD who were initially free of neurodegenerative disease, the severity of the REM atonia loss on the baseline PSG findings was associated with the development of PD [91]. Employing noninvasive imaging techniques such as transcranial sonography, single-photon emission computed tomography, and positron emission tomography may be helpful in identifying patients with iRBD potentially at future risk for PD [92].

Lesions of the locus coeruleus perialpha in cats and of the sublaterodorsal nucleus in rats have been shown to cause REM sleep without atonia with complex movements [93, 94]. The equivalent of these nuclei in humans is the subcoeruleus nucleus in the pons, which is first affected during the early stages of PD. In addition, other brainstem nuclei such as the cholinergic nuclei, pedunculopontine nucleus, and laterodorsal tegmental nucleus also play a role in regulating REM sleep [95]. In the study using neuromelanin-sensitive imaging, reduced signal intensity is found in the locus coeruleus/subcoeruleus area in patients with PD relative to controls, and that difference is more marked in patients with PSG-confirmed RBD than in those without RBD. A reduced signal intensity in those areas is found to be correlated with the percentage of abnormally increased muscle tone during REM sleep. This study first shows the involvement of the coeruleus/subcoeruleus complex in PD patients and, more markedly, in those with concomitant RBD [96].

The frequency of RBD is reported to be 15- 60% of PD patients (Table 7) [79]. Co-occurrence of RBD in PD may represent distinct characteristics of PD: akinetic rigid phenotype, an increased frequency of falls, and a poor response to dopaminergic medications, orthostatic hypotension, and impaired color vision have been described compared with PD patients without RBD [97, 98]. A decreased uptake of cardiac MIBG is also reported in PD patients with RBD compared with those without RBD [99, 100]. In a prospective study with 42 patients with PD (27 patients with PSG-confirmed RBD and 15 patients without RBD) for 4 years, 48% with RBD developed dementia, compared with 0% of those without RBD, suggesting that RBD was associated with an increased risk of dementia in patients with PD [101]. Similarly, Nomura et al found coexistence of clinical RBD, but not subclinical RBD, was associated with the development of dementia in PD. In their study, RBD, but not subclinical RBD, was associated with orthostatic hypotension and levodopa equivalent dose equivalents in patients with PD [102].

With respect to the clinical motor subtype, not all the studies support the akinetic rigid phenotype as the clinical phenotype associated with PD-RBD. A study of 457 PD patients with sleep disturbances did not find a characteristic clinical subtype for PD with RBD but did report a higher disease severity and longer disease duration in PD patients with RBD than in those without [103]. In early PD (disease duration ≤5 years and HY stage 1- 2.5), the RBD co-morbidity (confirmed by clinical history during the preceding 6 months and a cut-off score > 4 on the RBD screening questionnaire) was significantly higher (55%) in PD patients, but clinical subtype and disease severity did not differ between patients with and without RBD [104]. It has been reported that a tremor-dominant type may transition into a non-tremor dominant type over time and with increased age [105]. In our study including 93 patients with PD and controls using the Japanese version of the RBD screening questionnaire (RBDSQ-J) [106], 29% of PD patients had probable RBD (5≥RBDSQ-J) compared with 8.6% of controls [107]. Patients with probable RBD had a higher score of PDQ-39 cognition and emotional well-being and more frequent sleep onset insomnia, distressing dreams, and hallucinations. However, there were no differences between these two groups with respect to the clinical subtype, disease severity, or motor function. In the study consisting of 57 newly diagnosed drug-naïve patients with PD, 17 PD patients (30%) were diagnosed with RBD by overnight PSG. Non-RBD patients and RBD patients did not differ with respect to age, gender, disease duration, motor symptom subtype and severity, and cognitive performance. PSG parameters such as total sleep time, REM sleep percentage, apnea-hypopnea index, and mean oxygen saturation also did not differ [108]. Differences in clinical background factors between PD patients with and without RBD await confirmation in longitudinal studies. Interestingly, restored motor control (movements, speech, and facial expressions) during REM sleep with enacted dreams has been reported in PD patients with RBD [109].

Before starting treatment of RBD, it should be noted that RBD can be triggered or worsened by antidepressants [110]. Clonazepam (0.5 to 1.5 mg) at bedtime is the most effective treatment for RBD patients. Melatonin (3-12 mg) at bedtime has been shown to ameliorate RBD [111, 112]. Administration of Yi-Gan San, an herbal medication, at 2.5 g three times a day, alone or in conjunction with 0.25 mg clonazepam, may also be effective [113]. Some patients may respond to 1 evening or bedtime dose of 2.5g.

DISEASE	PREVALENCE (%)	
	RBD	RWA
Synucleinopathies		
Parkinson's disease	15-60	
Multiple system atrophy	90	
Dementia with Lewy bodies	86	
Tauopathies		
Progressive supranuclear palsy	10-11	0-33
Alzheimer's disease	7	29
Corticobasal degeneration	Case reports	
Frontotemporal dementia	None	
Pallidopontonigral degeneration	0	0
Guadeloupean parkinsonism	78	
Genetic Diseases		
Huntington's disease	12	
Spinocerebellar ataxia type 3	56	
Parkin mutation	60	

RBD, REM sleep behavior disorder; RWA, REM sleep without atonia

Table 7. RBD in neurodegenerative diseases (adapted from [79])

5.2. Restless leg syndrome

RLS is characterized by an urge to move the legs, uncomfortable leg sensations, and motor restlessness, typically occurring during the evening and night. The pathogenesis of RLS remains unclear; however, dysfunction of the dopaminergic A11 nucleus of the hypothalamus has been implicated [114]. The hypothalamic A11 nucleus has projections to the suprachiasmatic nuclei and dorsal raphe, and it provides descending projections to the preganglionic sympathetic neurons, dorsal horn region, interneurons, and somatic motor neurons [114]. Neurophysiological studies have revealed disinhibition of inhibitory cortical controls, decreased intracortical inhibition, and hyperexcitability of spinal pathways [115-117]. In view of a marked beneficial response to dopaminergic treatment observed in both PD and RLS, a shared dopaminergic dysfunction has been suggested in PD and RLS [118]. However, unlike RBD, there is no evidence suggesting RLS as a risk factor of PD, and the co-morbidity of RLS in PD patients varies widely from 0 to 50% [119]. In contrast to PD, which shows degeneration of the striatonigral dopaminergic neurons, confirmed by the reduced striatal uptake observed in neuroimaging studies, in idiopathic RLS, PET/SPECT studies have not produced consistent findings of striatonigral dopaminergic dysfunction [120, 121]. Postmortem studies of RLS patients have found an increased total and phosphorylated tyrosine hydroxylase in the putamen and substantia nigra [122]. Cerebrospinal fluid iron insufficiency has been demonstrated in idiopathic RLS independent of serum iron levels [123, 124]. The transcranial sonography findings of substantia nigra hypoechogenicity and brain imaging studies also suggest brain iron insufficiency in RLS patients [125, 126]. In contrast, the hyperechogenicity in the substantia nigra commonly observed in patients with PD may reflect increased levels of iron in the substantia nigra. No difference in the substantia nigra echogenicity has been reported between the PD with RLS and PD without RLS groups [127]. Thus, there are some similarities between PD and idiopathic RLS, including a marked response to dopamine agonist treatment, although the two disorders may have different pathogenic mechanisms [118, 128].

In PD, there are several conditions that mimic RLS, including sensory symptoms, pain, and the wearing-off phenomenon [118]. Moreover, the clinical overlap between RLS, wearing-off-related lower limb discomfort, and restlessness and akathisia has been suggested [129, 130]. In the study evaluating RLS in PD, 20.8% of PD patients had RLS, and patients with PD with RLS had an older age at onset and were much less likely to report a family history of RLS compared with patients with isolated RLS [131]. Complicatedly, dopaminergic treatment may either mask or augment coexisting RLS symptoms in PD [129], and there is an association between long-term dopaminergic treatment and RLS development in PD patients [132].

In addition, in recent studies, an increased frequency of leg motor restlessness (LMR) without fulfilling the criteria for RLS has been described in patients with PD [128]. A total of 200 early, drug-naive patients with PD derived from a population-based incident cohort and 173 age- and gender-matched control subjects were examined, and 31 (15.5%) of PD patients and 16 (9.2%) of control subjects met RLS criteria (p=0.07). However, LMR (OR 2.84, 95% CI 1.43–5.61, p=0.001) but not RLS (OR 1.76, 95% CI 0.90–3.43, p=0.089) occurs with a near 3-fold higher risk in early PD compared with controls [128]. Shimohata and Nishizawa reported that among 158 patients with PD, 11% had RLS and 19% had LMR without fulfilling the criteria for RLS (total LMR, 30%). The frequencies of insomnia and EDS in patients with LMR were lower than those of patients with RLS but higher than in patients without LMR or RLS, highlighting the impact of LMR and RLS on sleep disturbance in PD [133]. Likewise, our study showed that LMR was more frequent in patients with PD than in controls (32.3% vs. 14.0%; scores of PDSS-2 subitem 4 (restlessness of arms or legs) or subitem 5 (urge to move arms or legs) ≥2), although RLS frequency was similar between the patients with PD and controls (5.5% vs. 2.2%) [34].

For the treatment of RLS, iron replacement therapy should be considered when the serum levels of ferritin are lower than 50 μg / L. Using long-acting dopamine agonists at bedtime is effective.

5.3. Sleep apnea syndrome

Upper airway dysfunction associated with parkinsonism, such as bradykinesia and rigidity, and fluctuations in the respiratory muscles that occur with motor complications can contribute to obstructive sleep apnea in patients with PD [17]. A significant correlation between the apnea hypopnea index (AHI) and the severity of PD was reported [21]. Earlier studies suggested SAS is more frequent in patients with PD than in control subjects [17, 21]. However, in PD patients, lower levels of decline in the minimal or mean nocturnal oxygen saturation levels than in AHI-matched controls were observed [17, 21]. In contrast, recent studies suggest that the comorbidity of SAS is not more frequent in PD patients than in the general population, and thus, it may not a relevant issue in PD [10, 11, 134]. Moreover, it has been argued that SAS may not play a major role in EDS in PD. De Cock et al. [11] reported that sleep apnea (defined as an AHI > 5) was less frequent in the PD group than in the in-hospital control group (27% vs. 40%); however, PD patients with sleep apnea had greater motor disability than patients without sleep apnea. EDS was not correlated with sleep apnea.

In our questionnaire-based study, snoring was more frequent in PD patients than in controls (14.0% vs. 1.1%), and snoring in PD patients was associated with disease severity, impaired motor function, and a decreased quality of life, but it was not associated with EDS [135]. Table 8 shows the previous PSG studies that evaluated sleep-related breathing disorders in PD.

When a patient has severe obstructive SAS, continuous positive airway pressure therapy should be considered.

Authors	Year	Sample No. PD/Controls	Age (years) PD/ Controls	ESS score and EDS PD/Control	Frequency of SRBD PD/Controls	AHI (/h) PD/Controls
Arnulf et al [14]	2002	*54 (44 M)/NA	68±7.0/ NA	ESS; 14.3±4.1/NA EDS; 50%/NA (mean SL<5 min)	48.1%/NA (AHI>5) 20%/NA (AHI>15)	NA/NA
Maria et al [21]	2003	15 (12 M)/ 15 (12 M)	63±4 / 60±4	ESS; 12.3 / 6.1	66.7%/NA	11.7/5.7
De Cock et al [11]	2010	50 (35 M)/ 50 (35 M)	62.1 ± 9.8/ 62.4 ± 13.8	ESS; 9.2±4.7/5.8±4.0 EDS; 24%/72% (ESS>10)	20%/40% (AHI>5)	6±11/ 23±23
Trotti et al [134]	2010	**55 (37 M)/6132	63.9±9.1/ 62.9±11.0	NA/NA	43.6%/46.4% (AHI>5)	6.3-8.0(9.2-10.6)/ NA
Buskova et al [22]	2011	#15 (14 M)/ 15(14 M)	59.8±10.0/ 60.2±10.0	ESS; 5.6±3.0/6,1±2.0	26.7%/20.0%	9.5/4.6
Yong et al [13]	2011	56 (34 M)/ 68 (38 M)	65.4±9.1/ 59.3±9.1	EDS; 66.1%/2.9% (ESS≥10) EDS; 23.6%/39.4% (Mean SL<8 min.)	49.1%/65.1% (AHI≥5)	12.5/15.6/ 12.2±13.1

*Referred for sleepiness, **Controls were obtained from a population-based study, #drug-naïve PD patients

SL, sleep latency; SRBD, sleep-related breathing disorders

Table 8. Polysomnographic studies evaluating sleep-related breathing disorders in PD

6. Conclusion

Sleep disorders can occur in the early stages of PD and worsen as the disease progresses. The cause of sleep disorders in PD is multifactorial, reflecting PD-related pathology, various aspects of PD-related motor and non-motor symptoms, and comorbidity of primary sleep disorders. Early recognition of and active intervention for sleep disturbance is of great importance, as sleep disturbances significantly impair the quality of life of patients with PD.

Author details

Keisuke Suzuki[1], Tomoyuki Miyamoto[2], Masayuki Miyamoto[1], Ayaka Numao[1], Hideki Sakuta[1], Hiroaki Fujita[1], Yuji Watanabe[1], Masaoki Iwanami[2] and Koichi Hirata[1]

1 Department of Neurology, Dokkyo Medical University, Japan

2 Department of Neurology, Dokkyo Medical University Koshigaya Hospital, Japan

References

[1] Jankovic J. Parkinson's disease: clinical features and diagnosis. J Neurol Neurosurg Psychiatry 2008;79(4):368-376.

[2] Chaudhuri KR, Schapira AH. Non-motor symptoms of Parkinson's disease: dopaminergic pathophysiology and treatment. Lancet Neurol 2009;8(5):464-474.

[3] Parkinson J. An essay on the shaking palsy. 1817. J Neuropsychiatry Clin Neurosci 2002;14(2):223-236; discussion 222.

[4] Lees AJ, Blackburn NA, Campbell VL. The nighttime problems of Parkinson's disease. Clin Neuropharmacol 1988;11(6):512-519.

[5] Suzuki K, Miyamoto M, Miyamoto T, Iwanami M, Hirata K. Sleep disturbances associated with Parkinson's disease. Parkinsons Dis 2011;2011:219056.

[6] Kumar S, Bhatia M, Behari M. Sleep disorders in Parkinson's disease. Mov Disord 2002;17(4):775-781.

[7] Tandberg E, Larsen JP, Karlsen K. A community-based study of sleep disorders in patients with Parkinson's disease. Mov Disord 1998;13(6):895-899.

[8] Diederich NJ, McIntyre DJ. Sleep disorders in Parkinson's disease: many causes, few therapeutic options. J Neurol Sci 2012;314(1-2):12-19.

[9] Diederich NJ, Comella CL. Sleep disturbances in Parkinson's disease. In: Chokroverty S, Hening WA, Walters AS, editors. Sleep and Movement Disorders. Philadelphia:
Elsevier Science; 2003. p. 478–488.

[10] Peeraully T, Yong MH, Chokroverty S, Tan EK. Sleep and Parkinson's disease: a review of case-control polysomnography studies. Mov Disord 2012;27(14):1729-1737.

[11] De Cock VC, Abouda M, Leu S, Oudiette D, Roze E, Vidailhet M, et al. Is obstructive
sleep apnea a problem in Parkinson's disease? Sleep Med 2010;11(3):247-252.

[12] Happe S, Klosch G, Lorenzo J, Kunz D, Penzel T, Roschke J, et al. Perception of sleep:
subjective versus objective sleep parameters in patients with Parkinson's disease in
comparison with healthy elderly controls. Sleep perception in Parkinson's disease
and controls. J Neurol 2005;252(8):936-943.

[13] Yong MH, Fook-Chong S, Pavanni R, Lim LL, Tan EK. Case control polysomnographic studies of sleep disorders in Parkinson's disease. PLoS One 2011;6(7):e22511.

[14] Arnulf I, Konofal E, Merino-Andreu M, Houeto JL, Mesnage V, Welter ML, et al. Parkinson's disease and sleepiness: an integral part of PD. Neurology 2002;58(7):
1019-1024.

[15] Brunner H, Wetter TC, Högl B, Yassouridis A, Trenkwalder C, Friess E. Microstructure of the non-rapid eye movement sleep electroencephalogram in patients with
newly diagnosed Parkinson's disease: effects of dopaminergic treatment. Mov Disord
2002;17(5):928-933.

[16] Wetter TC, Brunner H, Högl B, Yassouridis A, Trenkwalder C, Friess E. Increased alpha activity in REM sleep in de novo patients with Parkinson's disease. Mov Disord
2001;16(5):928-933.

[17] Diederich NJ, Vaillant M, Leischen M, Mancuso G, Golinval S, Nati R, et al. Sleep apnea syndrome in Parkinson's disease. A case-control study in 49 patients. Mov Disord 2005;20(11):1413-1418.

[18] Wailke S, Herzog J, Witt K, Deuschl G, Volkmann J. Effect of controlled-release levodopa on the microstructure of sleep in Parkinson's disease. Eur J Neurol 2011;18(4):
590-596.

[19] Chaudhuri KR, Naidu Y. Early Parkinson's disease and non-motor issues. J Neurol
2008;255 Suppl 5:33-38.

[20] Shpirer I, Miniovitz A, Klein C, Goldstein R, Prokhorov T, Theitler J, et al. Excessive
daytime sleepiness in patients with Parkinson's disease: a polysomnography study.
Mov Disord 2006;21(9):1432-1438.

[21] Maria B, Sophia S, Michalis M, Charalampos L, Andreas P, John ME, et al. Sleep
breathing disorders in patients with idiopathic Parkinson's disease. Respir Med
2003;97(10):1151-1157.

[22] Buskova J, Klempir J, Majerova V, Picmausova J, Sonka K, Jech R, et al. Sleep disturbances in untreated Parkinson's disease. J Neurol 2011;258(12):2254-2259.

[23] Rye DB, Bliwise DL, Dihenia B, Gurecki P. FAST TRACK: daytime sleepiness in Parkinson's disease. J Sleep Res 2000;9(1):63-69.

[24] Chaudhuri KR, Pal S, DiMarco A, Whately-Smith C, Bridgman K, Mathew R, et al. The Parkinson's disease sleep scale: a new instrument for assessing sleep and nocturnal disability in Parkinson's disease. J Neurol Neurosurg Psychiatry 2002;73(6): 629-635.

[25] Högl B, Arnulf I, Comella C, Ferreira J, Iranzo A, Tilley B, et al. Scales to assess sleep impairment in Parkinson's disease: critique and recommendations. Mov Disord 2010;25(16):2704-2716.

[26] Abe K, Hikita T, Sakoda S. Sleep disturbances in Japanese patients with Parkinson's disease--comparing with patients in the UK. J Neurol Sci 2005;234(1-2):73-78.

[27] Margis R, Donis K, Schonwald SV, Fagondes SC, Monte T, Martin-Martinez P, et al. Psychometric properties of the Parkinson's Disease Sleep Scale--Brazilian version. Parkinsonism Relat Disord 2009;15(7):495-499.

[28] Martinez-Martin P, Salvador C, Menendez-Guisasola L, Gonzalez S, Tobias A, Almazan J, et al. Parkinson's Disease Sleep Scale: validation study of a Spanish version. Mov Disord 2004;19(10):1226-1232.

[29] Suzuki K, Okuma Y, Hattori N, Kamei S, Yoshii F, Utsumi H, et al. Characteristics of sleep disturbances in Japanese patients with Parkinson's disease. A study using Parkinson's disease sleep scale. Mov Disord 2007;22(9):1245-1251.

[30] Wang G, Cheng Q, Zeng J, Bai L, Liu GD, Zhang Y, et al. Sleep disorders in Chinese patients with Parkinson's disease: validation study of a Chinese version of Parkinson's disease sleep scale. J Neurol Sci 2008;271(1-2):153-157.

[31] Suzuki K, Miyamoto M, Miyamoto T, Okuma Y, Hattori N, Kamei S, et al. Correlation between depressive symptoms and nocturnal disturbances in Japanese patients with Parkinson's disease. Parkinsonism Relat Disord 2009;15(1):15-19.

[32] Dhawan V, Dhoat S, Williams AJ, Dimarco A, Pal S, Forbes A, et al. The range and nature of sleep dysfunction in untreated Parkinson's disease (PD). A comparative controlled clinical study using the Parkinson's disease sleep scale and selective polysomnography. J Neurol Sci 2006;248(1-2):158-162.

[33] Trenkwalder C, Kohnen R, Högl B, Metta V, Sixel-Döring F, Frauscher B, et al. Parkinson's disease sleep scale-validation of the revised version PDSS-2. Mov Disord 2011;26(4):644-652.

[34]   Suzuki K, Miyamoto M, Miyamoto T, Tatsumoto M, Watanabe Y, Suzuki S, et al. Nocturnal disturbances and restlessness in Parkinson's disease: using the Japanese version of the Parkinson's disease sleep scale-2. J Neurol Sci 2012;318(1-2):76-81.

[35]   Trenkwalder C, Kies B, Rudzinska M, Fine J, Nikl J, Honczarenko K, et al. Rotigotine effects on early morning motor function and sleep in Parkinson's disease: a double-blind, randomized, placebo-controlled study (RECOVER). Mov Disord 2011;26(1): 90-99.

[36]   van Hilten B, Hoff JI, Middelkoop HA, van der Velde EA, Kerkhof GA, Wauquier A, et al. Sleep disruption in Parkinson's disease. Assessment by continuous activity monitoring. Arch Neurol 1994;51(9):922-928.

[37]   Factor SA, McAlarney T, Sanchez-Ramos JR, Weiner WJ. Sleep disorders and sleep effect in Parkinson's disease. Mov Disord 1990;5(4):280-285.

[38]   Chaudhuri KR, Martinez-Martin P. Clinical assessment of nocturnal disability in Parkinson's disease: the Parkinson's Disease Sleep Scale. Neurology 2004;63(8 Suppl 3):S17-20.

[39]   Chaudhuri KR, Prieto-Jurcynska C, Naidu Y, Mitra T, Frades-Payo B, Tluk S, et al. The nondeclaration of nonmotor symptoms of Parkinson's disease to health care professionals: an international study using the nonmotor symptoms questionnaire. Mov Disord 2010;25(6):704-709.

[40]   Winge K, Fowler CJ. Bladder dysfunction in Parkinsonism: mechanisms, prevalence, symptoms, and management. Mov Disord 2006;21(6):737-745.

[41]   Kuno S, Mizuta E, Yamasaki S, Araki I. Effects of pergolide on nocturia in Parkinson's disease: three female cases selected from over 400 patients. Parkinsonism Relat Disord 2004;10(3):181-187.

[42]   Seif C, Herzog J, van der Horst C, Schrader B, Volkmann J, Deuschl G, et al. Effect of subthalamic deep brain stimulation on the function of the urinary bladder. Ann Neurol 2004;55(1):118-120.

[43]   Barone P, Antonini A, Colosimo C, Marconi R, Morgante L, Avarello TP, et al. The PRIAMO study: A multicenter assessment of nonmotor symptoms and their impact on quality of life in Parkinson's disease. Mov Disord 2009;24(11):1641-1649.

[44]   Starkstein SE, Preziosi TJ, Robinson RG. Sleep disorders, pain, and depression in Parkinson's disease. Eur Neurol 1991;31(6):352-355.

[45]   Goetz CG, Wilson RS, Tanner CM, Garron DC. Relationships among pain, depression, and sleep alterations in Parkinson's disease. Adv Neurol 1987;45:345-347.

[46]   Ford B. Pain in Parkinson's disease. Mov Disord 2010;25 Suppl 1:S98-103.

[47] Reuter I, Ellis CM, Chaudhuri KR. Nocturnal subcutaneous apomorphine infusion in Parkinson's disease and restless legs syndrome. Acta Neurol Scand 1999;100(3): 163-167.

[48] Arnulf I, Bejjani BP, Garma L, Bonnet AM, Houeto JL, Damier P, et al. Improvement of sleep architecture in PD with subthalamic nucleus stimulation. Neurology 2000;55(11):1732-1734.

[49] Chaudhuri KR, Martinez-Martin P, Rolfe KA, Cooper J, Rockett CB, Giorgi L, et al. Improvements in nocturnal symptoms with ropinirole prolonged release in patients with advanced Parkinson's disease. Eur J Neurol 2012;19(1):105-113.

[50] Comella CL, Morrissey M, Janko K. Nocturnal activity with nighttime pergolide in Parkinson disease: a controlled study using actigraphy. Neurology 2005;64(8): 1450-1451.

[51] Goetz CG. Hallucinations in Parkinson's disease: the clinical syndrome. Adv Neurol 1999;80:419-423.

[52] Goetz CG. New developments in depression, anxiety, compulsiveness, and hallucinations in Parkinson's disease. Mov Disord 2010;25 Suppl 1:S104-109.

[53] Nausieda PA, Weiner WJ, Kaplan LR, Weber S, Klawans HL. Sleep disruption in the course of chronic levodopa therapy: an early feature of the levodopa psychosis. Clin Neuropharmacol 1982;5(2):183-194.

[54] Reijnders JS, Ehrt U, Weber WE, Aarsland D, Leentjens AF. A systematic review of prevalence studies of depression in Parkinson's disease. Mov Disord 2008;23(2): 183-189; quiz 313.

[55] Borek LL, Kohn R, Friedman JH. Mood and sleep in Parkinson's disease. J Clin Psychiatry 2006;67(6):958-963.

[56] Happe S, Schrödl B, Faltl M, Müller C, Auff E, Zeitlhofer J. Sleep disorders and depression in patients with Parkinson's disease. Acta Neurol Scand 2001;104(5):275-280.

[57] Aarsland D, Pahlhagen S, Ballard CG, Ehrt U, Svenningsson P. Depression in Parkinson disease--epidemiology, mechanisms and management. Nat Rev Neurol 2012;8(1): 35-47.

[58] Cummings JL. Depression and Parkinson's disease: a review. Am J Psychiatry 1992;149(4):443-454.

[59] Barone P, Poewe W, Albrecht S, Debieuvre C, Massey D, Rascol O, et al. Pramipexole for the treatment of depressive symptoms in patients with Parkinson's disease: a randomised, double-blind, placebo-controlled trial. Lancet Neurol 2010;9(6):573-580.

[60] Mahowald M, Schenck C. REM sleep parasomnias. In: Kryger M, Roth T, Dement W, editors. Principles and Practice of Sleep Medicine. 5th ed. Philadelphia: Saunders; 2010. p. 1083-1097.

[61] Ondo WG, Dat Vuong K, Khan H, Atassi F, Kwak C, Jankovic J. Daytime sleepiness and other sleep disorders in Parkinson's disease. Neurology 2001;57(8):1392-1396.

[62] Suzuki K, Miyamoto T, Miyamoto M, Okuma Y, Hattori N, Kamei S, et al. Excessive daytime sleepiness and sleep episodes in Japanese patients with Parkinson's disease. J Neurol Sci 2008;271(1-2):47-52.

[63] Tandberg E, Larsen JP, Karlsen K. Excessive daytime sleepiness and sleep benefit in Parkinson's disease: a community-based study. Mov Disord 1999;14(6):922-927.

[64] Tan EK, Lum SY, Fook-Chong SM, Teoh ML, Yih Y, Tan L, et al. Evaluation of somnolence in Parkinson's disease: comparison with age- and sex-matched controls. Neurology 2002;58(3):465-468.

[65] Arnulf I, Leu S, Oudiette D. Abnormal sleep and sleepiness in Parkinson's disease. Curr Opin Neurol 2008;21(4):472-477.

[66] Overeem S, Scammell TE, Lammers GJ. Hypocretin/orexin and sleep: implications for the pathophysiology and diagnosis of narcolepsy. Curr Opin Neurol 2002;15(6): 739-745.

[67] Yasui K, Inoue Y, Kanbayashi T, Nomura T, Kusumi M, Nakashima K. CSF orexin levels of Parkinson's disease, dementia with Lewy bodies, progressive supranuclear palsy and corticobasal degeneration. J Neurol Sci 2006;250(1-2):120-123.

[68] Compta Y, Santamaria J, Ratti L, Tolosa E, Iranzo A, Munoz E, et al. Cerebrospinal hypocretin, daytime sleepiness and sleep architecture in Parkinson's disease dementia. Brain 2009;132(Pt 12):3308-3317.

[69] Fronczek R, Overeem S, Lee SY, Hegeman IM, van Pelt J, van Duinen SG, et al. Hypocretin (orexin) loss in Parkinson's disease. Brain 2007;130(Pt 6):1577-1585.

[70] Thannickal TC, Lai YY, Siegel JM. Hypocretin (orexin) cell loss in Parkinson's disease. Brain 2007;130(Pt 6):1586-1595.

[71] Brodsky MA, Godbold J, Roth T, Olanow CW. Sleepiness in Parkinson's disease: a controlled study. Mov Disord 2003;18(6):668-672.

[72] Paus S, Brecht HM, Koster J, Seeger G, Klockgether T, Wullner U. Sleep attacks, daytime sleepiness, and dopamine agonists in Parkinson's disease. Mov Disord 2003;18(6):659-667.

[73] Hobson DE, Lang AE, Martin WR, Razmy A, Rivest J, Fleming J. Excessive daytime sleepiness and sudden-onset sleep in Parkinson disease: a survey by the Canadian Movement Disorders Group. JAMA 2002;287(4):455-463.

[74] Kaynak D, Kiziltan G, Kaynak H, Benbir G, Uysal O. Sleep and sleepiness in patients with Parkinson's disease before and after dopaminergic treatment. Eur J Neurol 2005;12(3):199-207.

[75] Abbott RD, Ross GW, White LR, Tanner CM, Masaki KH, Nelson JS, et al. Excessive daytime sleepiness and subsequent development of Parkinson disease. Neurology 2005;65(9):1442-1446.

[76] Gjerstad MD, Alves G, Wentzel-Larsen T, Aarsland D, Larsen JP. Excessive daytime sleepiness in Parkinson disease: is it the drugs or the disease? Neurology 2006;67(5): 853-858.

[77] Monti JM, Monti D. The involvement of dopamine in the modulation of sleep and waking. Sleep Med Rev 2007;11(2):113-133.

[78] Bliwise DL, Trotti LM, Wilson AG, Greer SA, Wood-Siverio C, Juncos JJ, et al. Daytime alertness in Parkinson's disease: potentially dose-dependent, divergent effects by drug class. Mov Disord 2012;27(9):1118-1124.

[79] Trenkwalder C, Arnulf I. Principles and Practice of Sleep Medicine. In: Kryger MH, Roth T, Dement WC, editors. Parkinsonism. 5th ed. St. Louis: Saunders; 2010. p. 980-992.

[80] De Cock VC, Vidailhet M, Arnulf I. Sleep disturbances in patients with parkinsonism. Nat Clin Pract Neurol 2008;4(5):254-266.

[81] Schenck CH, Bundlie SR, Ettinger MG, Mahowald MW. Chronic behavioral disorders of human REM sleep: a new category of parasomnia. Sleep 1986;9(2):293-308.

[82] Postuma RB, Gagnon JF, Montplaisir JY. REM Sleep Behavior Disorder and Prodromal Neurodegeneration - Where Are We Headed? Tremor Other Hyperkinet Mov (N Y) 2013;3.

[83] Schenck CH, Bundlie SR, Mahowald MW. Delayed emergence of a parkinsonian disorder in 38% of 29 older men initially diagnosed with idiopathic rapid eye movement sleep behaviour disorder. Neurology 1996;46(2):388-393.

[84] Postuma RB, Gagnon JF, Vendette M, Fantini ML, Massicotte-Marquez J, Montplaisir J. Quantifying the risk of neurodegenerative disease in idiopathic REM sleep behavior disorder. Neurology 2009;72(15):1296-1300.

[85] Boeve BF, Silber MH, Ferman TJ, Lin SC, Benarroch EE, Schmeichel AM, et al. Clinicopathologic correlations in 172 cases of rapid eye movement sleep behavior disorder with or without a coexisting neurologic disorder. Sleep Med 2013;14(8):754-762.

[86] Gagnon JF, Vendette M, Postuma RB, Desjardins C, Massicotte-Marquez J, Panisset M, et al. Mild cognitive impairment in rapid eye movement sleep behavior disorder and Parkinson's disease. Ann Neurol 2009;66(1):39-47.

[87] Miyamoto T, Miyamoto M, Inoue Y, Usui Y, Suzuki K, Hirata K. Reduced cardiac 123I-MIBG scintigraphy in idiopathic REM sleep behavior disorder. Neurology 2006;67(12):2236-2238.

[88] Miyamoto T, Miyamoto M, Iwanami M, Hirata K. Olfactory dysfunction in Japanese patients with idiopathic REM sleep behavior disorder: comparison of data using the

university of Pennsylvania smell identification test and odor stick identification test for Japanese. Mov Disord 2010;25(10):1524-1526.

[89] Postuma RB, Gagnon JF, Vendette M, Montplaisir JY. Markers of neurodegeneration in idiopathic rapid eye movement sleep behaviour disorder and Parkinson's disease. Brain 2009;132(Pt 12):3298-3307.

[90] Iwanami M, Miyamoto T, Miyamoto M, Hirata K, Takada E. Relevance of substantia nigra hyperechogenicity and reduced odor identification in idiopathic REM sleep behavior disorder. Sleep Med 2010;11(4):361-365.

[91] Postuma RB, Gagnon JF, Rompre S, Montplaisir JY. Severity of REM atonia loss in idiopathic REM sleep behavior disorder predicts Parkinson disease. Neurology 2010;74(3):239-244.

[92] Miyamoto M, Miyamoto T. Neuroimaging of rapid eye movement sleep behavior disorder: transcranial ultrasound, single-photon emission computed tomography, and positron emission tomography scan data. Sleep Med 2013;14(8):739-743.

[93] Boissard R, Fort P, Gervasoni D, Barbagli B, Luppi PH. Localization of the GABAergic and non-GABAergic neurons projecting to the sublaterodorsal nucleus and potentially gating paradoxical sleep onset. Eur J Neurosci 2003;18(6):1627-1639.

[94] Sastre JP, Jouvet M. [Oneiric behavior in cats]. Physiol Behav 1979;22(5):979-989.

[95] Boeve BF. REM sleep behavior disorder: Updated review of the core features, the REM sleep behavior disorder-neurodegenerative disease association, evolving concepts, controversies, and future directions. Ann N Y Acad Sci 2010;1184:15-54.

[96] Garcia-Lorenzo D, Longo-Dos Santos C, Ewenczyk C, Leu-Semenescu S, Gallea C, Quattrocchi G, et al. The coeruleus/subcoeruleus complex in rapid eye movement sleep behaviour disorders in Parkinson's disease. Brain 2013;136(Pt 7):2120-2129.

[97] Postuma RB, Gagnon JF, Vendette M, Charland K, Montplaisir J. Manifestations of Parkinson disease differ in association with REM sleep behavior disorder. Mov Disord 2008;23(12):1665-1672.

[98] Postuma RB, Gagnon JF, Vendette M, Charland K, Montplaisir J. REM sleep behaviour disorder in Parkinson's disease is associated with specific motor features. J Neurol Neurosurg Psychiatry 2008;79(10):1117-1121.

[99] Miyamoto T, Miyamoto M, Iwanami M, Hirata K. Cardiac 123I-MIBG accumulation in Parkinson's disease differs in association with REM sleep behavior disorder. Parkinsonism Relat Disord 2011;17(3):219-220.

[100] Nomura T, Inoue Y, Hogl B, Uemura Y, Kitayama M, Abe T, et al. Relationship between (123)I-MIBG scintigrams and REM sleep behavior disorder in Parkinson's disease. Parkinsonism Relat Disord 2010;16(10):683-685.

[101] Postuma RB, Bertrand JA, Montplaisir J, Desjardins C, Vendette M, Rios Romenets S, et al. Rapid eye movement sleep behavior disorder and risk of dementia in Parkinson's disease: a prospective study. Mov Disord 2012;27(6):720-726.

[102] Nomura T, Inoue Y, Kagimura T, Nakashima K. Clinical significance of REM sleep behavior disorder in Parkinson's disease. Sleep Med 2013;14(2):131-135.

[103] Sixel-Döring F, Trautmann E, Mollenhauer B, Trenkwalder C. Associated factors for REM sleep behavior disorder in Parkinson disease. Neurology 2011;77(11):1048-1054.

[104] Bugalho P, da Silva JA, Neto B. Clinical features associated with REM sleep behavior disorder symptoms in the early stages of Parkinson's disease. J Neurol 2011;258(1): 50-55.

[105] Alves G, Larsen JP, Emre M, Wentzel-Larsen T, Aarsland D. Changes in motor subtype and risk for incident dementia in Parkinson's disease. Mov Disord 2006;21(8): 1123-1130.

[106] Miyamoto T, Miyamoto M, Iwanami M, Kobayashi M, Nakamura M, Inoue Y, et al. The REM sleep behavior disorder screening questionnaire: validation study of a Japanese version. Sleep Med 2009;10(10):1151-1154.

[107] Suzuki K, Miyamoto T, Miyamoto M, Watanabe Y, Suzuki S, Tatsumoto M, et al. Probable rapid eye movement sleep behavior disorder, nocturnal disturbances and quality of life in patients with Parkinson's disease: a case-controlled study using the rapid eye movement sleep behavior disorder screening questionnaire. BMC Neurol 2013;13:18.

[108] Plomhause L, Dujardin K, Duhamel A, Delliaux M, Derambure P, Defebvre L, et al. Rapid eye movement sleep behavior disorder in treatment-naive Parkinson disease patients. Sleep Med 2013.

[109] De Cock VC, Vidailhet M, Leu S, Texeira A, Apartis E, Elbaz A, et al. Restoration of normal motor control in Parkinson's disease during REM sleep. Brain 2007;130(Pt 2): 450-456.

[110] Schenck CH, Mahowald MW, Kim SW, O'Connor KA, Hurwitz TD. Prominent eye movements during NREM sleep and REM sleep behavior disorder associated with fluoxetine treatment of depression and obsessive-compulsive disorder. Sleep 1992;15(3):226-235.

[111] Boeve BF, Silber MH, Ferman TJ. Melatonin for treatment of REM sleep behavior disorder in neurologic disorders: results in 14 patients. Sleep Med 2003;4(4):281-284.

[112] Kunz D, Bes F. Melatonin effects in a patient with severe REM sleep behavior disorder: case report and theoretical considerations. Neuropsychobiology 1997;36(4): 211-214.

[113] Shinno H, Kamei M, Nakamura Y, Inami Y, Horiguchi J. Successful treatment with Yi-Gan San for rapid eye movement sleep behavior disorder. Prog Neuropsycho-pharmacol Biol Psychiatry 2008;32(7):1749-1751.

[114] Clemens S, Rye D, Hochman S. Restless legs syndrome: revisiting the dopamine hypothesis from the spinal cord perspective. Neurology 2006;67(1):125-130.

[115] Bara-Jimenez W, Aksu M, Graham B, Sato S, Hallett M. Periodic limb movements in sleep: state-dependent excitability of the spinal flexor reflex. Neurology 2000;54(8): 1609-1616.

[116] Tergau F, Wischer S, Paulus W. Motor system excitability in patients with restless legs syndrome. Neurology 1999;52(5):1060-1063.

[117] Tyvaert L, Houdayer E, Devanne H, Bourriez JL, Derambure P, Monaca C. Cortical involvement in the sensory and motor symptoms of primary restless legs syndrome. Sleep Med 2009;10(10):1090-1096.

[118] Iranzo A, Comella CL, Santamaria J, Oertel W. Restless legs syndrome in Parkinson's disease and other neurodegenerative diseases of the central nervous system. Mov Disord 2007;22 Suppl 18:S424-430.

[119] Möller JC, Unger M, Stiasny-Kolster K, Oertel WH. Restless Legs Syndrome (RLS) and Parkinson's disease (PD)-related disorders or different entities? J Neurol Sci 2010;289(1-2):135-137.

[120] Earley CJ, Kuwabara H, Wong DF, Gamaldo C, Salas R, Brasic J, et al. The dopamine transporter is decreased in the striatum of subjects with restless legs syndrome. Sleep 2011;34(3):341-347.

[121] Trenkwalder C, Walters AS, Hening WA, Chokroverty S, Antonini A, Dhawan V, et al. Positron emission tomographic studies in restless legs syndrome. Mov Disord 1999;14(1):141-145.

[122] Connor JR, Wang XS, Allen RP, Beard JL, Wiesinger JA, Felt BT, et al. Altered dopaminergic profile in the putamen and substantia nigra in restless leg syndrome. Brain 2009;132(Pt 9):2403-2412.

[123] Earley CJ, Connor JR, Beard JL, Malecki EA, Epstein DK, Allen RP. Abnormalities in CSF concentrations of ferritin and transferrin in restless legs syndrome. Neurology 2000;54(8):1698-1700.

[124] Mizuno S, Mihara T, Miyaoka T, Inagaki T, Horiguchi J. CSF iron, ferritin and transferrin levels in restless legs syndrome. J Sleep Res 2005;14(1):43-47.

[125] Allen RP, Barker PB, Wehrl F, Song HK, Earley CJ. MRI measurement of brain iron in patients with restless legs syndrome. Neurology 2001;56(2):263-265.

[126] Schmidauer C, Sojer M, Seppi K, Stockner H, Hogl B, Biedermann B, et al. Transcranial ultrasound shows nigral hypoechogenicity in restless legs syndrome. Ann Neurol 2005;58(4):630-634.

[127] Kwon DY, Seo WK, Yoon HK, Park MH, Koh SB, Park KW. Transcranial brain sonography in Parkinson's disease with restless legs syndrome. Mov Disord 2010;25(10): 1373-1378.

[128] Gjerstad MD, Tysnes OB, Larsen JP. Increased risk of leg motor restlessness but not RLS in early Parkinson disease. Neurology 2011;77(22):1941-1946.

[129] Poewe W, Högl B. Akathisia, restless legs and periodic limb movements in sleep in Parkinson's disease. Neurology 2004;63(8 Suppl 3):S12-16.

[130] Chaudhuri KR, Healy DG, Schapira AH, National Institute for Clinical E. Non-motor symptoms of Parkinson's disease: diagnosis and management. Lancet Neurol 2006;5(3):235-245.

[131] Ondo WG, Vuong KD, Jankovic J. Exploring the relationship between Parkinson disease and restless legs syndrome. Arch Neurol 2002;59(3):421-424.

[132] Lee JE, Shin HW, Kim KS, Sohn YH. Factors contributing to the development of restless legs syndrome in patients with Parkinson disease. Mov Disord 2009;24(4): 579-582.

[133] Shimohata T, Nishizawa M. Sleep disturbance in patients with Parkinson's disease presenting with leg motor restlessness. Parkinsonism Relat Disord 2013;19(5): 571-572.

[134] Trotti LM, Bliwise DL. No increased risk of obstructive sleep apnea in Parkinson's disease. Mov Disord 2010;25(13):2246-2249.

[135] Suzuki K, Miyamoto M, Miyamoto T, Suzuki S, Watanabe Y, Numao A, et al. Snoring is associated with an impaired motor function, disease severity and the quality of life but not with excessive daytime sleepiness in patients with Parkinson's disease. Intern Med 2013;52(8):863-869.

Current Use of Thalamic Vim Stimulation in Treating Parkinson's Disease

Naoki Tani, Ryoma Morigaki, Ryuji Kaji and
Satoshi Goto

1. Introduction

Recent advances in neuroimaging and neurosurgical techniques provide a growing body of evidence suggesting that deep brain stimulation (DBS) is a powerful and safe therapeutic option for medically intractable Parkinson's disease (PD). For more than half a century, the thalamic ventrolateral (VL) nucleus has been an anatomical target for stereotaxy in treating movement disorders that include PD. It plays a pivotal role in the basal ganglia-thalamo-cortical circuit that is associated with motor brain functions. The entire output of the basal ganglia is directed to the motor cortex via the VL nucleus where the cerebellar and pallidal afferents terminate predominantly in the ventralis intermedius (Vim) nucleus and ventralis oralis (Vo) nucleus, respectively. In accordance with the general concept that the cerebellothalamic fiber connections participate in tremor genesis, thalamic Vim DBS is now used in the treatment of a wide variety of tremor subtypes with different etiologies. Indeed, thalamic Vim DBS can exert a striking therapeutic impact on tremor-dominant PD that exhibits better clinical prognoses and slower disease progression with less cognitive decline as compared to akinesia/rigidity-dominant PD. In patients with tremor-dominant PD, tremor suppression can be achieved irrespective of age, disease duration, or baseline disease severity. Based on recent advances in the understanding of the pathophysiology of tremor-dominant PD, this review introduces the current use of thalamic Vim stimulation in treating patients with PD.

2. Surgical anatomy

The thalamic VL nucleus comprises 2 major functional territories [1-3]. Neurons in the VL thalamus that respond to voluntary movements are located largely within the Vo [4-6], and neurons that respond to kinesthetic/passive movements about a joint are mainly contained within the Vim [5, 7]. The pallidothalamic inhibitory afferents terminate preferentially in the ipsilateral Vo nucleus, with an anterior-to-posterior gradient of terminal densities through the VL nucleus. In contrast, the cerebellothalamic excitatory afferents terminate predominantly in the contralateral Vim nucleus, creating a posterior-to-anterior gradient of terminal densities through the VL nucleus [8-10]. Moreover, a somatotopic arrangement, i.e., a medial-to-lateral distribution of facial-, forelimb-, and hindlimb-receptive fields, also exists in the VL thalamic nucleus [11-14].

The cerebellothalamic pathway plays a role in the fine spatial and temporal tuning of coordinated movements, as well as in the learning and retention of new motor skills. Thus, functional interference might also be achieved in deep cerebellar nuclei and affect activities in the striatum and cerebral cortices via the VL nucleus, thereby affecting ongoing and intended movements [15-17].

3. Pathophysiology of parkinsonian tremor

The clinical heterogeneity of PD is well recognized, and patients can often be divided into tremor-dominant and akinesia/rigidity-dominant subgroups. Accumulating evidence suggests that akinesia/rigidity and tremor may be associated with functional impairments of different motor circuits. Striatal dopamine depletion and dysfunction of the basal ganglia seem to be more important in akinesia/rigidity than in tremor. It is generally thought that tremor is primarily related to the cerebello-thalamo-cortical pathway, while akinesia/rigidity is rooted in the basal ganglia-thalamo-cortical pathway. Recent results from clinicopathological, electrophysiological, and neuroimaging studies on patients with PD are discussed in the following sections.

3.1. Clinicopathological study

Although post-mortem studies are limited, patients with tremor-dominant PD appear to progress slowly despite a poorer therapeutic response to levodopa. A statistical analysis performed using the Unified Parkinson's Disease Rating Scale (UPDRS) showed that the motor score for tremor is independent of the scores for other motor symptoms in patients with PD [18]. Rajput et al. [19] reported that patients with tremor-dominant PD showed slower disease progression and lower incidence of dementia than did patients with akinesia/rigidity-dominant PD.

Patients with tremor-dominant PD have milder cell loss in the substantia nigra pars compacta and in the locus coeruleus than do patients with non-tremor PD [20]. This suggests that patients with tremor-dominant PD have less dopaminergic dysfunction than do patients with non-tremor PD. On the other hand, patients with tremor-dominant PD have considerably more cell loss in the retrorubral area of the midbrain [21]. The retrorubral area could produce tremor via its dopaminergic projection to the pallidum. Further, Selikhova et al. [22] reported that patients with the non-tremor subtype had more severe cortical Lewy body pathology and were more likely to develop dementia.

3.2. Positron emission tomography (PET) and single photon emission computed tomography (SPECT)

SPECT using Iodine-123 fluoropropyl-carbomethoxy-3 ([123I]FP-CIT SPECT) targets the dopamine transporter and is used to determine ongoing loss of dopaminergic neurons in patients with PD [23-25]. [123I]FP-CIT SPECT shows that patients with tremor-dominant PD had less striatal dopamine depletion than do patients with non-tremor PD [26-28].

The metabolic rate of glucose measured using (18F)fluoro-2-deoxy-D-glucose PET (FDG-PET) is known as a marker of integrated local synaptic activities and is sensitive to direct neuronal and synaptic damage and to the functional changes in synaptic activity distant from the primary site of pathology [29]. Using FDG-PET, Mure et al. [30] identified and validated that the PD tremor-related pattern is characterized by covarying metabolic increases in the cerebellum, motor cortex, and putamen. This network correlates specifically with clinical tremor ratings, but not with akinesia/rigidity. In patients with PD tremor, high-frequency stimulation of the Vim nucleus reduces regional metabolism and cerebral blood flow (CBF) in the ipsilateral sensorimotor cortex and contralateral dorsal cerebellar nucleus [30-33], and increases both measures in the Vim nucleus ipsilateral to the stimulation site [30, 34-37]. It should be noted that changes in CBF may not reflect the direct effects of DBS but rather may reflect sensory feedback from changes in motor activity [38].

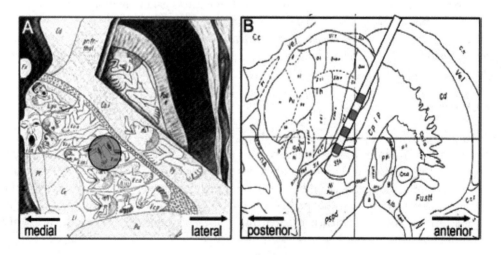

Figure 1. Schematic representations of the stereotactic targets for Vim-DBS on the axial (A) and sagittal (B) planes. The DBS lead implanted into the Vim nucleus is also shown in (B).

3.3. Functional magnetic resonance imaging (fMRI)

Intrinsic blood oxygen consumption detected by fMRI is correlated with low-frequency electrical amplitude fluctuations [64]. Patients with PD show increased overall activity in networks coupled to the primary motor cortex and cerebellum, and reduced functional connections in the supplementary motor area, dorsolateral prefrontal area, and putamen [65]. A recent study with simultaneous fMRI and EMG recording shows that the basal ganglia are transiently activated at the onset of tremor episodes, whereas tremor amplitude-related activity correlates with the cerebello-thalamo-cortical circuit [26]. The patients with tremor-dominant PD had increased functional connectivity between the basal ganglia and the cerebello-thalamo-cortical circuit.

3.4. Magnetoencephalography (MEG)

PD symptoms are related to alterations of oscillatory activity within the basal ganglia. Such pathologically increased oscillations have been demonstrated at several frequencies [56, 57]. In particular, those below 70 Hz have been shown to be antikinetic [56]. More specifically, oscillations at 4 to 12 Hz have been related to the origin of tremor symptoms in patients with PD [58]. Double tremor oscillations in the β range are not coherent with simultaneously recorded tremors [59-61]. However, a strong coherence in the β range is observed in the primary motor cortex, supplementary motor cortex, premotor cortex, diencephalon, and contralateral cerebellum [58]. Interestingly, this coupling can be successfully reduced by dopamine replacement therapy [62, 63]. These data indicate that PD resting tremor is associated with synchronous oscillatory coupling in a cerebello-thalamo-cortical loop and cortical motor and sensory areas contralateral to the tremor hand [58].

3.5. Cell recordings

So-called "kinesthetic" cells receive afferent inputs from muscle spindles and respond to passive joint movements. These cells are located just anterior to the nucleus ventralis caudalis (VC), which receives tactile sensory inputs [39, 40]. Percheron et al. [8] postulated that the kinesthetic zone is located in the latero-ventral part of the Vim nucleus, a region that sends a majority of its axons to the motor cortex. Vitek et al. [13] reported that in a monkey model of PD produced using 1-methyl-4 phenyl-1,2,3,6-tetrahydropyridine (MPTP), the kinesthetic zone expands anteriorly into regions that contain the active movement-related neurons. Kiss et al. [41] reported that in patients with tremor, there is an anterior expansion in the representation of the kinesthetic neurons without a change in their receptive field sizes. They suggested that tremor activates receptors responsive to deep sensations and, to a lesser degree, superficial sensations. Thus, repetitive tremor activities could result in a gradual increase in the synaptic efficacy of somatosensory inputs to kinesthetic neurons. Cells that respond to both somatosensory inputs and active movements are referred to as "combined" cells [42, 43] and have been identified only in patients with movement disorders.

Cells in the VL thalamic nucleus that demonstrate a discharge pattern with burst frequencies similar to that of tremor are called "tremor cells" [44, 45]. In a monkey model of resting tremor produced by a lesion of the ventral tegmentum, thalamic activity related to tremor frequency is unchanged following the interruption of sensory inputs [46, 47]. This finding has led to the hypothesis that the tremor cells may represent a central pacemaker for generating tremor, independent of sensory feedback [46, 48]. Tremor cells are reportedly located in the Vim nucleus and Vo complex [43, 49, 50]. The distribution of tremor cells is important for thalamic surgery, because tremor has been successfully treated when the radiofrequency lesion was centered within the cluster of tremor cells [39, 51, 52]. However, recent studies show that tremor cells are widely distributed in the Vim, Vo, and VC nuclei, and that they show no apparent differences in proportion within each nucleus [50]. These findings suggest that the ideal surgical target might not be determined by microelectrode recordings of tremor cells alone [49, 53]. The number of tremor cells in patients with PD is much higher than that in patients with other movement disorders, such as essential tremor (ET) and multiple sclerosis. This may play a role in the better surgical outcomes seen in patients with PD [50]. Based on their experiences, Katayama et al. [53] postulated that tremor cells might play a predominant role in the lateral portion of the Vim nucleus, an area that provides the most significant control of PD-associated tremor, in accordance with previous reports [54, 55].

3.6. Local field potentials (LFPs)

DBS procedures enable intraoperative micro-/macrorecordings and postoperative macrore-cordings. Local field potentials (LFPs) can be recorded via macro- as well as microrecordings [66]. The oscillatory activity in the β frequency range has clinical relevance to movement disorders. It is widely distributed throughout the motor system and is desynchronized by voluntary movement in both the Vim and subthalamic nucleus (STN) [67-69]. Levodopa and high-frequency STN stimulation reduce β band LFP oscillations. This reduction positively correlates with an improvement of akinesia and rigidity, but not with a decrease of tremor [70-72], and the β range STN stimulation causes further impairment of movement in patients with PD [73-76]. The α range oscillations in patients with tremor-dominant PD show finely segregated muscle-specific subloops that strongly correlate with the tremor-affected muscles, and tremor suppression can be achieved using STN-DBS in areas with pronounced α oscilla-tions [77, 78]. Given that basal ganglia β oscillation correlates with rigidity and akinesia and α oscillation correlates with tremor, these findings further suggest a differential pathophysi-ology between akinesia-rigidity and tremor.

In summary, the pathophysiological studies on parkinsonian tremor indicate that resting tremor may result from a pathological interaction between the basal ganglia and the cerebello-thalamo-cortical circuit. Tremor generation in the cerebello-thalamo-cortical circuit is likely triggered by activity in the basal ganglia.

4. Thalamic Vim DBS

4.1. Surgical procedures

The Vim DBS procedure is divided into the following five stages: (i) stereotactic imaging; (ii) thalamic mapping; (iii) electrode implantation; (iv) receiver of pulse generator implantation; and (v) programming. We perform the two successive steps of the procedure in the same operative session. The first step involves fixation of the stereotactic frame, stereotactic imaging, and placement of the thalamic electrode after application of local anesthesia. In the second step, the thalamic electrode is connected to the pulse generator while the patient is under general anesthesia. The intercommissural line-based coordinates for the tentative target in the thalamic Vim are determined 12 mm lateral to the midline, 5 mm anterior to the posterior commissure, and on the intercommissural line. In the operating room, a precoronal burr hole is placed 3 cm lateral to the midline, and a guiding cannula is inserted stereotactically. A quadripolar DBS electrode (Model 3387; Medtronic) is advanced directly through the guiding cannula. The characteristics of the tremor are assessed before, during, and immediately after the insertion of the electrode. Improvement of tremor at the time of insertion of the lead (the "microthalamotomy-like effect") is considered to indicate good positioning of the electrode. Thresholds for both intrinsic and extrinsic evoked responses are analyzed directly via the implanted electrode with a screening device (Model 3625; Medtronic). When a satisfactory electrode position has been achieved, the stylet of the lead and the guiding cannula are carefully removed. The lead is fixed to the cranium with the burr hole ring and cap. General anesthesia is induced while the stereotactic head frame is removed. The pulse generator is implanted in a subcutaneous infraclavicular pouch after being connected to the DBS electrode with a subcutaneous extension wire. In most patients, an Activa SC implantable pulse generator (Medtronic) is used.

The pulse generator can be programmed immediately after surgery. If a prolonged microthalamotomy-like effect is present, the pulse generator is programmed at the time of reappearance of the tremor. Routine postoperative CT scans are performed to rule out hemorrhage. Patients are instructed on how to switch their device on and off using a handheld magnet, and told to turn their device off at night when possible to maximize battery life. Some teams do not connect the pulse generator immediately and use this period to repeat some external stimulation to confirm that the stimulation improves tremor without side effects. This period can also be used to perform a brain MRI to check the electrode location and possible lesion. Many radiologists prefer this to be done before pulse generator implantation for safety reasons.

4.2. Programming challenges

The optimal stimulating parameters are determined using monopolar or bipolar stimulation. The easiest way to screen the parameters is to study each contact one after the other: the contact studied is programmed as the cathode, and the case is programmed as the anode. For example, first a constant pulse width of 90 µs and a constant frequency of 160 Hz are selected. Then the voltage is progressively increased to find the threshold for symptom suppression without adverse effects, using the contact(s) that gives the best effect. Best results are usually obtained at a pulse frequency of 130–185 Hz (no lower than 100 Hz), pulse width of 60–90 µs, and amplitude of 1.5–3.6 V.

If this screening does not reveal parameters to control tremor, other combinations can be tried. The pulse width and frequency can be increased. Stimulating more than one contact at the same time and using bipolar stimulation can also be tried. Bipolar stimulation is particularly useful if limiting side effects are obtained with a low voltage before reaching the threshold to stop tremor. If these measures are still not helpful, the position of the electrode can be checked using MRI or CT, and re-implantation can be discussed if necessary.

4.3. Mechanism of action

Similarities in the effectiveness of thalamic DBS and thalamotomy have led investigators to suggest that DBS acts as a reversible lesion of the thalamus, but the mechanism of action of thalamic DBS is yet unclear. With respect to tremor suppression, 4 different hypotheses of Vim DBS have been proposed: (1) conduction block—this hypothesis is supported by the fact that Vim thalamotomy has similar effects to Vim DBS [83]; (2) activation of inhibitory axon terminals that synapse onto and inhibit projection neurons [93]; (3) superimposition of continuous stimuli onto rhythmically oscillating subcortical-cortical loops [94]; and (4) inhibition of neuronal activity near the stimulation site while activating axonal elements that leave the target structure [95]. Recent reports have shown that during high-frequency stimulation, glutamate and adenosine are increased [96-99], and this elevated glutamate release could excite local interneurons, thereby increasing the production of inhibitory neurotransmitters (e.g., GABA and glycine) and resulting in a decrease in the firing rates of projection neurons [99].

4.4. Therapeutic impacts

Before the levodopa era, severe tremor was a main indication for surgery [79]. In the 1960s, thousands of patients with PD throughout the world received a thalamotomy [80] or other procedures such as pallidotomy, campotomy, or pedunculotomy [81]. During this period, it was observed that the high-frequency stimulation used for targeting during lesioning of the thalamus significantly reduced tremor [82]. In the 1980s, Benabid et al. demonstrated that DBS of the Vim significantly reduced tremor, and they have treated more than 100 patients with thalamic DBS [83-85]. Several studies have demonstrated that DBS of the thalamus has comparable control of tremor with fewer side effects than does thalamotomy. Vim DBS is highly beneficial for tremor control, but ineffective for the other disabling features of PD, including akinesia, rigidity, and gait and postural disturbances. Benabid et al. [85] showed that chronic Vim stimulation is highly effective for tremor in a group of 117 tremor patients; over 85% of patients had a very good or excellent response with little or no tremor evident in the contralateral arm. With a double-blind multicenter study to assess the efficacy of unilateral Vim DBS against placebo, Koller et al. [86] have shown an 80% reduction in contralateral arm tremor in 24 patients with PD tremor and 29 patients with ET with Vim DBS at the 1-year follow-up.

With respect to the long-term efficacy of Vim DBS, Schuurman et al. [87] reported that 88% of patients showed complete or nearly complete tremor suppression after a mean follow-up period of 5 years. Hariz et al. [88] reported 38 patients with PD who received Vim DBS with a follow-up period of 6 years. The long-term follow-up of Vim DBS revealed effective control of tremor 6 years postoperatively, while axial symptoms worsened. The initial improvement in activities of daily living (ADL) scores at the 1-year follow-up disappeared after 6 years. Hariz et al. [89] showed significant increases in stimulation parameters for up to 1 year; however, after the 1-year stimulation, the parameters seemed to stabilize. By contrast, Kumar et al. [90] reported that it was necessary to increase the current intensity over time to control tremor. This increase in amplitude is undesirable, as it often causes paresthesia and cerebellar adverse effects [83, 91]. During the follow-up, some tolerance (necessity to gradually increase the voltage to control tremor) and a rebound effect (tremor much worse than before when the stimulator is switched off) can develop [86, 89]. This affects an action tremor more frequently. Switching off the stimulator at night can sometimes limit the tolerance effect. Recurrence of tremor is seen in ~5% of patients several weeks or years after surgery [83, 92].

4.5. Adverse events

The stimulation-induced side effects of Vim DBS are reversible, and usually mild and acceptable. Incidences of stimulation-related complications reported at long-term (greater than 5 years) follow-up include paresthesia (4–38%), dysarthria (3–36%), dystonia/hypertonia (3–16%), gait disturbance (11–16%), balance disturbance (5%), and cognitive dysfunction (2%). Among these adverse effects, non-adjustable and long-lasting complications include dysarthria (10–27%), paresthesia (16%), gait disturbance (7%), dystonia (5%), upper limb ataxia (3–4%), and disequilibrium (3–4%) [88, 100, 101]. Pahwa et al. [101] described occurrences of persistent complications, including dysarthria, disequilibrium, and gait disturbance, after bilateral stimulation, even when the stimulus parameters were optimized.

The incidence of infection appears to be 0–11% during the early follow-up periods and 0–8% throughout the postoperative course [87, 88, 100]. Hardware failures are occasionally found in the stimulator (0–3%), the DBS lead (0–8%), or the cable (0–3%); skin erosion (0–4%) and hematoma requiring evacuation of the stimulator (0–3%) have also been reported [87, 88, 100].

5. Conclusions

Vim DBS is an appropriate first-line treatment for medically intractable tremor in patients with PD. Although its therapeutic effects on ADL outcome decreases gradually after the surgery, long-term tremor suppression remains stable. We suggest that Vim DBS is useful for patients with tremor-dominant PD, who manifest slow progression of disease and a good response of non-tremor PD symptoms to dopaminergic therapy.

Acknowledgements

This work was supported in part by the Grants from the Ministry of Education, Culture, Sports, Science and Technology of Japan (grant-in-aid for Scientific Research, 23500428; 21390269; 23659458; 24390223).

Author details

Naoki Tani[1], Ryoma Morigaki[2], Ryuji Kaji[3] and Satoshi Goto[2]

*Address all correspondence to: sgoto@clin.med.tokushima-u.ac.jp

1 Department of Neurosurgery, Otemae Hospital, Osaka, Japan

2 Department of Motor Neuroscience and Neurotherapeutics, Institute of Health Biosciences, Graduate School of Medical Sciences, University of Tokushima, Tokushima, Japan

3 Department of Clinical Neuroscience, Institute of Health Biosciences, Graduate School of
Medical Sciences, University of Tokushima, Tokushima, Japan

References

[1] Asanuma, C.; Thach, WT. & Jones EG. (1983). Distribution of cerebellar terminations
    and their relation to other afferent terminations in the ventral lateral thalamic region
    of the monkey. Brain Res. 286 (3): 237-265.

[2] Kultas-Ilinsky, K. & Ilinsky IA. (1991). Fine structure of the ventral lateral nucleus
    (VL) of the Macaca mulatta thalamus: cell types and synaptology. J Comp Neurol.
    314 (2): 319-349.

[3] Ilinsky, IA. & Kultas-Ilinsky, K. (2002). Motor thalamic circuits in primates with em-
    phasis on the area targeted in treatment of movement disorders. Mov Disord. 17
    (Suppl 3): S9-14.

[4] Hassler, R. Anatomy of the thalamus. In: Schaltenbrand G, Bailer, P., editor. An in-
    troduction to Stereotaxis With an Atlas of the Human Brain. Stuttgart: Thieme; 1959.
    p. 230-290.

[5] Krack, P.; Dostrovsky, J.; Ilinsky, I.; Kultas-Ilinsky, K.; Lenz, F.; Lozano, A. & Vitek, J.
    (2002). Surgery of the motor thalamus: problems with the present nomenclatures.
    Mov Disord. 17 (Suppl 3): S2-S8.

[6] Lenz, FA.; Jaeger, CJ.; Seike, MS.; Lin, YC. & Reich, SG. (2002). Single-neuron analysis
    of human thalamus in patients with intention tremor and other clinical signs of cere-
    bellar disease. J Neurophysiol. 87 (4): 2084-94.

[7] Ohye, C.; Maeda, T. & Narabayashi, H. (1976). Physiologically defined VIM nucleus.
    Its special reference to control of tremor. Appl Neurophysiol. 39 (3-4): 285-295.

[8] Percheron, G.; Francois, C.; Talbi, B.; Yelnik, J. & Fenelon, G. (1996). The primate mo-
    tor thalamus. Brain research Brain research reviews. 22 (2): 93-181.

[9]   Sakai, ST.; Inase, M. & Tanji, J. (1996). Comparison of cerebellothalamic and pallido-
      thalamic projections in the monkey (Macaca fuscata): a double anterograde labeling
      study. J Comp Neurol. 368 (2): 215-228.

[10] Gallay, MN.; Jeanmonod, D.; Liu, J. & Morel, A. (2008). Human pallidothalamic and
      cerebellothalamic tracts: anatomical basis for functional stereotactic neurosurgery.
      Brain Struct Funct. 212 (6): 443-463.

[11] Strick, PL. (1976). Activity of ventrolateral thalamic neurons during arm movement.
      Journal of neurophysiology. 39 (5): 1032-1044.

[12] Asanuma, C.; Thach, WR.; & Jones, EG. (1983). Anatomical evidence for segregated
      focal groupings of efferent cells and their terminal ramifications in the cerebellothala-
      mic pathway of the monkey. Brain Res. 286 (3): 267-297.

[13] Vitek, JL.; Ashe, J.; DeLong, MR. & Alexander, GE. (1994). Physiologic properties and
      somatotopic organization of the primate motor thalamus. J Neurophysiol. 71 (4):
      1498-1513.

[14] Vitek, JL.; Ashe, J,; DeLong, MR. & Kaneoke, Y. (1996). Microstimulation of primate
      motor thalamus: somatotopic organization and differential distribution of evoked
      motor responses among subnuclei. J Neurophysiol. 75(6): 2486-95.

[15] Rispal-Padel, L.; Harnois, C. & Troiani, D. (1987). Converging cerebellofugal inputs
      to the thalamus. I. Mapping of monosynaptic field potentials in the ventrolateral nu-
      cleus of the thalamus. Exp Brain Res. 68 (1): 47-58.

[16] Rispal-Padel, L.; Troiani, D. & Harnois, C. (1987). Converging cerebellofugal inputs
      to the thalamus. II. Analysis and topography of thalamic EPSPs induced by conver-
      gent monosynaptic interpositus and dentate inputs. Exp Brain Res. 68 (1): 59-72.

[17] Craig, AD. (2008). Retrograde analyses of spinothalamic projections in the macaque
      monkey: input to the ventral lateral nucleus. J Comp Neurol. 508 (2): 315-328.

[18] Stochl, J.; Boomsma, A.; Ruzicka, E.; Brozova, H. & Blahus, P. (2008). On the structure
      of motor symptoms of Parkinson's disease. Mov Disord. 23 (9): 1307-1312.

[19] Rajput, AH.; Voll, A.; Rajput, ML.; Robinson, CA. & Rajput, A. (2009). Course in Par-
      kinson disease subtypes: A 39-year clinicopathologic study. Neurology. 73 (3):
      206-212.

[20] Paulus, W. & Jellinger, K. (1991). The neuropathologic basis of different clinical sub-
      groups of Parkinson's disease. J Neuropathol Exp Neurol. 50 (6): 743-755.

[21] Hirsch, EC.; Mouatt, A.; Faucheux, B.; Bonnet, AM.; Javoy-Agid, F.; Graybiel, AM. &
      Agid, Y. (1992). Dopamine, tremor, and Parkinson's disease. Lancet. 340 (8811):
      125-126.

[22] Selikhova, M.; Williams, DR.; Kempster, PA.; Holton, JL.; Revesz, T. & Lees, AJ. (2009). A clinico-pathological study of subtypes in Parkinson's disease. Brain. 132 (Pt 11): 2947-2957.

[23] Kaufman, MJ. & Madras, BK. (1991). Severe depletion of cocaine recognition sites associated with the dopamine transporter in Parkinson's-diseased striatum. Synapse. 9 (1): 43-49.

[24] Niznik, HB.; Fogel, EF.; Fassos, FF. & Seeman, P. (1991). The dopamine transporter is absent in parkinsonian putamen and reduced in the caudate nucleus. J Neurochem. 56 (1): 192-198.

[25] Seibyl, JP.; Marek, K.; Sheff, K.; Zoghbi, S.; Baldwin, RM.; Charney, DS., van Dyck, CH. & Innis, RB. (1998). Iodine-123-beta-CIT and iodine-123-FPCIT SPECT measurement of dopamine transporters in healthy subjects and Parkinson's patients. J Nucl Med. 39 (9): 1500-1508.

[26] Helmich, RC.; Janssen, MJ.; Oyen, WJ.; Bloem, BR. & Toni, I. (2011). Pallidal dysfunction drives a cerebellothalamic circuit into Parkinson tremor. Ann Neurol. 69 (2): 269-281.

[27] Rossi C, Frosini D, Volterrani D, De Feo P, Unti E, Nicoletti V, et al. Differences in nigro-striatal impairment in clinical variants of early Parkinson's disease: evidence from a FP-CIT SPECT study. European journal of neurology : the official journal of the European Federation of Neurological Societies. 2010; 17(4): 626-30.

[28] Spiegel J, Hellwig D, Samnick S, Jost W, Mollers MO, Fassbender K, Kirsch, CM. & Dillmann, U. (2007). Striatal FP-CIT uptake differs in the subtypes of early Parkinson's disease. J Neural Transm. 114 (3): 331-335.

[29] Magistretti, PJ.; Pellerin, L.; Rothman, DL. & Shulman, RG. (1999). Energy on demand. Science. 283 (5401): 496-497.

[30] Mure, H.; Hirano, S.; Tang, CC.; Isaias, IU.; Antonini, A.; Ma, Y.; Dhawan, V. & Eidelberg, D. (2011). Parkinson's disease tremor-related metabolic network: characterization, progression, and treatment effects. Neuroimage. 54 (2): 1244-1253.

[31] Parker, F.; Tzourio, N.; Blond, S.; Petit, H. & Mazoyer, B. (1992). Evidence for a common network of brain structures involved in parkinsonian tremor and voluntary repetitive movement. Brain Res. 584 (1-2): 11-17.

[32] Boecker, H.; Wills, AJ.; Ceballos-Baumann, A.; Samuel, M.; Thomas, DG.; Marsden, CD. & Brooks, DJ. (1997). Stereotactic thalamotomy in tremor-dominant Parkinson's disease: an H2(15)O PET motor activation study. Ann Neurol. 41 (1): 108-111.

[33] Wielepp, JP.; Burgunder, JM.; Pohle, T.; Ritter, EP.; Kinser, JA. & Krauss, JK. (2001). Deactivation of thalamocortical activity is responsible for suppression of parkinsonian tremor by thalamic stimulation: a 99mTc-ECD SPECT study. Clin Neurol Neurosurg. 103 (4): 228-231.

[34] Rezai, AR.; Lozano, AM.; Crawley, AP.; Joy, ML.; Davis, KD.; Kwan, CL.; Dostrovsky, JO.; Tasker, RR. & Mikulis, DJ. (1999). Thalamic stimulation and functional magnetic resonance imaging: localization of cortical and subcortical activation with implanted electrodes. J Neurosurg. 90 (3): 583-590.

[35] Perlmutter, JS.; Mink, JW.; Bastian, AJ.; Zackowski, K.; Hershey, T.; Miyawaki, E.; Koller, W. & Videen, TO. (2002). Blood flow responses to deep brain stimulation of thalamus. Neurology. 58 (9): 1388-1394.

[36] Haslinger, B.; Boecker, H.; Buchel, C.; Vesper, J.; Tronnier, VM.; Pfister, R.; Alesch, F.; Moringlane, JR.; Krauss, JK.; Conrad, B.; Schwaiger, M. & Ceballos-Baumann, AO. (2003). Differential modulation of subcortical target and cortex during deep brain stimulation. Neuroimage. 18 (2): 517-524.

[37] Fukuda M, Barnes A, Simon ES, Holmes A, Dhawan V, Giladi N, Fodstad H, Ma Y, Eidelberg D. (2004). Thalamic stimulation for parkinsonian tremor: correlation between regional cerebral blood flow and physiological tremor characteristics. Neuroimage. 21 (2): 608-615.

[38] Perlmutter, JS. & Mink, JW. (2006). Deep brain stimulation. Ann Rev Neurosci. 29: 229-257.

[39] Ohye, C. & Narabayashi, H. (1979). Physiological study of presumed ventralis intermedius neurons in the human thalamus. J Neurosurg. 50 (3): 290-297.

[40] Ohye, C.; Shibazaki, T.; Hirai, T.; Wada, H.; Hirato, M. & Kawashima, Y. (1989). Further physiological observations on the ventralis intermedius neurons in the human thalamus. J Neurophysiol. 61 (3): 488-500.

[41] Kiss, ZH.; Davis, KD.; Tasker, RR.; Lozano, AM.; Hu, B. & Dostrovsky, JO. (2003). Kinaesthetic neurons in thalamus of humans with and without tremor. Exp Brain Res. 150 (1): 85-94.

[42] Lenz, FA.; Kwan, HC.; Dostrovsky, JO.; Tasker, RR.; Murphy, JT. & Lenz, YE. (1990). Single unit analysis of the human ventral thalamic nuclear group. Activity correlated with movement. Brain. 113 (Pt 6): 1795-1821.

[43] Lenz, FA.; Kwan, HC.; Martin, RL.; Tasker, RR.; Dostrovsky, JO. & Lenz, YE. (1994). Single unit analysis of the human ventral thalamic nuclear group. Tremor-related activity in functionally identified cells. Brain. 117 (Pt 3): 531-543.

[44] Lenz, FA.; Tasker, RR.; Kwan, HC.; Schnider, S.; Kwong, R.; Murayama, Y.; Dostrovsky, JO. & Murphy, JT. (1988). Single unit analysis of the human ventral thalamic nuclear group: correlation of thalamic "tremor cells" with the 3-6 Hz component of parkinsonian tremor. J Neurosci. 8 (3): 754-764.

[45] Ohye, C.; Saito, U.; Fukamachi, A. & Narabayashi, H. (1974). An analysis of the spontaneous rhythmic and non-rhythmic burst discharges in the human thalamus. J Neurol Sci. 22 (2): 245-259.

[46] Lamarre, Y. & Joffroy, A. Experimental tremor in monkey: activity of thalamic and precentral cortical neurons in the absence of peripheral feedback. In: Poirier LJ, Sourkes TI, Bedard P, editors. Adcances in Neurology. New York: Raven Press; 1979. p. 109-122.

[47] Ohye, C.; Bouchard, R.; Larochelle, L.; Bedard, P.; Boucher, R.; Raphy, B. & Poirier, LJ. (1970). Effect of dorsal rhizotomy on postural tremor in the monkey. Exp Brain Res. 10 (2): 140-150.

[48] Lee, RG. & Stein, RB. (1981). Resetting of tremor by mechanical perturbations: a comparison of essential tremor and parkinsonian tremor. Ann Neurol. 10 (6): 523-531.

[49] Kobayashi, K.; Katayama, Y.; Kasai, M.; Oshima, H.; Fukaya, C. & Yamamoto, T. (2003). Localization of thalamic cells with tremor-frequency activity in Parkinson's disease and essential tremor. Acta Neurochir. 87 (Suppl): 137-139.

[50] Brodkey, JA.; Tasker, RR.; Hamani, C.; McAndrews, MP.; Dostrovsky, JO. & Lozano, AM. (2004). Tremor cells in the human thalamus: differences among neurological disorders. J Neurosurg. 101 (1): 43-47.

[51] Hirai, T.; Shibazaki, T.; Nakajima, H.; Imai, S. & Ohye, C. (1979). Minimal effective lesion in the stereotactic treatment of tremor. Appl Neurophysiol. 42 (5): 307-308.

[52] Nagaseki, Y.; Shibazaki, T.; Hirai, T.; Kawashima, Y.; Hirato, M.; Wada, H.; Wada, H.; Miyazaki, M. & Ohye, C. (1986). Long-term follow-up results of selective VIM-thalamotomy. J Neurosurg. 65 (3): 296-302.

[53] Katayama, Y.; Kano, T.; Kobayashi, K.; Oshima, H.; Fukaya, C. & Yamamoto, T. (2005). Difference in surgical strategies between thalamotomy and thalamic deep brain stimulation for tremor control. Journal of neurology. 252 (Suppl 4): IV17-IV22.

[54] Hariz, MI. & Hirabayashi, H. (1997). Is there a relationship between size and site of the stereotactic lesion and symptomatic results of pallidotomy and thalamotomy? Stereotact Funct Neurosurg. 69 (1-4 Pt 2): 28-45.

[55] Atkinson, JD.; Collins, DL.; Bertrand, G.; Peters, TM.; Pike, GB. & Sadikot, AF. (2002). Optimal location of thalamotomy lesions for tremor associated with Parkinson disease: a probabilistic analysis based on postoperative magnetic resonance imaging and an integrated digital atlas. J Neurosurg. 96 (5): 854-866.

[56] Schnitzler, A. & Gross, J. (2005). Normal and pathological oscillatory communication in the brain. Nat Rev Neurosci. 6 (4): 285-296.

[57] Hutchison, WD.; Dostrovsky, JO.; Walters, JR.; Courtemanche, R.; Boraud, T.; Goldberg, J. & Brown, P. (2004). Neuronal oscillations in the basal ganglia and movement disorders: evidence from whole animal and human recordings. J Neurosci. 24 (42): 9240-9243.

[58] Timmermann, L.; Gross, J.; Dirks, M.; Volkmann, J.; Freund, HJ. & Schnitzler, A. (2003). The cerebral oscillatory network of parkinsonian resting tremor. Brain. 126 (Pt 1): 199-212.

[59] Raz, A.; Vaadia, E. & Bergman, H. (2000). Firing patterns and correlations of spontaneous discharge of pallidal neurons in the normal and the tremulous 1-methyl-4-phenyl-1,2,3,6-tetrahydropyridine vervet model of parkinsonism. J Neurosci. 20 (22): 8559-8571.

[60] Lemstra, AW.; Verhagen-Metman, L.; Lee, JI.; Dougherty, PM. & Lenz, FA. (1999). Tremor-frequency (3-6 Hz) activity in the sensorimotor arm representation of the internal segment of the globus pallidus in patients with Parkinson's disease. Neurosci Lett. 267 (2): 1291-32.

[61] Hurtado, JM.; Rubchinsky, LL.; Sigvardt, KA.; Wheelock, VL. & Pappas, CT. (2005). Temporal evolution of oscillations and synchrony in GPi/muscle pairs in Parkinson's disease. J Neurophysiol. 93 (3): 1569-1584.

[62] Salenius, S.; Avikainen, S.; Kaakkola, S.; Hari, R. & Brown, P. (2002). Defective cortical drive to muscle in Parkinson's disease and its improvement with levodopa. Brain. 125 (Pt 3): 491-500.

[63] Pollok, B.; Makhloufi, H.; Butz, M.; Gross, J.; Timmermann, L.; Wojtecki, L. & Schnitzler, A. (2009). Levodopa affects functional brain networks in Parkinsonian resting tremor. Mov Disord. 24 (1): 91-98.

[64] Logothetis, NK. & Wandell, BA. (2004). Interpreting the BOLD signal. Annu Rev Physiol. 66: 735-769.

[65] Wu, T.; Chan, P. & Hallett, M. (2010). Effective connectivity of neural networks in automatic movements in Parkinson's disease. Neuroimage. 49 (3): 2581-2587.

[66] Brown, P. (2003). Oscillatory nature of human basal ganglia activity: relationship to the pathophysiology of Parkinson's disease. Mov Disord. 18 (4): 357-363.

[67] Klostermann, F.; Nikulin, VV.; Kuhn, AA.; Marzinzik, F.; Wahl, M.; Pogosyan, A.; Kupsch, A.; Schneider, GH.; Brown, P. & Curio, G. (2007). Task-related differential dynamics of EEG alpha- and beta-band synchronization in cortico-basal motor structures. Eur J Neurosci. 25 (5): 1604-1615.

[68] Paradiso, G.; Cunic, D.; Saint-Cyr, JA.; Hoque, T.; Lozano, AM.; Lang, AE. & Chen, R. (2004). Involvement of human thalamus in the preparation of self-paced movement. Brain. 127 (Pt 12): 2717-2731.

[69] Kühn, AA.; Williams, D.; Kupsch, A.; Limousin, P.; Hariz, M.; Schneider, GH.; Yarrow, K. & Brown, P. (2004). Event-related beta desynchronization in human subthalamic nucleus correlates with motor performance. Brain. 127 (Pt 4): 735-746.

[70] Bronte-Stewart, H.; Barberini, C.; Koop, MM.; Hill, BC.; Henderson, JM. & Wingeier, B. (2009). The STN beta-band profile in Parkinson's disease is stationary and shows prolonged attenuation after deep brain stimulation. Exp Neurol. 215 (1): 20-28.

[71] Ray, NJ.; Jenkinson, N.; Wang, S.; Holland, P.; Brittain, JS.; Joint, C.; Stein, JF. & Aziz, T. (2008). Local field potential beta activity in the subthalamic nucleus of patients with Parkinson's disease is associated with improvements in bradykinesia after dopamine and deep brain stimulation. Exp Neurol. 213 (1): 108-113.

[72] Kühn, AA.; Kupsch, A.; Schneider, GH. & Brown, P. (2006). Reduction in subthalamic 8-35 Hz oscillatory activity correlates with clinical improvement in Parkinson's disease. Eur J Neurosci. 23 (7): 1956-1960.

[73] Brown, P.; Oliviero, A.; Mazzone, P.; Insola, A.: Tonali, P. & Di Lazzaro, V. (2001). Dopamine dependency of oscillations between subthalamic nucleus and pallidum in Parkinson's disease. J Neurosci. 21 (3): 1033-1038.

[74] Fogelson, N.; Kuhn, AA.; Silberstein, P.; Limousin, PD.; Hariz, M.; Trottenberg, T.; Kupsch, A. & Brown, P. (2005). Frequency dependent effects of subthalamic nucleus stimulation in Parkinson's disease. Neurosci Lett. 382 (1-2): 5-9.

[75] Chen, CC.; Litvak, V.; Gilbertson, T.; Kuhn, A.; Lu, CS.; Lee, ST.; Tsai, CH.; Tisch, S.; Limousin, P.; Hariz, M. & Brown, P. (2007). Excessive synchronization of basal ganglia neurons at 20 Hz slows movement in Parkinson's disease. Exp Neurol. 205 (1): 214-221.

[76] Eusebio, A.; Chen, CC.; Lu, CS.; Lee, ST.; Tsai, CH.; Limousin, P.; Hariz, M. & Brown, P. (2008). Effects of low-frequency stimulation of the subthalamic nucleus on movement in Parkinson's disease. Exp Neurol. 209 (1): 125-130.

[77] Reck, C.; Florin, E.; Wojtecki, L.; Krause, H.; Groiss, S.; Voges, J.; Maarouf, M.; Sturm, V.; Schnitzler, A. & Timmermann, L. (2009). Characterisation of tremor-associated local field potentials in the subthalamic nucleus in Parkinson's disease. Eur J Neurosci. 29 (3): 599-612.

[78] Reck, C.; Himmel, M.; Florin, E.; Maarouf, M.; Sturm, V.; Wojtecki, L.; Schnitzler, A.; Fink, GR. & Timmermann, L. (2010). Coherence analysis of local field potentials in the subthalamic nucleus: differences in parkinsonian rest and postural tremor. Eur J Neurosci. 32 (7): 1202-1214.

[79] Gildenberg, PL. History of Movement Disorder Surgery. In: Lozano A, editor. Movement Disorder Surgery Prog Neurol Surg. Basel: Karger; 2000. p. 1-20.

[80] Kelly PJ. Stereotactic thalamotomies. In: Koller W, Pulson G, editors. Therapy of Parkinson's Disease. 2nd ed. New York: Mecel Dekker; 1995. p. 331-351.

[81] Guridi, J. & Lozano, AM. (1997). A brief history of pallidotomy. Neurosurgery. 41(5): 1169-80.

[82] Hassler, R.; Riechert, T.; Mundinger, F.; Umbach, W. & Ganglberger, JA. (1960). Phys-iological observations in stereotaxic operations in extrapyramidal motor disturban-ces. Brain. 83: 337-350.

[83] Benabid, AL.; Pollak, P.; Gao, D.; Hoffmann, D.; Limousin, P.; Gay, E.; Payen, I. & Be-nazzouz, A. (1996). Chronic electrical stimulation of the ventralis intermedius nu-cleus of the thalamus as a treatment of movement disorders. J Neurosurg. 84 (2): 203-214.

[84] Benabid, AL.; Pollak, P.; Gervason, C.; Hoffmann, D.; Gao, DM.; Hommel, M.; Perret, JE. & de Rougemont, J. (1991). Long-term suppression of tremor by chronic stimula-tion of the ventral intermediate thalamic nucleus. Lancet. 337 (8738): 403-406.

[85] Pollak, P.; Benabid, AL.; Limousin, P. & Benazzouz, A. (1997). Chronic intracerebral stimulation in Parkinson's disease. Adv Neurol. 74: 213-20.

[86] Koller, W.; Pahwa, R.; Busenbark, K.; Hubble, J.; Wilkinson, S.; Lang, A.; Tuite, P.; Sime, E.; Lozano, A.; Hauser, R.; Malapira, T.; Smith, D.; Tarsy, D.; Miyawaki, E.; Norregaard, T.; Kormos, T. & Olanow, CW. (1997). High-frequency unilateral thala-mic stimulation in the treatment of essential and parkinsonian tremor. Ann Neurol. 42 (3): 292-299.

[87] Schuurman, PR.; Bosch, DA.; Merkus, MP. & Speelman, JD. (2008). Long-term fol-low-up of thalamic stimulation versus thalamotomy for tremor suppression. Mov Disord. 23 (8): 1146-1153.

[88] Hariz, MI.; Krack, P.; Alesch, F.; Augustinsson, LE.; Bosch, A.; Ekberg, L.; Johansson, F.; Johnels, B.; Meyerson, BA.; N'Guyen, JP.; Pinter, M.; Pollak, P.; von Raison, F.; Re-hncrona, S.; Speelman, JD.; Sydow, O. & Benabid, AL. (2008). Multicentre European study of thalamic stimulation for parkinsonian tremor: a 6 year follow-up. J Neurol Neurosurg Psychiatry. 79 (6): 694-699.

[89] Hariz, MI.; Shamsgovara, P.; Johansson, F.; Hariz, G. & Fodstad, H. (1999). Tolerance and tremor rebound following long-term chronic thalamic stimulation for Parkinso-nian and essential tremor. Stereotact Funct Neurosurg. 72 (2-4): 208-218.

[90] Kumar, K.; Kelly, M. & Toth, C. (1999). Deep brain stimulation of the ventral inter-mediate nucleus of the thalamus for control of tremors in Parkinson's disease and es-sential tremor. Stereotact Funct Neurosurg. 72 (1): 47-61.

[91] Yamamoto, T.; Katayama, Y.; Kano, T.; Kobayashi, K.; Oshima, H. & Fukaya, C. (2004). Deep brain stimulation for the treatment of parkinsonian, essential, and post-stroke tremor: a suitable stimulation method and changes in effective stimulation in-tensity. J Neurosurg. 101 (2): 201-209.

[92] Tasker, RR. (1998). Deep brain stimulation is preferable to thalamotomy for tremor suppression. Surg Neurol. 49 (2): 145-153.

[93]   Wu, YR.; Levy, R.; Ashby, P.; Tasker, RR. & Dostrovsky, JO. (2001). Does stimulation of the GPi control dyskinesia by activating inhibitory axons? Mov Disord. 16 (2): 208-216.

[94]   Montgomery, EBJr. & Baker, KB. (2000). Mechanisms of deep brain stimulation and future technical developments. Neurol Res. ogical research. 22 (3): 259-266.

[95]   Vitek, JL. (2002). Mechanisms of deep brain stimulation: excitation or inhibition. Mov Disord. 17 (Suppl 3): S69-S72.

[96]   Anderson, TR.; Hu, B.; Iremonger, K. & Kiss, ZH. (2006). Selective attenuation of afferent synaptic transmission as a mechanism of thalamic deep brain stimulation-induced tremor arrest. J Neurosci. 26 (3): 841-850.

[97]   Anderson, T.; Hu, B.; Pittman, Q. & Kiss, ZH. (2004). Mechanisms of deep brain stimulation: an intracellular study in rat thalamus. J Physiol. 559 (Pt 1): 301-313.

[98]   Bekar, L.; Libionka, W.; Tian, GF.; Xu, Q.; Torres, A.; Wang, X.; Lovatt, D.; Williams, E.; Takano, T.; Schnermann, J.; Bakos, R. & Nedergaard, M. (2008). Adenosine is crucial for deep brain stimulation-mediated attenuation of tremor. Nat Med. 14 (1): 75-80.

[99]   Tawfik, VL.; Chang, SY.; Hitti, FL.; Roberts, DW.; Leiter, JC.; Jovanovic, S. & Lee, KH. (2010). Deep brain stimulation results in local glutamate and adenosine release: investigation into the role of astrocytes. Neurosurgery. 67 (2): 367-375.

[100] Rehncrona, S.; Johnels, B.; Widner, H.; Tornqvist, AL.; Hariz, M. & Sydow, O. (2003). Long-term efficacy of thalamic deep brain stimulation for tremor: double-blind assessments. Mov Disord. 18 (2): 163-170.

[101] Pahwa, R.; Lyons, KE.; Wilkinson, SB.; Simpson, RKJr.; Ondo, WG.; Tarsy, D.; Norregaard, T.; Hubble, JP.; Smith, DA.; Hauser, RA. & Jankovic J. (2006). Long-term evaluation of deep brain stimulation of the thalamus. J Neurosurg. 104 (4): 506-512.   ·

7

Deep Brain Stimulation for Camptocormia Associated with Parkinson's Disease

Naoki Tani, Ryuji Kaji and Satoshi Goto

1. Introduction

Camptocormia, which is also known as bent spine syndrome, is characterized by abnormal posture of the trunk with marked forward flexion of the thoracolumbar spine, which increases during standing and walking and abates in the recumbent position (Azher & Jankovic, 2005). Camptocormia is a disabling symptom that occurs during the course of Parkinson's disease (PD), but the optimized medical and surgical therapy for PD-associated camptocormia remains to be established (Finsterer & Strobl, 2010; Doherty et al., 2011). PD-associated camptocormia is generally thought to be unresponsive to levodopa (Azher & Jankovic, 2005). In most patients with PD, the extreme anterior bending is not or poorly improved, or even worsened, in response to levodopa administration, and the severity of the bent spine is often unchanged during the medication-on and -off phases (Melamed & Djaldetti, 2006), although an exceptional case has been reported (Ho et al., 2007). Although some reports have shown that deep brain stimulation (DBS) in the subthalamic nucleus (STN) (Hellmann et al., 2006; Yamada et al., 2006; Sako et al., 2009; Umemura et al., 2010; Capelle et al., 2011; Asahi et al., 2011) and globus pallidus internus (GPi) (Micheli et al., 2005; Capelle et al., 2011; Thani et al., 2011) is effective in treating camptocormia, the overall efficacy of DBS in relieving PD-associated camptocormia has not been determined. This review introduces the use of DBS in the treatment of medically refractory camptocormia in patients with PD.

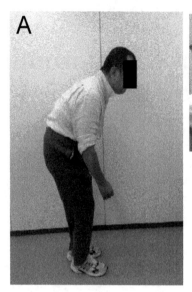
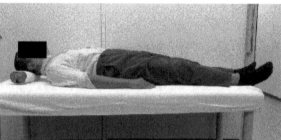

Figure 1. A patient having PD-associated camptocormia in the standing (A) and recumbent (B) positions.

2. Definition and diagnosis

Camptocormia was first described by Earle (1815) and Brodie (1818). Camptocormia, which is also referred to as "bent spine syndrome", was initially considered, especially in war times, to be a psychogenic disorder and a conversion reaction to war stress (Karbowski, 1999). Camptocormia is associated with various etiologies, including parkinsonian syndromes, dystonia, vascular lenticular lesions, and muscular and rheumatologic disorders. It was first described in association with PD by Djaldetti et al. (1999).

The term camptocormia is now used to describe marked forward flexion of the thoracolumbar spine that varies between 30 and 90 degrees, presents in a sitting position and typically increases during walking, and completely disappears in the recumbent position, but there are no criteria with a clear consensus for diagnosing camptocormia. Most of the diagnoses are made by subjectively assessing the patient's posture. Diagnosing camptocormia in PD patients is based on clinical examination alone. Nevertheless, some specific findings might suggest alternative diagnoses. For example, weakness of the truncal extension suggests concomitant myopathy or anterior horn cell disease. In addition, camptocormia can occur in other parkinsonian syndromes, such as multisystem atrophy, progressive supranuclear palsy, or corticobasal degeneration. Patients with psychogenic disorders sometimes develop movement disorders due to conversion syndromes or malingering. Bent spine that is due to simple kyphosis that is associated with degenerative vertebral spinal changes is easily ruled out, as this phenomenon remains largely unchanged when the patient is in the recumbent position.

3. Epidemiology

Among the 16 patients with camptocormia that have been described by Azher & Jankovic 2005, the most frequent etiology is PD. The reported prevalence of camptocormia in PD varies widely. Four studies have described the prevalence rates of camptocormia in patients with PD as being between 3% and 6-17% (Ashour & Jankovic, 2006; Lepoutre et al., 2006; Tiple et al., 2009; Abe et al., 2010). This wide range probably reflects the different thresholds that have been used for diagnosing camptocormia, the lack of a clear definition, and the different populations that have been studied. Most epidemiological studies show a positive association between camptocormia and disease severity (Ashour & Jankovic, 2006; Bloch et al., 2006; Tiple et al., 2009; Margraf et al., 2010), the male gender, older age, longer disease duration, prominent axial involvement, motor fluctuations, and autonomic symptoms (Lepoutre et al., 2006). In addition, camptocormia is associated with a high prevalence of lumbar or thoracolumbar scoliosis (in 61% of the patients) and mild to moderate low-back pain (in 77% of the patients). On average, camptocormia presents 7–8 years after the onset of parkinsonism in PD (Azher & Jankovic, Djaldetti et al., 1999; Bloch et al., 2006; Lepoutre et al., 2006; Margraf et al., 2010; Spuler et al., 2010).

4. Clinical features

Camptocormia occurs mostly in patients with PD in more advanced stages of disease progression, but, in a few cases, it appears even in the early stage (Melamed & Djaldetti, 2006). In some patients, the onset is subacute with the development of significant flexion over days to months (Lepoutre et al., 2006: Margraf et al., 2010; Spuler et al., 2010). In the majority of patients with camptocormia, the initial symptoms of PD are bradykinesia and rigidity and, less frequently, tremor. In almost all patients, the initial signs and symptoms are predominantly asymmetrical (Melamed & Djaldetti, 2006). The truncal forward flexion is more prominent when standing (see Fig. 1A) and walking, but complete straightening of the back in the recumbent position (see Fig. 1B). Normally, the strength in the abdominal and paravertebral muscles is normal. Some patients can, upon external command or strong self-will, straighten themselves up, but only for very short periods and at the expense of severe fatigue (Melamed & Djaldetti, 2006). In quite a number of cases, camptocormia is associated with lower back pain (Bloch et al., 2006; Lepoutre et al., 2006; Margraf et al., 2010), but, in others, it is painless (Melamed & Djaldetti, 2006). Some patients report a feeling of being pulled forward or a sensation of tightening in their abdomen (Azher & Jankovic, 2005). If the deformity is long established with secondary fixed changes, patients might complain of breathlessness due to restricted lung capacity or of difficulty lying flat in bed due to hip or knee contractures; the latter can be accompanied by skin irritation in the flexed segment (Bloch et al., 2006). Neuro-logical examination often reveals marked axial rigidity (Bloch et al., 2006; Lepoutre et al., 2006). The strength of the trunk and hip extension are normal unless testing is precluded by fixed posture or pain (Lepoutre et al., 2006). The paraspinal muscles can have a wooden consistency, and the rectus abdominis often feels tense (Azher & Jankovic, 2005). There might be compensatory hyperextension of the neck in order to obtain a normal visual field. There is often mixed deformity, with deviation also in the coronal plane.

5. Pathogenesis of camptocormia in PD

The pathophysiology of the axial postural abnormalities in PD is not well understood, and it seems to be heterogeneous. However, two possible causes for the camptocormia genesis in patients with PD have been proposed: dystonia and myopathy.

5.1. Dystonia

Axial or action dystonia is considered a possible etiology of camptocormia in patients with PD (Ponfick et al., 2011). The first report on camptocormia in PD patients has suggested that bent spine might represent an action dystonia resulting from dysfunction of the striatum (Djaldetti et al., 1999). Sławek et al. (2003) have described a PD patient who showed painful camptocor-mia that improved markedly after an unilateral pallidotomy, and the findings that DBS has a beneficial effect on camptocormia support a dystonic etiology (Micheli et al., 2005; Thani et al., 2011). Another study on camptocormia that was associated with lenticular lesions has also reported the critical role of the striatum and pallidum in the maintenance of axial posture (Nieves et al., 2001). Thus, it is possible that PD-associated camptocormia may serve as an axial dystonia, a result of dysfunction of the basal ganglia controlling the reticulospinal pathway that projects to the axial muscles (Djaldetti et al., 1999; Nieves et al., 2001; Azher & Jankovic, 2005; Bloch et al., 2006; Melamed & Djaldetti, 2006).

5.2. Myopathy

Recent studies have shown detailed evidence for camptocormia that is caused by a myopathy of the paraspinal muscles. Gdynia et al. (2009) have investigated paraspinal muscle biopsies in 19 patients with PD who presented with camptocormia or dropped head syndrome. Thirteen patients showed myopathic changes in electromyography recordings, and magnetic resonance imaging showed slight fatty degeneration of the erector spine musculature in three patients. Histopathological analyses of the patients with PD have demonstrated a wide spectrum of abnormalities in the skeletal muscles of those with camptocormia and dropped head syn-drome. Spuler et al. (2010) have examined 17 patients, 13 of whom had a myopathic pattern in electromyographic recordings. The authors found apparently folded proteins in the muscle biopsies, suggesting the possibility of a myopathy that was induced by an accumulation of aggregated proteins. Margraf et al. (2010) have examined 15 patients with PD and camptocormia with electromyography, muscle magnetic resonance imaging, and biopsy of the paravertebral muscles. They showed increased levels of creatine kinase in 9/15 patients, myogenic electromyographic changes in 8/15 patients, and myopathic changes in the muscle biopsies in 12/15 patients. They claimed that the cause of camptocormia in idiopathic PD is a focal myopathy and that the myopathy has a progressive course, resulting in degeneration of the paravertebral muscles.

6. Treatment

6.1. Pharmacotherapy

In the majority of cases with advanced PD, camptocormia is thought to be unresponsive to levodopa (Azher & Jankovic, 2005; Margraf et al., 2010). Depending on the investigated cohort, up to 20% of the patients with PD and camptocormia profit from levodopa therapy (Bloch et al., 2006). The adjustment of dopaminergic therapy by carbidopa-levodopa and entacapone has been shown to result in improvements in camptocormia. Fujimoto (2006) has described the deterioration of camptocormia in patients who were treated with dopamine agonists, thus suggesting that the withdrawal of these agents might lead to an improvement of camptocormia in some cases. The poor responses to these medical agents can be explained by the fact that, when postural abnormalities and postural instabilities appear, patients are already at an advanced stage of the disease with severe axial symptoms, and all of their symptoms are known to respond poorly to levodopa, suggesting the involvement of non-dopaminergic pathways (Campbell et al., 2003). Furthermore, postural reactions that support surface perturbations are resistant to dopaminergic therapy (Carpenter et al., 2004).

In patients who seem to have a predominantly dystonic element, another treatment option might be botulinum toxin injections in the rectus abdominis muscles (Azher & Jankovic, 2005; Jankovic, 2009; Bonanni et al., 2007; Lenoir et al., 2010). Azher and Jankovic (2005) have found this to be successful in selected patients, but few have reproduced their positive results.

6.2. Spinal surgery

Spinal surgery has been used to attenuate postural abnormalities in patients with camptocormia associated with PD, whereas it has significant complications, and often requires revision surgery (Babat et al., 2004; Peek et al., 2009; Koller et al., 2010; Wadia et al., 2011).

6.3. DBS

Stereotactic neurosurgery of the basal ganglia is a therapeutic alternative for patients with advanced PD. As DBS of the STN or GPi produces a significant improvement in the motor symptoms in patients with severe PD, it also can be effective in treating camptocormia associated with PD (see Table 1.).

DBS target	author/year	No of patients	age	duration of PD (years)	Improvement	follow up (months)
STN	Azher and JanKovic (2005)	1	n.a.	n.a.	0/1	n.a.
	Hellman et al. (2006)	1	53	25	1/1	10
	Yamada et al. (2006)	1	71	11	1/1	20
	Sako et al. (2009)	6	53-71	5-11	6/6	5-46
	Capelle et al (2010)	2	73/65	12/15	1/2	12-16
	Umemura et al. (2010)	8	59-79	8-20	6/8	12
	Upadhyaya et al (2010)	1	59	n.a.	0/1	2
	Asahi et al. (2011)	4	60-69	7-13	3/4	40
	Lyons et al. (2012)	1	63	19	1/1	3
GPi	Micheli et al. (2005)	1	62	10	1/1	14
	Upadhyaya et al. (2010)	1	59	n.a.	0/1	15
	Capelle et al. (2010)	1	64	10	1/1	36
	Thani et al. (2011)	1	57	13	1/1	14

n.a. = not applicable

Table 1. DBS for camptocormia: literature review

6.3.1. STN-DBS

STN-DBS is thought to be superior to GPi-DBS in improving the cardinal motor symptoms of PD and in reducing the dosage of dopaminergic medications in PD patients (Moro et al., 1999; Deep-Brain Stimulation for Parkinson's Disease Study Group, 2001; Krack et al., 2003). As far as we are aware, 25 patients in 9 reports have been reported as having undergone STN-DBS for PD with camptocormia, and 19 of the patients (76%) showed improvements of the camptocormia. Sako et al. (2009) have described 6 PD patients with severe camptocormia who underwent bilateral STN-DBS. In this series, improvements of the camptocormia were reported in all of the patients after STN-DBS (see Fig. 2). Improvement was defined as a change in the thoracolumbar angle that was sustained for a mean follow-up period of 17 months. Umemura et al. (2010) and Capelle et al. (2011) have shown a positive effect of STN-DBS on PD-associated camptocormia, but not in all of the patients. In their studies, only the severity of the postural abnormality was shown to be related to improvements in the postural abnormalities after STN-DBS; moderate, rather than severe, postural abnormalities tended to improve after surgery (Umemura et al., 2010; Capelle et al., 2011). Asahi et al. (2011) have described 4 cases with advanced PD with camptocormia that were treated with STN-DBS, with improvements of the camptocormia in 3 patients but no improvement in one patient. In their computed tomography study, the single patient who did not show improvement of the camptocormia exhibited marked muscle atrophy and degeneration of the fatty tissue in her paraspinal muscle (Asahi et al., 2011). Thus, STN-DBS is a potential treatment for camptocormia in patients with PD, but the outcomes have varied from excellent improvement to only mild improvement or no benefit. Camptocormia usually does not respond to levodopa treatment and STN-DBS is thought to be effective mainly for the dopa-responsive PD symptoms. The mechanisms by which STN-DBS improves camptocormia in some patients and not in others remain unclear. As the recent reports that have shown the beneficial effects of STN-DBS in the treatment of primary dystonias (Kleiner-Fisman et al., 2007; Novak et al., 2008; Ostrem et al., 2011; Fonoff et al., 2012), axial posturing could be controlled by the STN as a function of the basal ganglia.

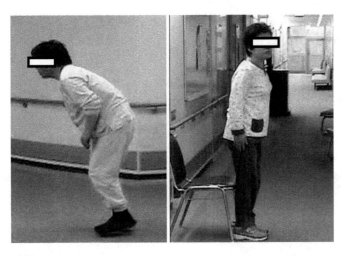

(A) Preoperative state; (B) Postoperative state

Figure 2. An impact of STN-DBS on camptocormia in a patient with PD.

6.3.2. GPi-DBS

The GPi is an alternative target that can be considered in the treatment of camptocormia. Previous research on patients with PD and camptocormia that was treated with GPi-DBS is limited to only four cases, with reports of no improvement in posture in one and improvement in posture in three (Micheli et al., 2005; Upadhyaya et al., 2010; Capelle et al., 2011; Thani et al., 2011). If camptocormia is considered a form of dystonia, then it is not surprising that high-frequency DBS of the GPi results in improvements because there is a large body of evidence of a dramatic effect of pallidal surgery on various forms of dystonia (for a review see Vidailhet et al., 2013). Micheli et al. (2005) have described a PD patient in whom bilateral GPi-DBS showed beneficial and sustained improvement of the PD symptoms and improvement of the camptocormia six months after surgery. In addition, Thani et al. (2011) have reported slow but steady improvement of camptocormia by six months, which was sustained at 14 months, after GPi-DBS in patients with PD. This progressive resolution of symptoms is reminiscent of the response that is expected in other forms of dystonia, with optimal improvement often requiring months.

7. Conclusion

Reports of success in controlling axial posturing in patients with camptocormia with both STN and GPi stimulation support the notion that the basal ganglia plays an important role in the maintenance of posture. Although both STN-DBS and GPi-DBS can be potential surgical means for treating camptocormia in patients with PD, further studies need to be performed in order to confirm this conclusion and to select PD patients with medically refractory camptocormia who are optimal candidates for STN or GPi DBS.

Acknowledgements

This work was supported in part by Grants from the Ministry of Education, Culture, Sports, Science and Technology of Japan (grant-in-aid for Scientific Research, 23500428; 21390269; 2365945800; 24390223).

Author details

Naoki Tani[1], Ryuji Kaji[2] and Satoshi Goto[3]

*Address all correspondence to: sgoto@clin.med.tokushima-u.ac.jp

1 Department of Neurosurgery, Otemae Hospital, Osaka, Japan

2 Department of Clinical Neuroscience, Institute of Health Biosciences, Graduate School of Medical Sciences, University of Tokushima, Tokushima, Japan

3 Department of Motor Neuroscience and Neurotherapeutics, Institute of Health Biosciences, G raduate School of Medical Sciences, University of Tokushima, Tokushima, Japan

References

[1] Abe, K..; Uchida, Y. & Notani M. (2010). Camptocormia in Parkinson's disease. Parkinson's Dis. 2010 Jun 30;2010. pii: 267640. doi: 10.4061/2010/267640

[2] Asahi, T.; Taguchi, Y.; Hayashi, N.; Hamada, H.; Dougu, N.; Takashima, S.; Tanaka, K. & Endo, S. (2011). Bilateral subthalamic deep brain stimulation for camptocormia associated with Parkinson's disease. Stereotact Funct Neurosurg. 89 (3): 173-177.

[3]   Ashour, R. & Jankovic, J. (2006). Joint and skeletal deformities in Parkinson's disease, multiple system atrophy, and progressive supranuclear palsy. Mov Disord. 21(11): 1856-1863.

[4]   Azher, SN. & Jankovic, J. Camptocormia: pathogenesis, classification, and response to therapy. (2005). Neurology. 65 (3): 355-359.

[5]   Babat, LB.; McLain, RF.; Bingaman, W.; Kalfas, I.; Young P. & Rufo-Smith C. (2004). Spinal surgery in patients with Parkinson's disease: construct failure and progressive deformity. Spine 29(18): 2006-12.

[6]   Bloch, F.; Houeto, JL.; Tezenas du Montcel, S.; Bonneville, F.; Etchepare F.; Welter, ML.; Rivaud-Pechoux, S.; Hahn-Barma, V.; Maisonobe, T.; Behar, C.; Lazennec, JY.; Kurys, E.; Arnulf, I.; Bonnet, AM. & Agid, Y. (2006). Parkinson's disease with camptocormia. J Neurol Neurosurg Psychiatry. 77(11): 1223-1228.

[7]   Bonanni, L.; Thomas, A.; Varanese, S.; Scorrano, V. & Onofrj, M. (2007).. Botulinum toxin treatment of lateral axial dystonia in Parkinsonism. Mov Disord. 22 (14): 2097-2103.

[8]   Bonneville, F.; Bloch, F.; Kurys, E.; du Montcel, ST.; Welter, ML.; Bonnet, AM.; Agid, Y.; Dormont, D. & Houeto, JL. (2008). Camptocormia and Parkinson's disease: MR imaging. Eur Radiol. 18 (8): 1710-1719.

[9]   Brodie BC. Pathological and surgical obsercations on diseases of the joints. London: Longman; 1818.

[10] Campbell, F.; Ashburn, A.; Thomas, P. & Amar, K. (2003). An exploratory study of the consistency of balance control and the mobility of people with Parkinson's disease (PD) between medication doses. Clin Rehabilitation. 17 (3): 318-324.

[11] Capelle, HH.; Schrader, C.; Blahak, C.; Fogel, W.; Kinfe, TM.; Baezner, H. & Krauss, JK. (2011). Deep brain stimulation for camptocormia in dystonia and Parkinson's disease. J Neurol. 258 (1): 96-103.

[12] Carpenter, MG.; Allum, JH.; Honegger, F.; Adkin, AL. & Bloem, BR. (2004). Postural abnormalities to multidirectional stance perturbations in Parkinson's disease. J Neurol Neurosurg Psychiatry. 75 (9): 1245-1254.

[13] Deep-Brain Stimulation for Parkinson's Disease Study Group. (2001). Deep-brain stimulation of the subthalamic nucleus or the pars interna of the globus pallidus in Parkinson's disease. N Engl J Med. 345 (13): 956-63.

[14] Djaldetti, R.; Mosberg-Galili, R.; Sroka, H.; Merims, D. & Melamed, E. (1999). Camptocormia (bent spine) in patients with Parkinson's disease--characterization and possible pathogenesis of an unusual phenomenon. Mov Disord. 14 (3): 443-447.

[15] Doherty, KM.; van de Warrenburg, BP.; Peralta, MC.; Silveira-Moriyama, L.; Azulay, JP.; Gershanik, OS. & Bloem, BR. (2011). Postural deformities in Parkinson's disease. Lancet Neurol. 10 (6): 538-49.

[16] Earle, H. Reply to the review of Mr. Bayton's essay on the cure of crooked spine. Edinburg Med Surg J. 1815; 11: 35-51.

[17] Finsterer, J. & Strobl, W. Presentation, etiology, diagnosis, and management of camptocormia. Eur Neurol . 2010; 64(1): 1-8.

[18] Fonoff, ET.; Campos, WK.; Mandel, M.; Alho, EJL. & Teixeira, MJ. (2012). Bilateral subthalamic nucleus stimulation for generalized dystonia after bilateral pallidotomy. Mov Disord. 27 (12):1559-1563.

[19] Fujimoto, K. (2006). Dropped head in Parkinson's disease. J Neurol. 253 (Suppl 7): VII21-26.

[20] Gdynia, HJ.; Sperfeld, AD.; Unrath, A.; Ludolph, AC.; Sabolek, M.; Storch, A. & Kassubek, J. (2009). Histopathological analysis of skeletal muscle in patients with Parkinson's disease and 'dropped head'/'bent spine' syndrome. Parkinsonism Relat Disord. 15 (9): 633-639.

[21] Gerton, BK.; Theeler, B. & Samii, A. Backpack treatment for camptocormia. (2010). Mov Disord. 25 (2): 247-248.

[22] Hellmann, MA.; Djaldetti, R.; Israel, Z. & Melamed, E. (2006). Effect of deep brain subthalamic stimulation on camptocormia and postural abnormalities in idiopathic Parkinson's disease. Mov Disord. 21 (11): 2008-2010.

[23] Ho, B.; Prakash, R.; Morgan, JC. & Sethi, KD. (2007). A case of levodopa-responsive camptocormia associated with advanced Parkinson's disease. Nat Clin Pract Neurol. 3 (9): 526-530.

[24] Jankovic, J. (2009). Disease-oriented approach to botulinum toxin use. Toxicon. 54 (5): 614-623.

[25] Karbowski, K. (1999). The old and the new camptocormia. Spine. 24 (14): 1494-1498.

[26] Kleiner-Fisman, G.; Liang, GS.; Moberg, PJ.; Ruocco, AC.; Hurtig, HI.; Baltuch, GH.; Jaggi, JL. & Stern, MB. (2007). Subthalamic nucleus deep brain stimulation for severe idiopathic dystonia: impact on severity, neuropsychological status, and quality of life. J Neurosurg. 107 (1): 29-36.

[27] Koller, H.; Acosta, F.; Zenner, J.; Ferraris, L.; Hitzl, W.; Meier, O.; Ondra, S.; Koski, T. & Schmidt, R. (2010). Spinal surgery in patients with Parkinson's disease: experiences with the challenges posed by sagittal imbalance and the Parkinson's spine. Eur Spine J. 19 (10): 1785-1794.

[28] Krack, P.; Batir, A.; Van Blercom, N.; Chabardes, S.; Fraix, V.; Ardouin, C.; Koudsie, A.; Limousin, PD.; Benazzouz, A.; LeBas, JF.; Benabid, AL. & Pollak, P. (2003). Five-

year follow-up of bilateral stimulation of the subthalamic nucleus in advanced Parkinson's disease. N Eng J Med. 349 (20): 1925-1934.

[29] Lenoir, T.; Guedj, N.; Boulu, P.; Guigui, P. & Benoist, M. Camptocormia: the bent spine syndrome, an update.(2010). Eur Spine J. 19 (8): 1229-1237.

[30] Lepoutre, AC.; Devos, D.; Blanchard-Dauphin, A.; Pardessus, V.; Maurage, CA.; Ferriby, D.; Hurtevent, JF.; Cotton, A.; Destée, A. & Defebvre L. (2006). A specific clinical pattern of camptocormia in Parkinson's disease. J Neurol Neurosurg Psychiatry. 77 (11): 1229-1234.

[31] Lyons, MK.; Birch, BD.; Hillman, RA.; Boucher, OK. & Evidente, VG. (2010). Long-term follow-up of deep brain stimulation for Meige syndrome. Neurosurg focus. 29 (2): E5.

[32] Lyons, M.; Boucher, O.; Patel, N.; Birch, B. & Evidente, V. (2012). Long-term benefit of bilateral subthalamic deep brain stimulation on camptocormia in Parkinson's disease. Turkish Neurosurg. 22 (4): 489-492.

[33] Margraf, NG.; Wrede, A.; Rohr, A.; Schulz-Schaeffer, WJ.; Raethjen, J.; Eymess, A.; Volkmann, J.; Mehdorn, MH.; Jansen, O. & Deuschl, G. (2010). Camptocormia in idiopathic Parkinson's disease: a focal myopathy of the paravertebral muscles. Mov Disord 25 (5): 542-551.

[34] Melamed, E. & Djaldetti, R. Camptocormia in Parkinson's disease. (2006). J Neurol. 253 (Suppl 7): VII14-16.

[35] Micheli, F.; Cersosimo, MG. & Piedimonte, F. (2005). Camptocormia in a patient with Parkinson disease: beneficial effects of pallidal deep brain stimulation. Case report. J Neurosurg. 103 (6): 1081-1083.

[36] Moro, E.; Scerrati, M.; Romito, LM.; Roselli, R.; Tonali, P. & Albanese, A. (1999). Chronic subthalamic nucleus stimulation reduces medication requirements in Parkinson's disease. Neurology. 53 (1): 85-90.

[37] Nieves, AV.; Miyasaki, JM. & Lang, AE. (2001). Acute onset dystonic camptocormia caused by lenticular lesions. Mov Disord. 16 (1): 177-180.

[38] Novak, KE.; Nenonene, EK.; Bernstein, LP.; Vergenz, S.; Cozzens, JW. & Rezak, M. (2008). Successful bilateral subthakamic nucleus stimulation for segmental dystonia after unilateral pallidotomy. Stereotact Funct Neurosurg. 86 (2):80-86.

[39] Ostrem, J L.; Racine, CA.; Glass, GA.; Grace, JK.; Volz, MM.; Heath, SL. & Starr PA. (2011). Subthalamic nucleus deep brain stimulation in primary cervical dystonia. Neurology. 76 (10): 870-878.

[40] Peek, AC.; Quinn, N.; Casey, AT. & Etherington, G. (2009). Thoracolumbar spinal fixation for camptocormia in Parkinson's disease. J Neurol Neurosurg Psychiatry. 80 (11): 1275-1278.

[41] Ponfick, M.; Gdynia, HJ.; Ludolph, AC. & Kassubek, J. (2011). Camptocormia in Par-
      kinson's disease: a review of the literature. Neurodegenerative Dis. 8 (5): 283-288.

[42] Sako, W.; Nishio, M.; Maruo, T.; Shimazu, H.; Matsuzaki, K.; Tamura, T.; Mure, H.;
      Ushio, Y.; Nagahiro, S.; Kaji, R. & Goto, S. (2009). Subthalamic nucleus deep brain
      stimulation for camptocormia associated with Parkinson's disease. Mov Disord. 24
      (7): 1076-1079.

[43] Slawek, J.; Derejko, M. & Lass P. (2003). Camptocormia as a form of dystonia in Par-
      kinson's disease. Eur J Neurol. 10 (1): 107-108.

[44] Spuler, S.; Krug, H.; Klein, C.; Medialdea, IC.; Jakob, W.; Ebersbach, G.; Gruber, D;
      Hoffmann, KT.; Trottenberg, T. & Kupsch, A. (2010). Myopathy causing camptocor-
      mia in idiopathic Parkinson's disease: a multidisciplinary approach. Mov Disord. 25
      (5): 552-559.

[45] Thani, NB.; Bala, A.; Kimber, TE. & Lind CR. (2011). High-frequency pallidal stimula-
      tion for camptocormia in Parkinson disease: case report. Neurosurgery. 68 (5): E1501-
      E1505.

[46] Tiple, D.; Fabbrini, G.; Colosimo, C.; Ottaviani, D.; Camerota, F.; Defazio, G. & Berar-
      delli, A. (2009). Camptocormia in Parkinson disease: an epidemiological and clinical
      study. J Neurol Neurosurg Psychiatry. 80 (2): 145-148.

[47] Umemura, A.; Oka, Y.; Ohkita, K.; Yamawaki, T. & Yamada, K. (2010). Effect of sub-
      thalamic deep brain stimulation on postural abnormality in Parkinson disease. J Neu-
      rosurg. 112 (6): 1283-1288.

[48] Upadhyaya, CD.; Starr, PA. & Mummaneni, PV. (2010). Spinal deformity and Parkin-
      son disease: a treatment algorithm. Neurosurg Focus. 28 (3): E5.

[49] Vidailhet, M.; Jutras, M-F.; Grabli, D. & Rose, E. (2013). Deep brain stimulation for
      dystonia. J Neurol Neurosurg Psychiatry. 84: 1029-1042.

[50] von Coelln, R.; Raible, A.; Gasser, T. & Asmus, F. (2008). Ultrasound-guided injection
      of the iliopsoas muscle with botulinum toxin in camptocormia. Mov Disord. 23 (6):
      889-892.

[51] Wadia, PM.; Tan, G.; Munhoz, RP.; Fox, SH.; Lewis, SJ. & Lang, AE. (2011). Surgical
      correction of kyphosis in patients with camptocormia due to Parkinson's disease: a
      retrospective evaluation. J Neurol Neurosurg Psychiatry. 82 (4): 364-368.

[52] Yamada, K.; Goto, S.; Matsuzaki, K.; Tamura, T.; Murase, N.; Shimazu, H.; Nagahiro,
      S.; Kuratsu, J. & Kaji, R. (2006). Alleviation of camptocormia by bilateral subthalamic
      nucleus stimulation in a patient with Parkinson's disease. Parkinsonism Relat Disord.
      12 (6): 372-375.

8

Melatonin in Parkinson's Disease

Alessia Carocci, Maria Stefania Sinicropi,
Alessia Catalano, Graziantonio Lauria and
Giuseppe Genchi

1. Introduction

Parkinson's disease (PD) is characterized by the progressive depletion of pigmented neurons containing dopamine (DA) in the region known as substantia nigra pars compacta (SNpc) and by the presence of intraneuronal aggregates called Lewy bodies, which are enriched in filamentous α-synuclein and other proteins, that are often ubiquitinated before being destroyed [1]. The locus coeruleus, the dorsal motor nucleus, the autonomic nervous system and the cerebral cortex are additional neuronal fields and neurotransmitter systems involved in PD with consequent loss of noradrenergic, serotonergic and cholinergic neurons. These neuronal changes led to progressive non-motor symptoms like sleep abnormalities, depression and cognitive decline in the later stages of PD [2].

Currently, levodopa is widely prescribed for the treatment of PD. Although it is highly effective as a symptomatic treatment, levodopa is incapable of providing the long-term protection that is needed to impair the onset or progress of the disease [3]. In fact, in addition to a few specific mutations, oxidative stress and generation of free radicals from both mitochondrial impairment and DA metabolism play critical and important roles in PD etiology. Deficits in mitochondrial functions, oxidative and nitrosative stress, accumulation of aberrant and misfolded proteins, and ubiquitin-proteasome system dysfunction can represent the main molecular pathways that trigger the pathogenesis of sporadic and familiar forms of PD [4].

It is known that about 15% of PD patients has a family background of the disease and few specific mutations have been identified to be responsible for rare familial forms of the pathology: α-synuclein, parkin, UCH-L1, DJ-1, and PINK1 are genes found to be related to PD [5]. These genetic defects seem to affect a common molecular pathway related to the ubiquitin-proteasome system with exception of PINK1, which is related to mitochondrial metabolism [6].

Some, if not all, of these mutations are partially related to free-radical generation. High levels of free-radical, reactive oxygen species (ROS) and reactive nitrogen species (RNS) damage not only phospholipids and polyunsaturated fatty acids of mitochondrial bilayers but also mitochondrial DNA (mtDNA) and mitochondrial proteins [7]. Uncontrolled increase in these metabolites lead to free radical-mediated chain reactions which indiscriminately target proteins, lipids and DNA resulting in cell death [8], producing neurodegeneration, at least in part, through the mitochondrial apoptotic pathway [9]. Several experimentally PD models are used to study the pathogenesis of the disease. 1-Methyl-4-phenyl-1,2,3,6-tetrahydropyridine (MPTP) is a neurotoxin able to produce experimentally Parkinson's disease in humans and monkeys (Figure 1). When administered to animals, MPTP readily crosses the blood-brain barrier (BBB), where it selectively destroys DA neurons in the substantia nigra (SN). Once MPTP crosses the BBB, it enters astrocytes, where it is converted into the active metabolite 1-methyl-4-phenylpyridinium (MPP$^+$) by the action of the enzyme monoamine oxidase B (MAO B) [10]. MPP$^+$ leaves the astrocytes and via the DA transporter enters the dopaminergic neurons. First of all, MPP$^+$ accumulates into mitochondrial matrix, where it inhibits the Krebs cycle enzyme α-ketoglutarate dehydrogenase [11]. In addition, this metabolite inhibits complex I of the electron transport chain (ETC), causing increased generation of ROS, decreased adenosine triphosphate (ATP) production and nigral cell death [12,13]. MPP$^+$, by inducing nitric oxide synthase (NOS) expression in SNpc, has been shown to produce large amounts of nitric oxide (NO) that, reacting with O_2^- generates the highly toxic peroxynitrite (ONOO$^-$), a molecule that impairs mitochondrial functions causing irreversible inhibition of all ETC complexes [14] and neuronal cell death [15].

Together with MPTP, other toxin-based models frequently used to induce dopaminergic neurodegeneration include the neurotoxin 6-hydroxydopamine (6-OHDA), the herbicides paraquat (N,N'-dimethyl-4,4'-bipyridinium dichloride) and rotenone, and the fungicide maneb (Figure 1). They are capable of inducing the pathological hallmark of PD, the neuronal cell loss in the SN. The main contributing factor to this cell loss is mitochondrial dysfunction by inhibiting complex I, resulting in oxidative stress and eventually cell death [16]. In particular, neurotoxin 6-OHDA induces reduction of the antioxidant glutathione (GSH) and antioxidant enzyme superoxide dismutase (SOD) [17], increase of iron levels in SN [18] and inhibition of complexes I and IV in mitochondria [19] which lead to further oxidative stress. The herbicide paraquat having a structural similarity to MPP$^+$ directly inhibits complex I [20] and produces oxidative stress through redox cycling. The herbicide rotenone, extracted from tropical plants, easily crosses the BBB and accumulates inside the mitochondrial dopaminergic neuron, where it inhibits complex I. Maneb, on the other hand, induces the nigrostriatal dopaminergic neurodegeneration by inhibiting complex III [16].

Actually, considering that the existence of mitochondrial damage, due to oxidative stress, is the base of the disease which may lead to a decrease in the activities of mitochondrial complexes and ATP production, and as a consequence, a further increase in free radical generation, with the final consequence being cell death by necrosis or apoptosis, the use of antioxidants as an important co-treatment with traditional therapies has been suggested.

There are several agents that are currently under investigation for their potential neuroprotective effects based on their capacity to modify mitochondrial dysfunction. These include creatine, melatonin (MLT), nicotine, nicotinamide, lipoic acid, acetyl-L-carnitine, resveratrol etc. (Table 1) [21]. Among these compounds, melatonin has shown to be effective in preventing neuronal cell death and ameliorating PD symptoms in several *in vivo* and *in vitro* PD models.

MLT is a natural hormone secreted by the pineal gland that easily crosses BBB. This hormone regulates and modulates a wide variety of physiological functions. Besides the well-known chronobiotic and sleep inducing properties [22], many other physiological effects have been ascribed to MLT, such as the modulation of cardiovascular [23] and immune [24] systems and the influence on hormone secretion and metabolism [25]. Other effects of MLT described in the literature include antitumor [26,27], anti-inflammatory [28], pain modulator [29], neuroprotective [30,31], and antioxidant [32] activities.

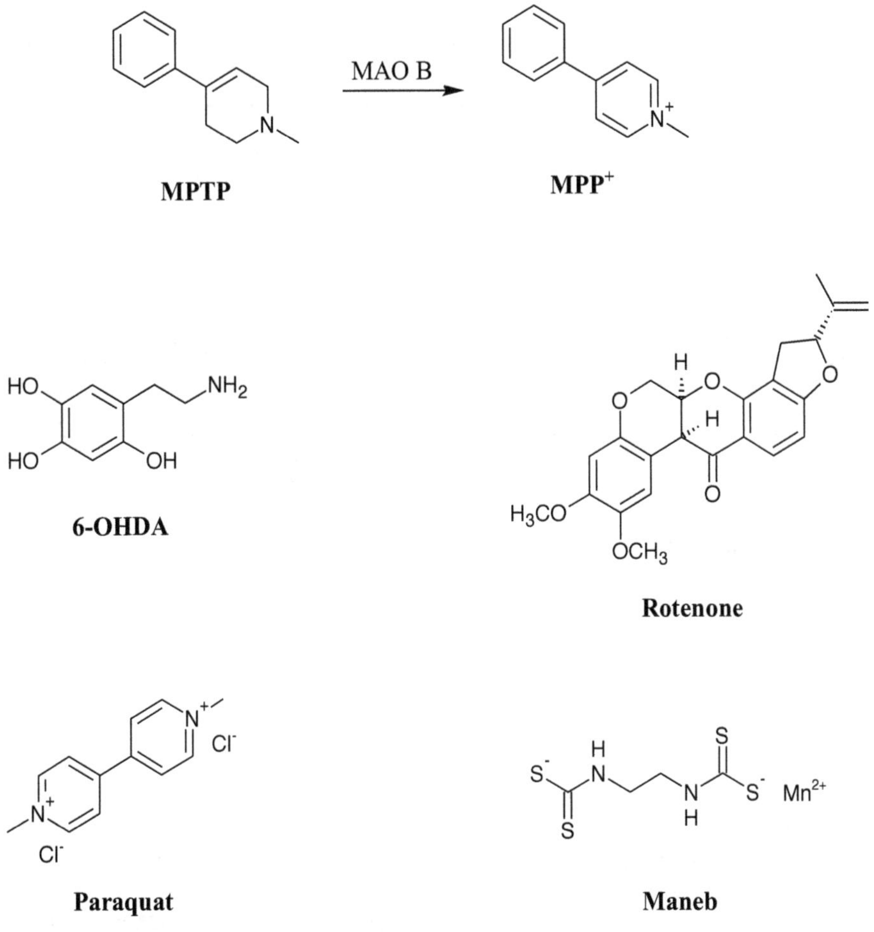

Figure 1. Toxins in experimental PD models.

Many *in vitro* and *in vivo* experimental models have contributed to demonstrate the role of MLT as an efficient radical scavenger against several reactive oxygen species (ROS), for example, the hydroxyl radical, the peroxynitrite anion, the superoxide anion, and singlet oxygen [33]. MLT has also been shown to enhance the production and the activity of several antioxidant enzymes, including superoxide dismutase (SOD), glutathione peroxidase (GPx), glutathione reductase (GRd), catalase, and glucose-6-phosphate dehydrogenase [34,35]. Furthermore, *in vivo* observations on the protective role of MLT in ischemic brain injury [36] or in animal models of PD [37] emphasize the therapeutic potential of this compound as a neuroprotective agent [38]. Moreover, MLT increases the efficiency of the electron transport chain thereby limiting electron integrity of the mitochondria and helps to maintain cell functions and survival [39]. Treatment with MLT counteracts the effects of MPTP in brain nuclei, increasing complex I activity, and the effects of MPTP on lipid peroxidation and nitrite levels in the cytosol and in the mitochondria of mice brain [40]. There is growing evidence that MLT antiapoptotic effects play an important role in neurodegeneration as well [41].

Agent	Structure
Acetyl-L-carnitine	
Aspirin (acetylsalicylic acid)	
Carnitine	
Caffeine	
Creatine	
Curcumin	

Agent	Structure
(–)-Epigallocatechin gallate (EGCG)	
(R)-Lipoic acid	
Melatonin (MLT)	
(–)-Nicotine	
Nicotinamide	
Resveratrol	
Riluzole	

Table 1. Neuroprotective agents in PD models.

2. Neuroprotective agents for Parkinson's disease

Relevant preclinical studies have identified several compounds such as MLT, estrogen, nicotine, caffeine, riluzole, curcumin, aspirin, epigallocatechin-3-gallate (EGCG) and resveratrol, as neuroprotective agents in PD [42] (Table 1). Various prospective studies have suggested a strong association between tobacco smoking and a decreased risk of PD. Nicotine is one of the main constituents of tobacco and is known for its pharmacological effects, exerted by interaction with cholinergic nicotinic receptors in both central and peripheral nervous systems [43]. A recent clinical trial among six male PD patients demonstrated that chronic high doses of nicotine improved motor scores, reduced dopaminergic treatment and had a potential beneficial effect on striatal dopamine transporter density [44]. Chronic nicotine treatment partly protects against the MPTP-induced degeneration of nigrostriatal dopamine neurons in the black mouse, counteracts the disappearance of tyrosine-hydroxylase-immunoreactive nerve cell bodies, dendrites and terminals in the mesostriatal dopamine system and prevent striatal dopamine loss provoked by 6-OHDA administration in the substantia nigra [45-47].

17β-estradiol (E2) is a predominant sex hormone that acts on the whole body. Since several epidemiological studies have shown a greater incidence of PD in men than women, extensive research have investigated the possible neuroprotective effects of E2 in MPTP mice models and in 6-OHDA-injury model [48,49]. Estrogens alters MPTP-induced neurotoxicity in female mice with effects on striatal DA concentrations and release [50]. E2 prevents loss of dopamine transporter (DAT) and vesicular monoamine transporter (VMAT2) in substantia nigra, induces regulation of striatal preproenkephalin mPRNA levels in MPTP-lesioned mice, protects the SNpc of female rats from lesion induced by 6-OHDA and interacts with the insulin-like growth factor-1 (IGF-1) system to protect nigrostriatal dopamine and maintain motoric behavior after 6-OHDA lesions [51-53].

Caffeine is the most widely used psychoactive substance in the world due to its presence in coffee and other beverages. Several epidemiological studies have linked coffee intake with a lower incidence of PD, suggesting neuroprotective properties for caffeine and demonstrating its strong neuroprotective role in rodents for various injury models [54,55]. In particular, Chen and co-authors found that caffeine (10 mg/kg) was neuroprotective when administered 10 min prior to four injections of MPTP [56], attenuating the depletions in striatal DA, 3,4-dihydrox-yphenylacetic acid (DOPAC) and DAT-binding sites. The same effects were also established in a 6-OHDA model [57]. Several epidemiological studies suggested an interaction between estrogen and caffeine. It has been reported that caffeine attenuated the toxic effects of MPTP in male mice in a dose-dependent manner. In contrast, this results was not found in female mice and estrogen treatment also prevented this effect in young male mice [58].

Riluzole is a selective Na^+-channel blocker and some researchers have demonstrated its neuroprotective effects in rodents and in a primate model. Boireau and co-authors reported that riluzole neuroprotection in combination with MPTP was due to interference with MPP^+ production by MAO-B inhibition. The protective effect was confirmed in MPTP- treated mice, partially due to astrocyte activation [59].

Many evidences reported that an important risk factor for the disease is aging [60]. It contributes to PD progression because of accumulative oxidative damage and decrease of antioxidant capacity. Genetic studies have also revealed that aging can be controlled by changes in intracellular NAD/NADH ratio regulating sirtuins, a group of proteins linked to aging, metabolism and stress tolerance in several organisms. Consistently, the neuroprotective roles of dietary antioxidants including for example, acetyl-L-carnitine, curcumin, epigallocatechin-3-gallate (EGCG), carnosine, resveratrol, etc. have been demonstrated through the activation of these redox-sensitive intracellular pathways.

In particular, acetyl-L-carnitine has been proposed to have beneficial effects in preventing the loss of brain function which typically occurs during aging and neurodegenerative disorders [21]. In fact, acetyl-L-carnitine treatment has been shown to prevent age-related changes in mitochondrial respiration and decrease oxidative stress biomarkers through the up-regulation of HO-1 (heme oxygenase-1), Hsp70 (heat shock protein 70) and superoxide dismutase-2 in senescent rats [61]. Acetyl-L-carnitine has shown to be neuroprotective through a variety of other effects such as the increase in protein kinase C (PKC) activity [62]. Moreover acetyl-L-carnitine has also been reported to attenuate the occurrence of parkinsonian symptoms associated with MPTP *in vivo*, and protects *in vitro* against the toxicity of neurotoxic MPP$^+$ [63].

Curcumin is an active polyphenolic compound of Turmeric (*Curcuma longa*), which is extensively used as dietary spice in Indian food. Curcumin is used as a food additive because of its yellow colouring properties and presents anti-inflammatory and antioxidant properties. Recent studies demonstrated the neuroprotective effects of pretreatment with curcumin in the 6-OHDA model in rats. Both motor deficits and neuronal damage were prevented by curcumin and by one of its main metabolites, tetrahydrocurcumin, which also had beneficial effects on the antioxidant status, with increasing GSH levels and activity of antioxidant enzymes. Curcumin inhibited, in fact, MAO-B activity which prevents the conversion of MPTP to its toxic metabolite MPP+ [64].

EGCG is a catechin ubiquitously found in plants and is an important substance in green tea. Interestingly, there are several epidemiological studies that investigated an association between tea and PD. Among tea drinkers, the risk of developing PD was lower than in non-tea drinkers [65]. This effect was thought to be especially influenced by EGCG, to which has been ascribed a wide range of therapeutic properties, including neuroprotection. In fact, green tea and EGCG prevented MPTP-induced neuron loss and inhibited the upregulation of striatal SOD and catalase enzymes [66].

Inflammation is believed to be one of the important factors in the pathogenesis of PD. Moreover, it had been demonstrated that the enzyme cyclooxygenase (COX) and other inflammatory proteins are elevated in PD. Therefore, there is a significant interest in non-steroidal anti-inflammatory drugs (NSAIDs), especially aspirin [42]. The aspirin has an additional free radical scavenging property in addition to COX2 inhibition. In a study reported by Marahaj and co-authors, aspirin (100 mg/kg) and paracetamol (100 mg/kg) prevented KCN-induced superoxide generation and lipid peroxidation. While paracetamol was a more effective antioxidant, aspirin completely blocked the debilitating effects of MPP$^+$ on striatal DA in rats, whereas paracetamol was only able to partially block this effect [67].

Also resveratrol, a polyphenol compound, found in grapes and in red wine, has shown anti-inflammatory, anti-oxidant, and neuroprotective properties. The effects of resveratrol on the 6-OHDA injury in rats were studied by Khan ànd colleagues [68]. They have demonstrated that resveratrol was not only capable to protect neurons, but also to increase the activity of antioxidant enzymes and decrease the levels of thiobarbituric acid reactive substances (TBARS), protein carbonyl (PC), and phospholipase A2 (PA2), providing evidence for a possible antioxidant property. Then, pretreatment with resveratrol (50 and 100 mg/kg) prevented neuronal cell loss in the SN and striatal DA depletion, in 6-OHDA-injury model in rats it was neuroprotective and it has been shown to decrease mRNA and protein levels of TNF-α in COX2, suggesting that an anti-inflammatory mechanism underlies the protective effects of this polyphenol [69,70].

3. Melatonin

Melatonin (N-acetyl-5-methoxy triptamine, MLT), a triptophan derivative, is a highly conservative naturally occurring molecule present in a wide spectrum of organisms, including bacteria, fungi, plants, protozoa, invertebrates [71] and vertebrates. In vertebrates, MLT is primarily produced by the pineal gland with a marked circadian rhythm that is governed by the central circadian pacemaker in the suprachiasmatic nuclei (SCN) of the hypothalamus, the highest levels occurring during the period of darkness [72]. Extrapineal sites of MLT production include retina, Harderian gland, gut, bone marrow [74], platelets, and skin [75]. However, with the exception of retina, the physiological significance of these extrapineal sites is still a matter of debate. MLT was first isolated and identified in the bovine pineal gland by Lerner and coworkers in 1958 [76].

MLT acts as time-giver (*Zeitgeber*) in the regulation of circadian rhythms [77,78] and in synchronizing the reproductive cycle with the appropriate season of the year in photoperiodic species [8]. In non-photoperiodic species such as humans, MLT actions consist in consolidation of sleep and regulation of the circadian rhythm [9]. MLT actions, however, are not restricted to its role in the neuroendocrine physiology. Many other physiological effects have been ascribed to MLT, such as the modulation of cardiovascular [23] and immune [24] systems and the influence on hormone secretion and metabolism [25]. Other effects of MLT described in the literature include antitumor [26, 27], anti-inflammatory [28], pain modulator [29], neuroprotective [30, 31] and antioxidant [32] properties. MLT have also been associated with the cellular antioxidant defence since it is a powerful free radical scavenger, and it is able to induce the expression and/or the activity of the main antioxidant enzymes [79].

MLT exerts its actions by multiple mechanisms. Many of its physiological actions are mediated through activation of distinct MLT receptors expressed in a wide variety of tissues. Cloning studies have revealed at least three MLT receptor subtypes, two of which (MT_1 and MT_2) have been found in mammals and are localized in different areas of the central nervous system (CNS) as well as in peripheral tissues [80]. Moreover, a non-mammalian MLT binding site with a lower affinity profile (MT_3) has been found in hamster brain and characterized as a MLT-sensitive form of the human enzyme quinine reductase 2 [81]. MLT is also a ligand for retinoid orphan nuclear hormone receptors referred to as RZRα and RZRβ at concentrations in the low nanomolar range. Both receptors are present in the central and peripheral nervous system and have been associated with cell differentiation and immune response regulation [82,83]. The melatonin MT_1 receptor is coupled to different G proteins that mediate the inhibition of adenylyl cyclase and the activation of phospholipase C [84], while the MT_2 receptor is coupled to a number of signal transduction mechanisms, among them phosphoinositide production, inhibition of adenylyl cyclase and guanylyl cyclase [80].

Tryptophan serves as the precursor for the biosynthesis of MLT (Figure 2). It is converted into serotonin via 5-hydroxytryptophan. Serotonin is then acetylated to form N-acetylserotonin by arylalkylamine N-acetyltransferase (AANAT or NAT), one of the key enzyme in MLT synthesis. N-acetylserotonin is then converted to MLT by hydroxyindole-O-methyltransferase (HIOMT) which has been identified as the rate-limiting enzyme in the biosynthesis of pineal MLT [85]. In all mammals pineal MLT biosynthesis is synchronized to light/dark cycle by the SCN, which receives its input from the retinohypothalamic tract. Special photoreceptive retinal ganglion cells containing melanopsin as a photopigment are involved in the projection from retina [86]. Fibers from the SCN pass through a circuitous route involving the paraventricular nucleus of the hypothalamus and then proceed to innervate pineal gland as postganglionic sympathetic fibers. Norepinephrine released from these fibers binds to postsynaptic adreno-ceptors whose activation induces an increase in cyclic adenosine-3′,5′-monophosphate (cyclic AMP) accumulation and a subsequent activation of NAT [87].

MLT has two important functional groups which determine its specificity and amphiphilicity: the 5-methoxy group and the N-acetyl side chain. Due to its lipophilic nature and pK_a, MLT readily crosses the BBB. Once formed within the pineal gland, the majority of MLT diffuses directly towards the cerebrospinal fluid of the brain's third ventricle, while another fraction is released into the blood stream where it is distributed to all tissues. The brain has much higher concentrations of MLT than any other tissue in the body [88].

Circulating MLT is partially bound to albumin and can also binds to hemoglobin [89,90]. MLT is mainly metabolized in the liver via hydroxylation reaction by cytochrome P450 mono-oxygenases. This reaction is followed by conjugation with sulfuric or glucuronic acid, to produce the principal urinary metabolite, 6-sulfatoxymelatonin. Conjugated MLT and minute quantities of unmetabolized MLT are eliminated through the kidney. In addition to hepatic metabolism, oxidative pyrrole-ring cleavage appears to be the major metabolic pathway in other tissues, including CNS [91].

MLT seems to function via a number of means to reduce oxidative stress. It can develop its action at two levels: as a direct antioxidant, due its ability to act as a free radical scavenger, and as an indirect antioxidant, since it is able to induce the expression and/or the activity of the main antioxidant enzymes.

MLT is a powerful free radical scavenger since it is able to remove H_2O_2, $^{\bullet}OH$, peroxinitrite anion ($ONOO^-$), singlet oxygen ($^1O_2$), $O_2^{\bullet-}$ and peroxyl radical ($LOO^{\bullet}$). MLT, as an electron-rich molecule, is able to interact with free radicals through consecutive reactions giving rise to

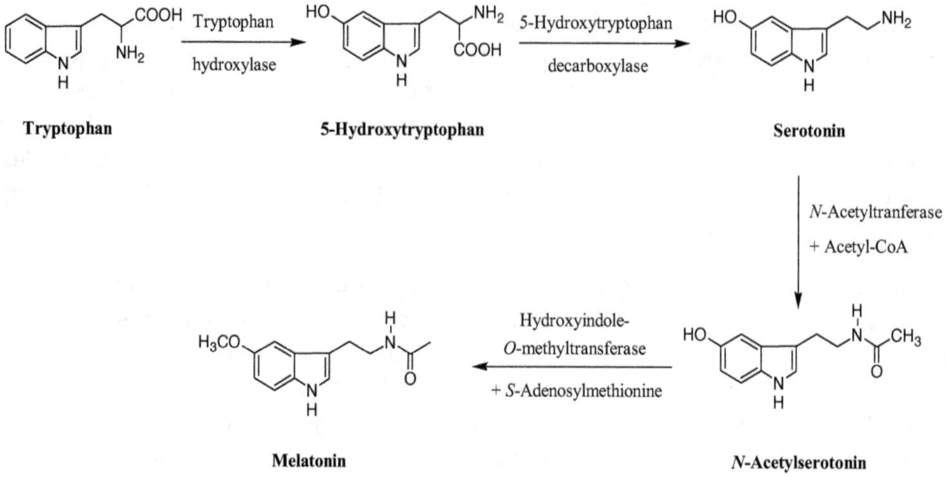

Figure 2. Biosynthetic pathway of melatonin.

many stable compounds that can be excreted by urine. In fact, the MLT antioxidant mechanism implied a free radical scavengers cascade, since secondary, and even tertiary metabolites are also efficient free radicals scavengers, like N-acetyl-N-formyl-5-methoxykynuramine (AFMK) and N-acetyl-methoxykynuramine (AMK) (Figure 3) [92,93]. The formation of such metabolites from MLT implies that, unlike classic antioxidants, melatonin does not produce prooxidant reactions and, even more, AMK and AFMK, in all the mitochondrial studies where comparisons were made, were more potent than MLT itself [94].

The large subcellular distribution of MLT allows its interaction with almost any kind of molecule, diminishing oxidative damage in both lipid and aqueous environments. This is supported experimentally by numerous data that show that MLT is able to protect lipids in the cellular membranes, proteins in the cytosol and DNA in the nucleus from free radical damage [95]. MLT gets free access to all cell components especially in the nucleus [96] and mitochondria [97], where it seems to accumulate in high concentration. In addition, MLT interacts with lipid bilayers of mitochondria, stabilizing its inner membrane [98], an effect that improves ETC activity [99].

Apart from its direct scavenging activity, MLT confers indirect protection against oxygen species through its capability to increase the gene expression and/or activities of antioxidant enzymes. This regulatory role is also mediated by the metabolites of MLT [34,35]. The expression of enzymes, such as GPx, GRd and SOD, related to the endogenous antioxidant system of the cells and the mitochondria, are under genomic regulation of MLT [100,101]. Some antioxidant properties of MLT are attributable to a genomic effect in the regulation of the activities of other antioxidant enzymes such as inducible (iNOS) and mitochondrial (mtNOS) isoforms of nitric oxide synthase [102]. MLT also inhibits neuronal nitric oxide synthase (nNOS) activity because of its binding to the calcium-calmodulin complex [103].

The pineal production of MLT exhibits an unambiguous circadian rhythm with its peak near the middle of scotophase and basal levels during the photophase. The amount of MLT produced by the pineal gland of mammals changes as animals age. The tendency is that pineal MLT production wanes with advanced age. In humans, MLT production not only decreases in the aged but also is significantly lower in many age-related diseases as Alzheimer's, Parkinson's and Huntington's disease [104,105] and cardiovascular disease [106,107].

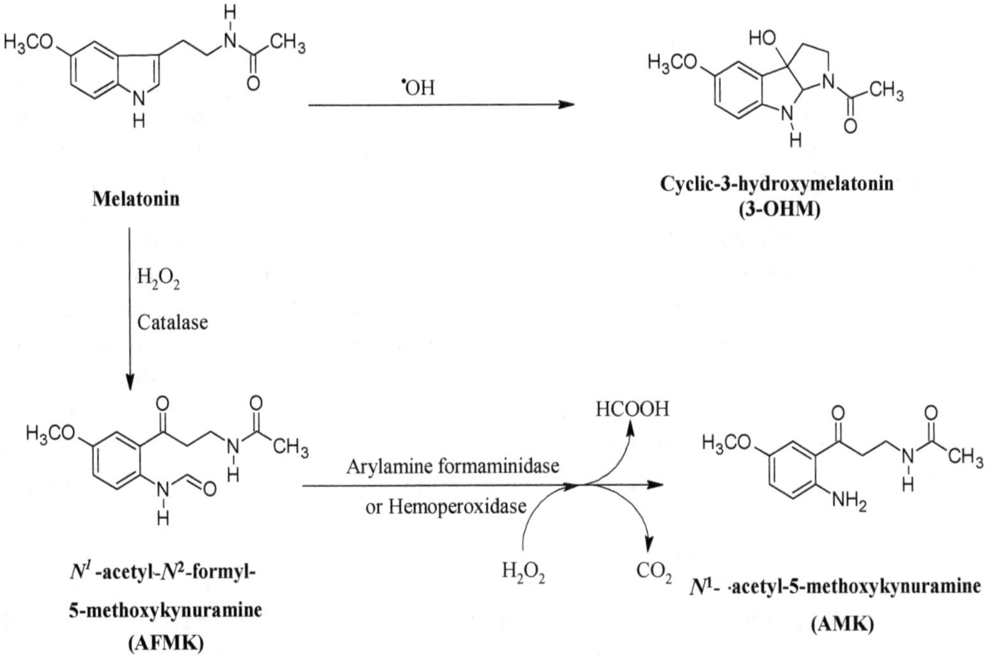

Figure 3. Melatonin oxidation.

4. Mitochondria and melatonin

Mitochondria are organelles found almost ubiquitously in eukaryotes, that play a central role in the cell physiology; in fact, besides their classic function of energy metabolism, these organelles perform many other functions including the distribution of energy through the cells, energy/heat modulation, ROS regulation, calcium homeostasis, and apoptosis control. In mitochondria important metabolic pathways take place including fatty acids β-oxidation, pyruvate oxidation, Krebs cycle, lipids and cholesterol biosynthesis. Many of these processes are functions required for the wellbeing of the cells and of the human beings. The inner mitochondrial membrane is rich in proteins, half of which are involved in oxidation-reduction reactions with transport of electrons and in oxidative phosphorylation (OXPHOS). The oxidative phosphorylation, coupled to electron transport chain (ETC), allows the synthesis of adenosine triphosphate (ATP), a molecule rich in energy, via the enzyme complex ATP synthase.

Human mitochondria contain their own genome (mitochondrial DNA, mtDNA), a circular double stranded-molecule. The human mitochondrial chromosome contains 37 genes (16,569 base pairs), including 13 that encode subunits of respiratory chain/oxidative phosphorylation proteins; the remaining genes code for rRNA and tRNA molecules necessary to the protein-synthesizing complex of mitochondria. About 99% of the mitochondrial proteins are encoded by nuclear DNA (nDNA); so these proteins have to be imported into mitochondria. Mito-chondrial proteins synthesized in the cytosol possess mitochondrial targeting signals that direct them to the appropriate compartment (outer or inner membranes, intermembranes space and matrix) within the organelle. Transport across outer and inner membranes needs a complex machinery including the presence of ATP, docking proteins, chaperonins and proteases, and it involves unfolding and refolding of the proteins to be translocated.

NADH produced in the cytosol by glycolysis and in the mitochondria by oxidation of pyruvate, fatty acids β-oxidation, and Krebs cycle, are oxidized by respiratory chain transferring electrons to O_2, that is converted to water. The primary function of mitochondria is to generate ATP (from ADP and phosphate by adenin nucleotide and phosphate translocators and FoF1 ATP synthase) through the ETC resulting in OXPHOS. The ETC, located in the inner mito-chondrial membrane, comprises a series of electron carriers grouped into four enzyme complexes: complex I or NADH ubiquinone reductase, complex II or succinate ubiquinone reductase, complex III or ubiquinol cytochrome c reductase, and complex IV or cytochrome c oxidase. The end product of the respiratory chain is water generated after reduction of O_2 by mitochondrial complex IV; this process needs the addition of four electrons to each oxygen molecule. However, about 5-10% of the oxygen is involved in production of hydrogen peroxide (H_2O_2), superoxide anion radical ($O_2{}^{\bullet-}$), and the extremely reactive hydroxyl radical ($^{\bullet}OH$) [108]. These three molecules are ROS and represent endogenous oxidotoxins. The mitochon-dria for action of the enzyme nitric oxide synthase (mtNOS) can also produce nitric oxide ($NO^{\bullet}$) from L-arginine [109], which can be converted into various reactive nitrogen species (RNS), such as nitrosonium cation (NO^+), nitroxyl anion (NO^-) and peroxynitrite ($ONOO^-$) [110]. These free radicals are detoxified or their peroxidation products are decomposed by the natural antioxidant defense system as SOD, glutathione redox cycle, catalase and coenzyme Q. Mitochondria not only generate ROS/RNS, but are also the main target of their actions [111]. Small fluctuations in the steady-state concentration of ROS/RNS may play a role in intracellular signaling [112]. Several mechanisms take part in the control of ROS/RNS production. Among these the enzyme SOD, localized in the inner side of the inner mitochondrial membrane, remove $O_2{}^{\bullet-}$ [113]. When formed, $O_2{}^{\bullet-}$ is immediately dismutated to H_2O_2 by cytosolic or mitochondrial superoxide dismutase. As H_2O_2 is the precursor of the highly damaging $^{\bullet}OH$, it is imperative that H_2O_2 is removed very quickly.

The enzyme GPx metabolizes H_2O_2 to water and O_2; GPx in this reaction also converts reduced GSH to its oxidized form (GSSG). In turn, GSSG is reduced to GSH by the action of the enzyme glutathione reductase (GRd) in the presence of NADPH [114,115]. These enzymes form part of the endogenous antioxidant defense system suppressing ROS/RNS levels both in the cells and in the mitochondria. Under normal conditions, MLT reduces mitochondrial hydroperoxide levels and stimulates the activity of GPx and GRd, enzymes involved in the GSH-GSSG balance [116]. The indoleamine MLT is also able to neutralize the oxidative stress induced by high doses of t-butyl hydroperoxide, restoring GSH levels and GPx and GRd activities. However, vitamins C and E have no such effect under the same conditions [116].

Other antioxidants such as ascorbate, ubiquinone and α-tocopherol can participate in the mitochondrial antioxidative defense system, but without to be able to convert $O_2{}^{\cdot-}$ to O_2. However, uncontrolled increase in these metabolites leads to a series of reactions which target proteins, lipids and DNA resulting in cell death by necrosis or apoptosis. In recent years, several findings support the antioxidant effect of MLT in mitochondrial homeostasis [99,117,118].

Apoptosis and necrosis are two types of cell death occurring in neurodegeneration. Apoptosis (programmed cell death) occurs naturally under normal physiological conditions; on the contrary, necrosis is caused by external factors such as toxins, infections and trauma. Apoptosis is characterized by cell shrinkage, cytoplasm contraction, nuclear fragmentation, chromatin condensation, and chromosomal DNA fragmentation, plasma membrane bleb formation and apoptotic body formation [119]. Many of these changes are activated by a family of caspases, i.e. proteases that in their active site possess a cysteine and cleaves the substrates after aspartate residues. Apoptotic cells are rapidly sequestered by phagocytosis before they can lyse and cause an inflammatory process [120]. Necrosis does not involve any DNA or protein degradation and is accompanied by swelling of the cytoplasm and of the mitochondria with membrane ruptures. Both apoptosis and necrosis involve a change in mitochondrial membrane permeabilization (MMP) [121].

MMP causes the opening of a nonspecific pore in the mitochondrial membranes, known as the mitochondrial transition pore (MTP), that allows the passage of any molecules of >1500 Da across this membrane. This pore can be rapidly closed by chelation of calcium ion. Because MTP allows also rapid passage of protons (H^+), its opening causes depolarization of mitochondria and uncoupling of oxidative phosphorylation without synthesis of ATP. If the MTP remains open, ATP levels can be totally depleted; on the contrary, transient opening of the MTP can be involved in the mitochondrial-mediated apoptosis through the proteins released from mitochondria. Among these apoptogenic proteins we know cytochrome c [122], the serine protease HtrA2/Omi [123], and endonuclease G [124].

Permeabilization events, which occur at points where outer and inner mitochondrial membranes are in contact, involve association of several proteins from different districts of the cell and the mitochondria [125]: cytosol (hexokinase), outer mitochondrial membrane (peripheral benzodiazepine receptor and voltage dependent anion channel or VDAC), mitochondrial inner membrane space (creatine kinase), inner mitochondrial membrane (adenine nucleotide translocator or ANT) and mitochondrial matrix (cyclophilin D).

Two main considerations suggest a role for MLT in mitochondrial homeostasis. As it is known, mitochondria produce high amounts of ROS and RNS. Besides, mitochondria depend on the GSH uptake from the cytosol, even if they have GPx and GRd to maintain redox cycling. Thus, the anti-oxidant effect of melatonin and its ability to increase the levels of GSH may be of great importance for mitochondrial physiology [126]. The fact that the inhibition of CN$^-$ on complex IV of the mitochondrial ETC is removed by MLT, also supports its intramitochondrial role [127]. A protective effect of MLT against MPP$^+$-induced inhibition of complex I of ETC has been also shown [128].

The effects of MLT on mitochondrial ETC have been also studied on submitochondrial particles from rat liver and brain mitochondria [129]. MLT at 1 nM concentration significantly increased the activity of the complexes I and IV of ETC in rat liver submitochondrial particles, whereas 10-100 nM MLT stimulated the activity of the same complexes but in brain submitochondrial particles. The indoleamine counteracted CN$^-$-induced inhibition of complex IV, restoring the levels of Cyt aa3. This effect was of physiological significance, since the MLT increased the ETC and OXPHOS activities with a consequent increase of ATP synthesis [129]. In addition, due the high redox potential of MLT (-0.98 V), this molecule can donate directly electrons to complex I of the ETC [130].

The effect of MLT (10 mg/kg) on ETC complexes from rat liver and brain mitochondria has been also studied in vivo. Martin et al. [116] have found that MLT increases the activity of the respiratory chain complexes I and IV and ATP synthesis in a time-dependent manner after mitochondrial damage induced by ruthenium red [116].

Recently, the role of MLT on cardiolipin and mitochondrial biogenesis was studied [131]. Cardiolipin, a phospholipid located in inner mitochondrial membrane, is required for several mitochondrial bioenergetic processes as well as for the activity of transport proteins. Alterations in cardiolipin structure and acyl chain composition have been associated with mitochondrial dysfunction under a variety of pathological dysfunctions. The authors [131] reported that MLT protects the mitochondrial membranes from oxidation-reduction damage by preventing cardiolipin oxidation.

5. Melatonin and Parkinson's

In the last decade, many research findings provide scientific evidence for the protective role of MLT in a number of oxidative stress related diseases, especially Alzheimer's [132] and Parkinson's diseases [133], being the protective actions of the indoleamine attributable to its direct and indirect antioxidative properties. The first evidence of a significant relationship between Parkinson's disease and MLT derived from the evidence of a reduction in the concentration of circulating MLT in PD patients as a consequence of a decreased activity of the pineal gland [134]. After its antioxidant properties were uncovered, melatonin has been successfully tested in several *in vivo* and *in vitro* PD models.

MLT was found to inhibit *in vitro* the prooxidant effects of dopamine and L-dopa [135] and to be more effective than the vitamin E analog, trolox, in preventing dopamine autooxidation [136]. Melatonin was also reported to prevent in the MPTP model the rise in lipid peroxidation products in the substantia nigra (SN) of MPP$^+$-treated rats and, additionally, to preserve tyrosine hydroxylase (TH) activity, which is normally decreased after toxin treatment [69].

When the 6-OHDA model was used instead of MPTP ones to induce dopaminergic degeneration, MLT administration restored the motor deficits elicited by apomorphine co-treatment with 6-OHDA [137] and also completely prevented the rise in neural lipid peroxidation products and partially rescued striatal dopaminergic levels after lesioning with 6-OHDA [138]. The protective action of MLT against dopaminergic neuronal degeneration was also expressed by reduction of the DNA fragmentation induced by MTPT [139] and of mitochondrial complex I deficiency observed after 6-OHDA administration [140]. MLT also counters MPTP-induced c-Jun-N-terminal kinase and caspase-dependent signaling leading to the dopaminergic neurodegeneration [141]. It has been reported that MLT partially preserves the GSH concentrations in SN of MPTP-treated rats [142,143]. The antioxidant activity of MLT was supposed to be the major mechanism underlying MLT's protection in these PD models. The protective function of MLT also include its antiapoptotic effects. MLT has been reported to rescue dopamine neurons from spontaneous cell death in low-density seeding culture [144].

PD epidemiological studies have suggested an association with the environmental toxin rotenone, a mitochondrial complex I inhibitor. In recent years, *Drosophila melanogaster* has been used as a model for several neurodegenerative diseases, including PD. Coulom and Birman studied for several days the neurodegenerative effects of a chronic exposure to rotenone in *Drosophila melanogaster*. After several days of treatment, flies presented characteristic locomotor impairments that increased with the dose of herbicide. Immunocytochemistry analysis demonstrated a dramatic and selective loss of dopaminergic neurons in the brain of all treated flies. The addition of L-dopa into the feeding medium rescued the behavioral deficits but not neuronal death, as is the case in human PD patients. On the contrary, the antioxidant MLT alleviated both symptomatic impairment and neuronal loss, supporting the idea that this agent may be beneficial in the treatment of parkinsonism [145].

MLT has been shown to protects PC12 cells from both apoptosis and necrosis induced by high doses of 6-OHDA [146,147]. Since 6-OHDA induced cellular toxicity is mediated by increased free-radical generation, the antioxidant properties of MLT presumably account for its ability to suppress both necrosis and apoptosis. Numerous data suggest a role for MLT in mitochondrial homeostasis [148]. It has been reported that MLT increases the activities of respiratory complexes I and IV in a time-dependent manner after *in vivo* administration to rats [129] and maintains GSH homeostasis in the mitochondrial matrix under increased oxidative stress; these actions are not shared by either vitamin C or vitamin E [117]. Mitochondria in the cell are the major source of ROS, owing to the leakage of electrons through the electron transport chain. Due the critical role of mitochondria in programmed cell death and PD, it is conceivable that actions at the mitochondrial level mediate at least some of MLT apoptotic effects. It has been reported that MLT induces ATP production, increasing the activity of the mitochondrial oxidative phosphorylation (OXPHOS) enzymes [129]. The indoleamine also protects mitochondrial DNA, which is particularly vulnerable to oxidative damage, thus indirectly helping to preserve mitochondrial metabolism.

Since mitochondria play a critical role in the pathogenesis of PD, it is conceivably that actions at mitochondria level mediate some of MLT antiapoptotic effects. The beneficial actions of MLT in PD has been widely investigated not only on the basis of its neuroprotective efficacy assessment but also because of the down regulation of MLT receptors in the nigrostriatal region of PD brain [149]. There is growing evidence of sleep–wake boundary dysfunction in PD. REM sleep behavior disorder (RBD) which is characterized by loss of normal skeletal muscle tone with prominent motor activity and dreaming, has been associated with PD and/or other forms of dementia, with a tendency for RBD to precede the onset of parkinsonism. There is some clinical evidence that MLT can be a useful add-on therapy for RBD in PD [150].

6. Conclusions

PD is a highly debilitating condition that concerns thousands of family in the world and annually cost millions of euro for treatment. This disease has occasionally a genetic basis, but the signs of PD develop after free-radical damage to the substantia nigra pars compacta. Moreover, neuroinflammation and mitochondrial dysfunction participate in the ethiology of this neurodegenerative disorder and contribute to the increase of oxidative damage to the dopaminergic neurons.

The mitochondria in cells play a myriad of different and important functions, so any alteration in these organelles could have a considerable impact on the functionality of the cells and also the entire body. Mitochondria are also the site of generation of reactive oxygen and nitrogen species (ROS/RNS) and the subsequent widespread deleterious effects (oxidation and/or nitrosylation of mtDNA, oxidation of phospholipids and proteins) of these intermediates. These effects lead also to the opening of the mitochondrial transition pore, release of Cyt c and the activation of the events that culminate in apoptosis.

Abnormal mitochondrial functions (decreased respiratory complexes activities, increased electron leakage, opening of the mitochondrial transition pore) have all been shown to play a role in the pathophysiology of neurodegenerative disorders such as PD, AD and HD. Mitochondrial involvement in PD is revealed by deficiency of mitochondrial complexes I and IV, decreased ATP production with a parallel reduction in GSH levels.

Among the substances involved in maintaining mitochondrial biogenetics, a number of *in vivo* and *in vitro* studies indicate that MLT may emerge as a major therapeutic candidate to preserve bioenergetic function of mitochondria.

MLT is a molecule present in all creatures from prokaryotes to human beings. It is an antioxidant that protected organisms from oxidative stresses and apoptosis and mediates seasonal physiological functions, is a signal of dark/light promoting also sleep, modulates the immune system, and inhibits the growth of several cancer. Indoleamine is an antioxidant that directly scavenges ROS/RNS produced during the normal metabolism of mitochondria and it indirectly promotes the activity of the antioxidant enzymes including SOD, catalase, GPx and GRd.

It has also been documented that the ability of MLT to quell the oxidation-reduction processes, with the formation of free radicals, is due to its conversion to metabolites, such as cyclic 3-OHM, AFMK and AMK. Considering the cascade of reactions that include AFMK and AMK, a MLT can scavenge about ten ROS/RNS. MLT increases the activity of ETC and the ATP synthesis, reducing at the same time the oxygen consumption; then, it avoids an excess of ROS/RNS, preventing PTP opening and apoptosis.

Considering that this hormone is an endogenous, nontoxic, antioxidant molecule without known side-effects, it should be considered as a useful agent in PD patients as a treatment with other conventional therapies. Although MLT is an important molecule and possibly has a great future in PD research, it should be extensively tested across multiple populations for efficacy and real effects along with the side effects at the efficacious doses. Future therapeutic strategies could be directed at identifying and developing MLT analogues as drugs with more powerful inhibitory effects on the mitochondrial cell death pathway, slowing the progression of neurodegenerative diseases.

Author details

Alessia Carocci[1], Maria Stefania Sinicropi[2*], Alessia Catalano[1], Graziantonio Lauria[2] and Giuseppe Genchi[2]

*Address all correspondence to: s.sinicropi@unical.it; genchi@unical.it

1 Department of Pharmacy-Drug Sciences, University of Bari "Aldo Moro", Bari, Italy

2 Department of of Pharmacy, Health and Nutritional Sciences, University of Calabria, Cosenza, Italy

References

[1] Lee VM, Trojanowsky JQ. Mechanisms of Parkinson's disease linked to pathological alpha-synuclein: new targets for drug discovery. Neuron 2006;52(1): 33-38.

[2] Braak H, Del Tredici K, Rub U, de Vos RA, Jansen Steur EN, Braak E. Staging of brain pathology related to sporadic Parkinson's disease. Neurobiology of Aging 2003;24(2): 197-211.

[3] Yacoubian TA, Standaert DG. Targets for neuroprotection in Parkinson's disease 2009;1792(7): 676-687.

[4] Schapira AHV. Mitochondria in the aetiology and pathogenesis of Parkinson's disease. The Lancet Neurology 2008;7(1): 97-109.

[5] Huang Y, Cheung L, Rowe D, Halliday G. Genetic contributions to Parkinson's disease. Brain Research Brain Research Reviews 2004;46(1): 44-70.

[6] Vila M, Przedborski S. Genetic clues to the pathogenesis of Parkinson's disease. Nature Medicine 2004;10(7s): S58-S62.

[7]   Dexter DT, Holley AE, Flitter WD, Slater TF, Wells FR, Daniel SE, Lees AJ, Jenner P, Marsden CD. Increased levels of lipid hydroperoxides in the Parkinsonian substantia nigra: an HPLC and ESR study. Movement Disorders 1994;9(1): 92-97.

[8]   Fleury C, Mignotte B, Vayssiere JL. Mitochondrial reactive oxygen species in cell death signaling. Biochimie 2002;84(2-3): 131-141.

[9]   Vila M, Przedborski S. Targeting programmed cell death in neurodegenerative diseases. Nature Reviews Neuroscience 2003;4(5): 365-375.

[10] Javitch JA, D'Amato RJ, Strittmatter SM, Snyder SH. Parkinsonism-inducing neurotoxin, N-methyl-4-phenyl-1,2,3,6-tetrahydropyridine: uptake of the metabolite N-methyl-4-phenylpyridine by dopamine neurons explains selective toxicity. Proceedings of the National Academy of Sciences of the United States of America 1985;82(7): 2173-2177.

[11] Mizuno Y, Saitoh T, Sone N. Inhibition of mitochondrial alpha-ketoglutarate dehydrogenase by 1-methyl-4-phenylpyridinium ion. Biochemical and Biophysical Research Communications 1987;143(3): 971-976.

[12] Schober A. Classic toxin-induced animal models of Parkinson's disease: 6-OHDA and MPTP. Cell and Tissue Research 2004;318(1): 215-224.

[13] Terzioglu M, Galter D. Parkinson's disease: genetic versus toxin-induced rodent models. The FEBS Journal 2008; 275(7): 1384-1391.

[14] Brown GC, Borutaite, V. Inhibition of mitochondrial respiratory complex I by nitric oxide, peroxynitrite and S-nitrosothiols. Biochimica et Biophysica Acta (BBA) - Bioenergetics 2004;1658(1-2): 44-49.

[15] Zhang L, Dawson VL, Dawson TM. Role of nitric oxide in Parkinson's disease. Pharmacological Therapy 2006;109(1-2): 33-41.

[16] Duty S, Jenner P. Animal models of Parkinson's disease: a source of novel treatments and clues to the cause of the disease. British Journal of Pharmacology 2011;164(4): 1357-1391.

[17] Perumal AS, Gopal VB, Tordzro WK, Copper TB, Cadet JL. Vitamine E attenuates the toxic effects of 6-hydroxydopamine on free radical scavenging systems in rat brain. Brain Research Bulletin 1992;29(5): 699-701.

[18] Oestreicher E, Sengstock GJ, Riederer P, Olanow CW, Dunn AJ, Arendash GW. Degeneration of nigrostriatal dopaminergic neurons increases within the substantia nigra: a histochemical and neurochemical study. Brain Research 1994;660(1): 8-18.

[19] Glinka Y, Gassen M, Youdim MB. Mechanism of 6-hydroxydopamine neurotoxicity. Journal of Neural Transmission. Supplementa 1997;50: 55-56.

[20] Miller GW. Paraquat: the red herring of Parkinson's disease research. Toxicological Sciences 2007; 100(1): 1-2.

[21] Sinicropi M.S., Rovito N., Carocci A., Genchi G. Acetyl-L-carnitine in Parkinson's disease. In: Dushanova J. (ed.) Mechanisms in Parkinson's Disease - Models and Treatments. Rijeka: Intech; 2011. p367-392.

[22] Pevet P, Bothorel B, Slotten H, Saboureau M. The chronobiotic properties of melatonin. Cell Tissue Research 2002;309(1): 183-191.

[23] Sewerynek E. Melatonin and the cardiovascular system. Neuroendocrinology Letters 2002;23(Suppl 1): 79-83.

[24] Carillo-Vico A, Reiter RJ, Lardone PJ, Herrera JL, Fernandez-Montesinos R. Guerrero JM, Pozo D. The modulatory role of melatonin on immune responsiveness. Current Opinion in Investigational Drugs 2006;7(5): 423-431.

[25] Barrenetxe J, Delagrange P, Martinez JA. Physiological and metabolic functions of melatonin. Journal of Physiological Biochemistry 2004;60(1): 61-72.

[26] Blask DE, Sauer LA, Dauchy RT. Melatonin as a chronobiotic/anticancer agent: cellular, biochemical, and molecular mechanisms of action and their implications for circadian-based cancer therapy. Current Topics in Medicinal Chemistry 2002;2(2): 113–132

[27] Millis E, Wu P, Seely D, Guyatt G. Melatonin in the treatment of cancer: a systematic review of randomized controlled trials and meta-analysis. Journal of Pineal Research 2005;39(4): 360-366.

[28] Genovese E, Mazzon C, Muia P, Bramanti P, De Sarro A, Cuzzocrea S. Attenuation in the evolution of experimental spinal cord trauma by treatment with melatonin. Journal of Pineal Research 2005;38(3): 198-208.

[29] Peres MFP. Melatonin, the pineal gland and their implications for headache disorders. Cephalalgia 2005;25(6): 403-411.

[30] Srinivasan V, Pandi-Perumal SR, Cardinali DP, Poeggeler B, Hardeland R. Melatonin in Alzheimer's disease and other neurodegenerative disorders. Behavioral and Brain Functions 2006;2: 15.

[31] Medeiros CA, Carvalhedo de Bruin PF, Lopes LA, Megalhães MC, de Lourdes Seabra M, de Bruin VM. Effect of exogenous melatonin on sleep and motor dysfunction in Parkinson's disease. A randomized, double blind, placebo-controlled study Journal of Neurology 2007;254(4): 459-464.

[32] Sofic E, Rimpapa Z, Kundurovic Z, Sapcanin A, Tahirovic I, Rustencbegovic A, Cao G. Antioxidant capacity of the neurohormone melatonin. Journal of Neural Transmission 2005;112(3): 349-358.

[33] Reiter RJ. Oxidative damage in the central nervous system: protection by melatonin. Progess in Neurobiology 1998,56(3): 359-384.

[34] Rodriguez C, Mayo JC, Sainz RM, Antolín I, Herrera F, Martín V, Reiter RJ. Regulation of antioxidant enzymes: a significant role for melatonin. Journal of Pineal Research 2004;36(1): 1-9.

[35] Tomas-Zapico C, Coto-Montes A. A proposed mechanism to explain the stimulatory effect of melatonin on antioxidative enzymes. Journal of Pineal Research 2005; 39(2): 99-104.

[36] Cuzzocrea S, Costantino C, Gitto E, Mazzon E, Fulia F, Serraino I, Cordaro S, Barberi I, De Sarro A, Caputi AP. Protective effects of melatonin in ischemic brain injury. Journal of Pineal Research 2000; 29(4): 217-227.

[37] Mayo JC, Sainz RM, Tan DX, Antolín I, Rodríguez C, Reiter RJ. Melatonin and Parkinson's disease. Endocrine 2005;27(2):169–178.

[38] Savaskan, E. Melatonin in aging and neurodegeneration. Drug Development Research 2002;56(3): 482-490.

[39] Leon J, Acuña-Castroviejo D, Sainz RM, Mayo JC, Tan DX, Reiter RJ. Melatonin and mitochondrial function. Life Sciences 2004;75(7): 765-790.

[40] Tapias V, Escames G, López LC, López A, Camacho E, Carrión MD, Entrena A, Gallo MA, Espinosa A, Acuña-Castroviejo D. Melatonin and its brain metabolite N1-acetyl-5-methoxykynuramine prevent mitochondrial nitric oxide synthase induction in parkinsonian mice. Journal of Neuroscience Research 2009;87(13): 3002-3010.

[41] Wang X. The antiapoptotic activity of melatonin in neurodegenerative disease. CNS Neuroscience & Therapeutics 2009;5(4): 345-357.

[42] Douna H, Bavelaar BM, Pellikaan H, Olivier B, Pieters T. Neuroprotection in Parkinson's disease: a systematic review of the preclinical data. The Open Pharmacology Journal 2012;6: 12-26.

[43] Allam MF, Campbell MJ, Hofman A, Del Castillo AS, Fernàndez-Crehuet Navajas R. Smoking and Parkinson's disease: systematic review of prospective studies. Movement Disorders 2004;19(6): 614-621.

[44] Itti E, Villafane G, Malek Z, Brugières P, Capacchione D, Itti L, Maison P, Cesaro P, Meignan M. Dopamine transporter imaging under high-dose transdermal nicotine therapy in Parkinson's disease: an observational study. Nuclear Medicine Communications 2009;30(7): 513-518.

[45] Janson AM, Fuxe K, Agnati LF, Kitayama I, Härfstrand A, Andersson K, Goldstein M. Chronic nicotine treatment counteracts the disappearance of tyrosine-hydroxylase-immunoreactive nerve cell bodies, dendrites and terminals in the mesostriatal dopamine system of the male after partial hemitransection. Brain Research 1988;455(2): 332-345.

[46] Costa G, Abin-Carriquiry JA, Dajas F. Nicotine prevents striatal dopamine loss produced by 6-hydroxydopamine lesion in the substantia nigra. Brain Research 2001;888(2): 336-342.

[47] Abin-Carriquiry JA, McGregor-Armas R, Costa G, Urbanavicius J, Dajas F. Presynaptic involvement in the nicotine prevention of the dopamine loss provoked by 6-OH-DA administration in the substantia nigra. Neurotoxicity Research 2002;4(2): 133-139.

[48] Taylor KSM, Cook JA, Counsell CE. Heterogeneity in male to female risk for Parkinson's disease. Journal of Neurology, Neurosurgery & Psychiatry 2007;78: 905-906.

[49] Murray HE, Pillai AV, McArthur SR, Razvi N, Datla KP, Dexter DT, Gillies GE. Dose and sex-dependent effects of the neurotoxin 6-hydroxydopamine on the nigrostriatal dopaminegic pathway of adult rats: differential actions of estrogen in males and females. Neuroscience 2003;116(1): 213-222.

[50] Dluzen DE, McDermott JL, Liu B. Estrogen alters MPTP-induced neurotoxicity in female mice: effects on striatal dopamine concentrations and release. Journal of Neurochemistry 1996;66(2): 658-666.

[51] Quesada A, Micevych PE. Estrogen interacts with the IGF-1 system to protect nigrostriatal dopamine and maintain motoric behavior after 6-hydroxdopamine lesions. Journal of Neuroscience Research 2004;75(1): 200-205.

[52] D'Astous M, Morisette M, Callier S, Di Paolo T. Regulation of striatal preproenkephalin mRNA levels in MPTP-lesioned mice treated with estradiol. Journal of Neuroscience Research 2005;80(1): 138-144.

[53] Jourdain S, Morissette M, Morin N, Di Paolo T. Oestrogens prevent loss of dopamine transporter (DAT) and vesicular monoamine transporter (VMAT2) in substantia nigra of 1-methyl-4-phenyl-1,2,3,6-tetrahydropyridine mice. Journal of Neuroendocrinology 2005;17(8): 509-517.

[54] Kachroo A, Irizarry MC, Schwarzschild MA. Caffeine protects against combined paraquat and maneb-induced dopaminergic neuron degeneration. Experimental Neurology 2010;223(2): 657-661.

[55] Xu K, Xu Y-H, Chen J-F, Schwarzschild MA. Neuroprotection by caffeine: time course and role of its metabolites in the MPTP model of Parkinson's disease. Neuroscience 2010;167(2): 475-481.

[56] Chen JF, Xu K, Petzer JP, Staal R, Xu YJ, Beilstein M, Sonsalla PK, Castagnoli K, Castagnoli N, Schwarzschild MA. Neuroprotection by caffeine and A(2A) adenosine receptor inactivation in a model of Parkinson's disease. The Journal of Neuroscience 2001;21(10) RC143.

[57] Joghataie MT, Roghani M, Negahdar F, Hashemi L. Protective effect of caffeine against neurodegeneration in a model of Parkinson's disease in rat: behavioral and histochemical evidence. Parkinsonism & Related Disorders 2004;10(8): 657-661.

[58] Xu K, Xu Y, Brown-Jermyn D, Chen J-F, Ascherio A, Dluzen DE, Schwarzschild MA. Estrogen prevents neuroprotection by caffeine in the mouse 1-methyl-4-phenyl-1,2,3,6-tetrahydropyridine model of Parkinson's disease. The Journal of Neuroscience 2006;26(2): 535-541.

[59] Boireau A, Bubedat P, Bordier F, Imperato A, Moussaoui S. The protective effect of riluzole in the MPTP model of Parkinson's disease in mice is not due to a decrease in MPP+ accumulation. Neuropharmacology 2000;39(6): 1016-1020.

[60] Parris MK. Parkinson's disease as multifactorial oxidative neurodegeneration: implications for integrative management. Alternative Medicine Review 2000;5(6): 502-545.

[61] Calabrese V, Colombrita C, Sultana R, Scapagnani G, Calvani M, Butterfield DA, Giuffrida Stella AM. Redox modulation of heat shock protein expression by acetylcarnitine in aging brain: relationship to antioxidant status and mitochondrial function. Antioxidants and Redox Signaling 2006;8(3-4): 404-416.

[62] McDaniel MA, Maier SF, Einstein GO. "Brain-specific" nutrients: a memory cure? Nutrition 2003;19(11-12): 957-975.

[63] Hongyu Z, Haiqun J, Jianghai L. Ni A, Bing Y, Weili S, Xuemin W, Xin L, Cheng L, Jiankang L. Combined R-α-lipoic acid and acetyl-L-carnitine exerts efficient preventative effects in a cellular model of Parkinson's disease. Journal of Cellular and Molecular Medicine 2010;14(1-2): 215-225.

[64] Rajeswari A, Sabesan M. Inhibition of monamine oxidase-B by the polyphenolic compound, curcumin and its metabolite tetrahydrocurcumine, in a model of Parkinson's disease induced by MPTP neurodegeneration in mice. Inflammopharmacology 2008;16(2): 96-99.

[65] Hu G, Bidel S, Jousilahti P, Antikainen R, Tuomilehto J. Coffee and tea consumption and the risk of Parkinson's disease. Movement Disorders 2007;22(1): 2242-2248.

[66] Levites Y, Weinreb O, Maor G, Youdim MB, Mandel S. Green tea polyphenol (-) epigallocatechin-3-gallate prevents N-methyl-4-phenyl-1,2,3,6-tetrahydropyridine-induced dopaminergic neurodegeneration. Journal of Neurochemistry 2001;78(5): 1073-1082.

[67] Maharaj DS, Saravanan KS, Maharaj H, Mohanakumar KP, Daya S. Acetaminophen and aspirin inhibit superoxide anion generation and lipid peroxidation, and protect against 1-methyl-4-phenyl pyridinium-induced dopaminergic neurotoxicity in rats. Neurochemistry International 2004;44(5): 355-360.

[68] Khan M, Ahmad A, Ishrat T, Khan MB, Hoda MN, Khuwaja G, Raza SS, Khan A, Javed H, Vaibhav K, Islam F. Resveratrol attenuates 6-hydroxydopamine-induced oxidative damage and dopamine depletion in rat model of Parkinson's disease. Brain Research 2010;1328(139-151): 139-151.

[69] Jin BK, Shin DY, Jeong MY, Gwag MR, Baik HW, Yoon KS, Cho YH, Joo WS, Kim YS, Baik HH. Melatonin protects nigral dopaminergic neurons from 1-methyl-4-phenyl-pyridinium (MPP+) neurotoxicity in rats. Neuroscience Letters 1998;245(2): 61-64.

[70] Blanchet J, Longpré F, Bureau G, Morisette M, Di Paolo T, Bronchti G, Martinoli MG. Resveratrol, a red wine polyphenol, protects dopaminergic neurons in MPTP-treated mice. Progress in Neuropsychopharmacology and Biological Psychiatry 2008;32(5): 1243-1250.

[71] Hardeland R, Coto-Montes A, Poeggeler B. Circadian rhythms, oxidative stress and antioxidative defense mechanisms. Chronobiology International 2003;20(6): 921-962.

[72] Berson DM, Dunn FA, Takao M. Phototransduction by retinal ganglion cells that set the circadian clock. Science 2002;295(5557): 1070-1073.

[73] Iuvone PM, Tosini G, Pozdeyev N, Haque R, Klein DC, Chaurasia SS. Circadian clocks, clock networks, arylalkylamine N acetyltransferase, and melatonin in the retina. Progress in Retinal and Eye Research 2005; 24(4): 433-456.

[74] Conti A, Conconi S, Hertens E, Skwarlo-Sonta K, Markowska M, Maestroni JM. Evidence for melatonin synthesis in mouse and human bone marrow cells. Journal of Pineal Research 2000;28(4): 193-202.

[75] Slominski A, Tobin DJ, Zmijewski MA, Wortsman J, Paus R. Melatonin in the skin: synthesis, metabolism and functions. Trends Endocrinolology & Metabolism 2007;19(1) 17-24.

[76] Lerner AB, Case JD, Takahashi Y, Lee TH, Mori W. Isolation of melatonin, the pineal gland factor that lightens melanocytes. Journal of the American Chemical Society 1958;80(10): 2587-2587.

[77] Reiter RJ. Melatonin: the chemical expression of darkness. Molecular and Cellular Endocrinology 1991;79(1-3): C153-C158.

[78] Reiter RJ. The melatonin rhythm: both a clock and a calendar. Experientia 1993;49(8) 654-664.

[79] Tomas-Zapico C, Coto-Montes A. Melatonina as antioxidant under pathological processes. Recent Patents on Endocrine, Metabolic & Immune Drug Discovery 2007;1: 63-82

[80] Dubocovich ML, Delagrange P, Krause DN, Sugden D, Cardinali DP, Olcese J. International union of basic and clinical pharmacology. LXXV. Nomenclature, classification, and pharmacology of G protein-coupled melatonin receptors. Pharmacological Reviews 2010; 62: 343-380.

[81] Nosjean O, Ferro M, Coge F, Beauverger P, Henlin JM, Lefoulon F, Fauchere JL, Delagrange P, Canet E, Boutin JA. Identification of the melatonin-binding site MT as the quinone reductase 2, Journal of Biological Chemistry 2000;275(40): 31311-31317.

[82] Wiesenberg I, Missbach M, Kahlen JP, Schrader M, Carlberg C. Transcriptional activation of the nuclear receptor RZRα by the pineal gland hormone melatonin and identification of CGP 52608 as a synthetic ligand. Nucleic Acids Research 1995;23(3): 327-333.

[83] Smirnov AN. Nuclear melatonin receptors. Biochemistry 2001;66(1): 19-26.

[84] Dubocovich ML, Delagrange P, Krause DN, Sugden D, Cardinali DP, Olcese J. International union of basic and clinical pharmacology. LXXV. Nomenclature, classification, and pharmacology of G protein-coupled melatonin receptors. Pharmacological Reviews 2010;62(3): 343-380.

[85] Liu T, Borjigin J. N-acetyltransferase is not the ratelimiting enzyme of melatonin synthesis at night. Journal of Pineal Research 2005;39(1): 91-96.

[86] Berson, DM, Dunn FA, Takao M. Phototransduction by retinal ganglion cells that set the circadian clock. Science 2002;295: 1070-1073.

[87] Sugden D. Melatonin biosynthesis in the mammalian pineal gland. Experientia 1989;45(10): 922-932.

[88] Tan DX, Manchester LC, Sanchez-Barcelo E, Mediavilla MD, Reiter RJ. Significance of high levels of endogenous melatonin in mammalian cerebrospinal fluid and in the central nervous system. Current Neuropharmacology 2010;8(3): 162-167.

[89] Cardinali DP, Lynch HJ, Wurtman RJ. Binding of melatonin to human and rat plasma proteins. Endocrinology 1972;91(5): 1213-1218.

[90] Gilad E, Zisapel N. High-affinity binding of melatonin to hemoglobin. Biochemical and Molecular Medicine 1995;56(2): 115-120.

[91] Hirata F, Hayaishi O, Tokuyama T, Senoh S. In vitro and in vitro formation of two new metabolites of melatonin. Journal of Biological Chemistry 1974;249(4):1311-1313.

[92] Tan DX, Manchester LC, Burkhardt S, Sainz RM, Mayo JC, Kohen R, Shohami E, Huo Y-S, Hardeland R, Reiter RJ. N1-acetyl-N2- formyl-5-methoxykynuramine, a biogenic amine and melatonin metabolite, functions as a potent antioxidant. The FASEB Journal 2001; 15(12): 2294-2296.

[93] Ressmeyer AR, Mayo JC, Zelosko V, et al. Antioxidant properties of the melatonin metabolite N1-acetyl-5-methoxykynuramine (AMK): scavenging of free radicals and prevention of protein destruction. Redox Report 2003; 8(4): 205-213.

[94] Acuña-Castroviejo D, Escames G, Leon J, Carazo A, Khaldy H. Mitochondrial regulation by melatonin and its metabolites. Advances in Experimetal Medicine and Biology 2003; 527: 549-557.

[95] Reiter RJ, Tan DX, Gitto E, Sainz RM, Mayo JC, Leon J, Manchester LC, Vijayalaxmi, Kilic E, Kilic U. Pharmacological utility of melatonin in reducing oxidative cellular and molecular damage. Polish Journal of Pharmacology 2004; 56(2): 159-170.

[96] Menendez-Pelaez A, Poeggeler B, Reiter RJ, Barlow-Walden L, Pablos MI, Tan DX. Nuclear localization of melatonin in different mammalian tissues: immunocytochemical and radioimmunoassay evidence. Journal of Cellular Biochemistry 1993;53: 373-382.

[97] Escames G, López A, García JA, García L, Acuña-Castroviejo D, García JJ, López LC. The role of mitochondria in brain aging and the effects of melatonin. Current Neuropharmacology 2010;8(3): 182-193.

[98] García JJ, Reiter RJ, Pié J, Ortiz GG, Cabrera J, Sáinz RM, Acuña-Castroviejo D. Role of pinoline and melatonin in stabilizing hepatic microsomal membranes against oxidative stress. Journal of Bioenergetics and Biomembranes 1999;31(6): 609-616.

[99] Acuña-Castroviejo D, Martin M, Macias M, Escames G, Leon J, Khaldy H, Reiter RJ. Melatonin, mitochondria, and cellular bioenergetics. Journal of Pineal Research 2001;30(2): 65-74.

[100] Antolín I, Rodríguez C, Sáinz RM, Mayo JC, Uría H, Kotler ML, Rodríguez-Colunga MJ, Tolivia D, Menéndez-Peláez A. Neurohormone melatonin prevents cell damage: effect on gene expression for antioxidant enzymes. The FASEB Journal 1996;10(8): 882-890.

[101] Crespo E, Macias M, Pozo D, Escames G, Martin M, Vives F, Guerrero JM, Acuña-Castroviejo D. Melatonin inhibits expression of the inducible NO synthase II in liver and lung and prevents endotoxemia in lipopolysaccharide-induced multiple organ dysfunction syndrome in rats. The FASEB Journal. 1999;13(12): 1537-1546.

[102] Escames G, Leon J, Macias M, Khaldy H, Acuña-Castroviejo D. Melatonin counteracts lipopolysaccharide-induced expression and activity of mitochondrial nitric oxide synthase in rats. The FASEB Journal 2003;17(8): 932–934.

[103] León J, Macías M, Escames G, Camacho E, Khaldy H, Martín M, Espinosa A, Gallo MA, Acuña-Castroviejo D. Structure-related inhibition of calmodulin-dependent neuronal nitric-oxide synthase activity by melatonin and synthetic kynurenines. Molecular Pharmacology 2000;58(5): 967-975.

[104] Liu RY, Zhou JN, van Heerikhuize J, Hofman MA, Swaab DF. Decreased melatonin levels in postmortem cerebrospinal fluid in relation to aging, Alzheimer's disease, and apolipoprotein E-epsilon4/4 genotype. The Journal of Clinical Endocrinology & Metabolism 1999;84(1): 323-327.

[105] SrinivasanV, Spence DW, Pandi-Perumal SR, Brown GM, Cardinali DP. Melatonin in mitochondrial dysfunction and related disorders. International Journal of Alzheimer's Disease 2011: 1-16.

[106] Domínguez-Rodríguez A, Abreu-González P, García MJ, Sanchez J, Marrero F, de Armas-Trujillo D. Decreased nocturnal melatonin levels during acute myocardial infarction. Journal of Pineal Research 2002;33(4): 248-252.

[107] Yaprak M, Altun A, Vardar A, Aktoz M, Ciftci S, Ozbay G. Decreased nocturnal synthesis of melatonin in patients with coronary artery disease. International Journal of Cardiology 2003;89(1): 103-107.

[108] Lenaz G. The mitochondrial production of reactive oxygen species: mechanisms and implications in human pathology. IUBMB Life 2001;52(3-5): 159-164.

[109] Giulivi C, Poderoso JJ, Boveris A. Production of nitric oxide by mitochondria. The Journal of Biological Chemistry 1998;273(18): 11038-11043.

[110] Stamler JS, Singel DJ, Loscalzo, J. Biochemistry of nitric oxide and its redox-activated forms. Science 1992;258(5090): 1898-1902.

[111] Raha S, Robinson BH. Mitochondria, oxygen free radicals, disease and ageing. Trends in Biochemical Sciences 2000;25(10): 502-508.

[112] Droge W. Free radicals in the physiological control of cell function. Physiological Reviews 2002;82(1): 47-95.

[113] Liochev SI, Fridovich I. Mechanism of the peroxidase activity of Cu, Zn superoxide dismutase. Free Radical Biology and Medicine 2010;48(12): 1565-1569.

[114] Chance B, Sies H, Boveris A. Hydroperoxide metabolism in mammalian organs. Physiological Reviews 1979;59(3): 527-605.

[115] Fernandez-Checa JC, Kaplowski N. Hepatic mitochondrial glutathione: transport and role in disease and toxicity. Toxicology and Applied Pharmacology 2005;204(3): 263-273.

[116] Martín M, Macías M, Escames G, Leon J, Acuña-Castroviejo D. Melatonin but not vitamins C and E maintains glutathione homeostasis in t-butyl hydroperoxide-induced mitochondrial oxidative stress. The FASEB Journal 2000;14(12): 1677-1679.

[117] Martín M, Macías M, Escames G, Reiter RJ, Agapito MT, Ortiz GG, Acuña-Castroviejo D. Melatonin-induced increased activity of the respiratory chain complexes I and IV can prevent mitochondrial damage induced by ruthenium red in vivo. Journal of Pineal Research 2000;28(4): 242-248.

[118] Acuña-Castroviejo D, Escames G, Carazo A, Leon J, Khaldy H, Reiter RJ. Melatonin, mitochondrial homeostasis and mitochondrial-related diseases. Current Topics in Medicinal Chemistry 2002;2(2): 133-151.

[119] Kerr J.F.R., Harmon B.V. Definition and incidence of apoptosis: an historical perspective. In: Tomei L.D., Cope F.O. (ed.) Apoptosis: the Molecular Basis of Cell Death. Cold Spring Harbor Laboratory Press, Cold Spring Harbor, NY, 1991. p5-29.

[120] Ren Y, Savill J. Apoptosis: the importance of being eaten. Cell Death & Differentiation; 1998;5(7): 563-568.

[121] Kroemer G, Dallaporta B, Resche-Rigon M. The mitochondrial death/life regulator in apoptosis and necrosis. Annual Review of Physiology 1998;60: 619-642.

[122] Yang J, Liu X, Bhalla K, Kim CN, Ibrado AM, Cai J, Peng TI, Jones DP, Wang X. Prevention of apoptosis by Bcl-2: release of cytochrome c from mitochondria blocked. Science 1997;275(5303): 1129-1132.

[123] Suzuki Y, Imai Y, Nakayama H, Takahashi K, Takio K, Takahashi R. A serine protease, HtrA2, is released from the mitochondria and interacts with XIAP, inducing cell death. Molecular Cell 2001;8(3): 613-621.

[124] Li LY, Luo X, Wang X. Endonuclease G is an apoptotic DNase when released from mitochondria. Nature 2001;412(6842): 95-99.

[125] Halestrap AP, Mcstay GP, Clarke SJ. The permeability transition pore complex: another view. Biochimie 2002;84(2-3): 153-166.

[126] Urata Y, Honma S, Goto S, Todoriki S, Ueda T, Cho S, Honma K, Kondo T. Melatonin induces-glutamylcysteine synthase mediated by activator protein-1 in human vascular endothelial cells. Free Radical Biology & Medicine 1999;27(7-8): 838-847.

[127] Yamamoto HA, Tang HW. Preventive effects of melatonin against cyanide-induced seizures and lipid peroxidation in mice. Neuroscience Letters 1996;207(2): 89-92.

[128] Absi E, Ayala A, Machado A, Parrado J. Protective effect of melatonin against the 1-methyl-4-phenylpyridinium-induced inhibition of Complex I of the mitochondrial respiratory chain. Journal of Pineal Research 2000;29(1): 40-47.

[129] Martín M, Macías M, León J, Escames G, Khaldy H, Acuña-Castroviejo D. Melatonin increases the activity of the oxidative phosphorylation enzymes and the production of ATP in rat brain and liver mitochondria. The International Journal of Biochemistry & Cell Biology 2002;34(4): 348-357.

[130] Reiter RJ, Tan DX, Qi, W, Manchester LC, Karbownik M, Calvo JR. Pharmacology and physiology of melatonin in the reduction of oxidative stress in vivo. Biological Signals and Receptors 2000;9(3-4): 160-171.

[131] Paradies G, Petrosillo G, Paradies V, Reiter RJ, Ruggiero FM. Melatonin, cardiolipin and mitochondrial bioenergetics in health and disease. Journal of Pineal Research 2010;48(4): 297-310.

[132] Pappolla MA, Simovich MJ, Bryant-Thomas T, Chyan Y-J, Poeggeler B, Dubocovich M, Bick R, Perry G, Cruz-Sanchez F, Smith MA. The neuroprotective activities of melatonin against the Alzheimer β-protein are not mediated by melatonin membrane receptors. Journal of Pineal Research 2002;32(3): 135-142.

[133] Antolín I, Mayo JC, Sainz RM, de los Angeles del Brío M, Herrera F, Martín V, Rodríguez C. Protective effect of melatonin in a chronic experimental model of Parkinson's disease. Brain Research 2002;943(2): 163-173.

[134] Sandik R. Pineal melatonin functions: possible relevance to Parkinson's disease. International Journal of Neuroscience 1990;50(1-2): 37-53.

[135] Miller JW, Selhub J, Joseph JA. Oxidative damage caused by free radicals produced during catecholamine autoxidation: protective effects of O-methylation and melatonin. Free Radical Biology & Medicine 1996;21(2): 241-249.

[136] Khaldy H, Escames G, Leon J, Vives F, Luna JD, Acuna-Castroviejo D. Comparative effects of melatonin, L-deprenyl, Trolox and ascorbate in the suppression of hydroxyl radical formation during dopamine autoxidation in vitro. Journal of Pineal Research 2000;29(2): 100-107.

[137] Kim YS, Joo WS, Jin BK, Cho YH, Baik HH, Park CW. Melatonin protects 6-OHDA-induced neuronal death of nigrostriatal dopaminergic system. Neuroreport 1998;9(10): 2387-2390.

[138] Joo WS, Jin BK, Park CW, Maeng SH, Kim YS. Melatonin increases striatal dopaminergic function in 6-OHDA-lesioned rats. NeuroReport 1998;9: 4123-4126.

[139] Ortiz GG, Crespo-Lopez ME, Moran-Moguel C, Garcia JJ, Reiter RJ, Acuna-Castroviejo D. Protective role of melatonin against MPTP-induced mouse brain cell DNA fragmentation and apoptosis in vivo. Neuroendocrinology Letters 2001;22(2): 101-108.

[140] Dabbeni-Sala F, Di Santo S, Franceschini D, Skaper SD, Giusti P. Melatonin protects against 6-OHDA-induced neurotoxicity in rats: a role for mitochondrial complex I activity. The FASEB Journal 2001;15(1): 164-170.

[141] Chetsawang J, Govitrapong P, Chetsawang B. Melatonin inhibits MPP$^+$-induced caspase-mediated death pathway and DNA fragmentation factor-45 cleavage in SK-N-SH cultured cells. Journal of Pineal Research 207;43(2): 115-120.

[142] Khaldy H, Escames G, Leon J, Bikjdaouene L, Acuna-Castroviejo D. Synergistic effects of melatonin and deprenyl against MPTP-induced mitochondrial damage and DA depletion. Neurobiology of Aging 2003;24(3): 491-500.

[143] Chen ST, Chuang JI, Hong MH, Li EI. Melatonin attenuates MPP+-induced neurodegeneration and glutathione impairment in the nigrostriatal dopaminergic pathway. Journal of Pineal Research 2002;32(4): 262-269.

[144] Stull ND, Polan DP, Iacovitti L. Antioxidant compounds protect dopamine neurons from death due to oxidative stress in vitro. Brain Research 2002;931(2): 181-185.

[145] Coulom H, Birman S. Chronic exposure to rotenone models sporadic Parkinson's disease in Drosophila melanogaster. Journal of Neuroscience 2004;24(48):10993-10998.

[146] Mayo JC, Sainz RM, Uria H, Antolin I, Esteban MM, Rodriguez C. Melatonin prevents apoptosis induced by 6-hydroxydopamine in neuronal cells: implications for Parkinson's disease. Journal of Pineal Research 1998; 24(3): 179-192.

[147] Mayo JC, Sainz RM, Antolin I, Rodriguez C. Ultrastructural confirmation of neuronal protection by melatonin against the neurotoxin 6-hydroxydopamine cell damage. Brain Research 1999;818(2): 221-227.

[148] León J, Acuña-Castroviejo D, Escames G, Tan DX, Reiter RJ. Melatonin mitigates mitochondrial malfunction. Journal of Pineal Research 2005;38(1): 1-9.

[149] Adi N, Mash DC, Ali Y, Singer C, Shehadeh L, Papapetropoulos S. Melatonin MT_1 and MT_2 receptor expression in Parkinson's disease. Medical Science Monitor 2010;16(2): BR61-BR67.

[150] Aurora RN, Zak RS, Maganti RK, Auerbach SH, Casey KR, Chowdhuri S, Karippot A, Ramar K, Kristo DA, Morgenthaler TI. Best practice guide for the treatment of REM sleep behavior disorder (RBD). Journal of Clinical Sleep Medicine 2010;6(1): 85-95.

9

Role of Autophagy in Parkinson's Disease

Grace G.Y. Lim, Chengwu Zhang and
Kah-Leong Lim

1. Introduction

Parkinson's disease (PD) is a prevalent neurodegenerative movement disorder whose occurrence crosses geographic, racial and social boundaries affecting 1-2% of the population above the age of 65 (Dorsey et al., 2007). Clinically, the disease is attended by a constellation of motoric deficits that progressively worsen with age, which ultimately leads to near total immobility. Although pathological changes are distributed in the PD brain (Braak et al., 2003), the principal lesion that underlies the characteristic motor phenotype of PD patients is unequivocally the loss of dopaminergic neurons in the *substantia nigra pars compacta* (SNpc) of the midbrain. This neuronal loss results in a severe depletion of striatal dopamine (DA) and thereby an impaired nigrostriatal system that otherwise allows an individual to execute proper, coordinated movements. Accordingly, pharmacological replacement of brain DA via L-DOPA administration represents an effective symptomatic recourse for the patient (especially during the initial stages of the disease) and remains a clinical gold standard treatment for PD. However, neither L-DOPA nor any currently available therapies could slow or stop the insidious degenerative process in the PD brain. Thus, PD remains an incurable disease. Invariably, the debilitating nature and morbidity of the disease present significant healthcare, social, emotional and economic problems. As the world population rapidly ages, these problems undoubtedly would also increase. According to a recent report, more than 4 million individuals in Europe's five most and the world's ten most populous countries are currently afflicted with PD (Dorsey et al., 2007). In less than 20 years' time, the number of PD sufferers is projected to increase to close to 10 million (i.e. in 2030). This is definitely a worrying trend, and one that aptly emphasizes the urgency to develop more effective treatment modalities for the PD patient. Towards this endeavour, a better understanding of the molecular mechanism(s) that underlies the pathogenesis of PD would definitely be helpful, as the illumination of which would allow the identification and therapeutic exploitation of key molecules/events involved in the pathogenic process.

Although a subject of intense research, the etiology of PD unfortunately remains incompletely understood. However, a broad range of studies conducted over the past few decades, including epidemiological, genetic and post-mortem analysis, as well as *in vitro* and *in vivo* modelling, have contributed significantly to our understanding of the pathogenesis of the disease. In particular, the recent identification and functional characterization of several genes, including *α-synuclein, parkin, DJ-1, PINK1* and *LRRK2*, whose mutations are causative of rare familial forms of PD have provided tremendous insights into the molecular pathways underlying dopaminergic neurodegeneration (Lim and Ng, 2009; Martin et al., 2011). Collectively, these studies implicate aberrant protein and mitochondrial homeostasis as key contributors to the development of PD, with oxidative stress likely acting an important nexus between the two pathogenic events.

2. Aberrant protein homeostasis & PD

Perhaps the most glaring evidence suggesting that protein homeostasis has gone awry in the PD brain is the presence of intra-neuronal inclusions, known as Lewy Bodies (LBs), in affected regions of the diseased brain in numbers that far exceed their occasional presence in the normal brain (Lewy, 1912). These signature inclusions of PD comprise of a plethora of protein constituents that include several PD-linked gene products such as α-synuclein, parkin, DJ-1, PINK1 and LRRK2. In a recent report, Wakabayashi and colleagues have documented more than 90 components of the LB and have grouped them into 13 functional groups (Table 1) (Wakabayashi et al., 2012). Among these, α-synuclein is recognized as the major component of LB and thought to be the key initiator of LB biogenesis.

However, whether LB biogenesis represents a cytoprotective or pathogenic mechanism in PD remains debatable. Notwithstanding this, how proteins aggregate to form LB is intriguing in the first place, as the cell is endowed with several complex surveillance machineries to detect and repair faulty proteins, and also destroy those are beyond repair rapidly (Fig. 1). In this surveillance system, the chaperones (comprising of members of the heat-shock proteins) represent the first line of defense in ensuring the correct folding and refolding of proteins (Liberek et al., 2008). When a native folding state could not be attained, the chaperones will direct the misfolded protein for proteolyic removal typically by the proteasome. Proteins that are destined for proteasome-mediated degradation are usually added a chain of ubiquitin via a reaction cascade that involves the ubiquitin-activating (E1), -conjugating (E2) and -ligating (E3) enzymes, whereby successive iso-peptide linkages are formed between the terminal residue (G76) of one ubiquitin molecule and a lysine (K) residue (most commonly K48) within another. The (G76-K48) polyubiquitinated substrate is then recognized by the 26S proteasome as a target for degradation (Pickart and Cohen, 2004). It is noteworthy to mention that although the G76-K48 chain linkage is the most common form of polyubiquitin, ubiquitin self-assembly can occur at any lysine residues within the molecule (at positions 6, 11, 27, 29, 33, 48 and 63)

(Pickart, 2000; Peng et al., 2003). In addition, proteins can also be monoubiquitinated. Notably, both K63-linked polyubiquitination and monoubiquitination of proteins are not typically associated with proteasome-mediated degradation (Pickart, 2000; Peng et al., 2003).

Group	Components	Remarks
1	α-synuclein; Neurofilaments	Structural Elements
2	Agrin; 14-3-3; Synphilin-1; Tau	α-synuclein-binding proteins
3	Dorfin; GSK-3β; NUB1; Parkin; Pin1; SIAH-1	Synphilin-1-binding proteins
4	Ubiquitin; E1; UbcH7; TRAF6; TRIM9; Proteasome subunits; PA700; PA28; β-TrCP; Cullin-1; HDAC4; NEDD8; p38; p62 (Sequestosome 1); ROC1; UCHL1	UPS-related proteins
5	LC3; GABARAP; GATE-16; Glucocerebrosidase; NBR-1	Autophagosome-lysosome system
6	γ-tubulin; HDAC6; Peri-centrin	Aggresome-related proteins
7	DJ-1; CHIP; Clusterin/apolipoprotein J; DnaJB6; Heat Shock Proteins; Torsin A; SOD1 & 2; FOXO3a	Stress response-related proteins
8	CaMKII; Casein Kinase II; CDK5, G-Protein Coupled Receptor Kinase 5; LRRK2; PINK1; IκBα; NFκB; p35; phospho-lipase C-δ; Tissue Transglutaminase	Signal transduction-related proteins
9	MAP1B; MAP2; Sept4/H5	Cytoskeletal proteins
10	Cox IV; Cytochrome C; Omi/HtrA2	Mitochondria-related proteins
11	Cyclin B; Retinoblastoma Protein	Cell cycle proteins
12	Amyloid Precursor Protein; Calbindin; Choline Acetyltransferase; Chromogranin A; Synaptophysin; Synaptotagmin; Tyrosine Hydroxylase; VMAT2	Cytosolic Proteins
13	Complement Proteins; Immunoglobulin	Immune-related proteins

Table 1. Components of Lewy Body (Wakabayashi et al., 2012)

Whilst the coupling of chaperone and ubiquitin protein system (UPS) provides an efficient way for the cell to deal with protein misfolding, there are times when the capacity of these systems may be exceeded by the production of misfolded proteins (e.g. under conditions of cellular stress). In such cases, aggregation-prone proteins that failed to be degraded may be transported along microtubules in a retrograde fashion to the microtubule organizing center to form an "aggresome", a term originally coined by Johnston and Kopito more than a decade ago (Johnston et al., 1998). According to the model, aggresome formation represents a cellular response towards proteasome impairments and their localization to the juxta-nuclear region is to facilitate their capture by lysosomes and thereby their clearance by macroautophagy (hereafter referred to as autophagy). Consistent with this, aggregation-prone proteins often generate aggresome-like structures when ectopically expressed in cultured cells in the presence of proteasome inhibition (Wong et al., 2008). Moreover, several groups including ours have demonstrated that autophagy induction promotes the clearance of aggresomes whereas the reverse is true when the bulk degradation system is inhibited (Fortun et al., 2003; Iwata et al., 2005b; Opazo et al., 2008; Wong et al., 2008).

Together, the chaperone, ubiquitin-proteasome and autophagy systems thus function in synergism to effectively counterbalance the threat of protein misfolding and aggregation. Accordingly, aberrations in one or more of these systems would be expected to promote protein aggregation and inclusion body formation, as in the case of affected neurons in the PD brain where LBs occur.

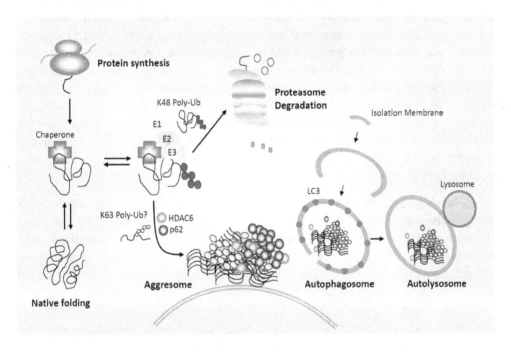

Figure 1. Schematic depiction of the collaboration among the chaperone, ubiquitin-proteasome and autophagy systems in the maintenance of intracellular protein homeostasis.

3. Biogenesis of Lewy bodies – An aggresome-related process reflecting failed autophagy?

As mentioned earlier, α-synuclein is a major component of LBs, suggesting that aberrant α-synuclein homeostasis contributes to the biogenesis of these inclusion bodies in the PD brain. The presynaptic terminal-enriched α-synuclein protein is an interesting molecule in that it is typically unfolded (or intrinsically disordered) in its native state, although the protein is extremely sensitive to its environment and can be moulded into an assortment of structurally unrelated conformations including a fibrillization-prone partially folded structure as well as various α-helical and β-sheet species occurring in both monomeric and oligomeric states (Uversky, 2007). Along with this conformation flexibility, α-synuclein also tends to misfold and becomes aggregated in the process. PD-associated mutations, including missense substitutions (A53T, A30P and E46K), duplication or triplication are known to enhance α-synuclein accumulation and aggregation (Giasson et al., 1999; Narhi et al., 1999; Conway et al., 2000; Uversky, 2007). Further, several groups have demonstrated in different experimental models that various exogenous neurotoxicants linked to PD, including pesticides, herbicides and metal ions, significantly accelerate the aggregation of α-synuclein (Manning-Bog et al., 2002; Uversky et al., 2002; Sherer et al., 2003). Not surprisingly, α-synuclein accumulation and aggregation can lead to impairments of the chaperone and UPS systems [For a recent review, see (Tan et al., 2009)]. Under such conditions, the isolation of α-synuclein aggregates into an aggresome would represent an alternative way by which the protein could be cleared, i.e. via autophagy. Indeed, emerging evidence suggest that LB biogenesis may be an aggresome-related process (Olanow et al., 2004). Because the protofibrillar, oligomeric forms of α-synuclein are thought to be more toxic than fibrillar, aggregated α-synuclein species, aggresome formation may also be regarded as a "protective" response that serves as a trap to immobilize soluble toxic forms of α-synuclein. However, this process has to be coupled to the active removal of the aggresomes by autophagy, as the unregulated growth of an inclusion body could conceivably affect cellular functions, physically or otherwise.

The relevance of aggresome formation to LB biogenesis in PD is exemplified by their striking similarities to each other in terms of structural organization, protein composition and intracellular localization (Olanow et al., 2004). For example, aggresome-related proteins such as γ-tubulin and HDAC6 can be found in LB (Table 1). HDAC6 plays an important role during aggresome formation by facilitating the retrograde transport of ubiquitinated misfolded proteins along the microtubule network to the γ-tubulin-positive MTOC by the dynein motor complex (Kawaguchi et al., 2003). Moreover, LBs are also immunopositive for p62 and NBR1, which are autophagy adapter proteins capable of binding to ubiquitinated substrates and the autophagosome protein LC3 (Bjorkoy et al., 2005; Pankiv et al., 2007; Kirkin et al., 2009). By virtue of this binding property, p62 and NBR1 may provide a link between aggresome-related proteins and their clearance by the autophagy machinery. Interestingly, all the three ubiquitin-binding autophagy receptors, i.e. p62, HDAC6 and NBR1, show preference for K63-linked polyubiquitin chains (Olzmann et al., 2007; Tan et al., 2008a; Kirkin et al., 2009), suggesting that this form of ubiquitin modification may underlie the formation as well as autophagic degradation of protein aggregates. Consistent with this, we found that K63-linked ubiquitination promotes the formation of inclusion bodies associated with PD and other neurodegenerative diseases and importantly, acts as a cargo selection signal for their subsequent removal by autophagy (Tan et al., 2008a; Tan et al., 2008b). As per our original proposal (Lim et al., 2006), it is tempting to think that the cell may switch to an alternative, proteasome-independent form of ubiquitination under conditions of proteasome-related stress that could help divert cargo proteins away from an otherwise overloaded proteasome. All these would culminate to the ultimate clearance of these proteins by autophagy (Fig. 1).

What remains curious about LB biogenesis is that it apparently takes place in the presence of constitutive autophagy, which is a characteristic of post-mitotic neurons (Wong and Cuervo, 2010). Moreover, α-synuclein is itself a substrate for autophagy (Webb et al., 2003).

Although α-synuclein can also be degraded by the proteasome, the aggregates of which appear to be preferentially cleared by the autophagy system (Petroi et al., 2012). Consistent with this, autophagy is recruited as the primary removal system in transgenic mice over-expressing oligomeric species of α-synuclein (Ebrahimi-Fakhari et al., 2011). Further, the protein can also be removed via chaperone-mediated autophagy (CMA), a specialized form of lysosomal degradation by which proteins containing a particular pentapeptide motif related to KFERQ are transported across the lysosomal membrane via the action of the integral membrane protein LAMP-2A and both cytosolic and lumenal hsc70 (Klionsky et al., 2011). Notably, the intralysosomal level of α-synuclein is significantly increased along with LAMP-2A and hsc70 in mice treated with the herbicide paraquat (which induces parkinsonism) or expressing α-synuclein as a transgene (Mak et al., 2010). Thus in theory, the level of α-synuclein, whether present as soluble or aggregated species, should be effectively managed in neurons under normal conditions or even when they are undergoing stress. Indeed, even in the PD brain, LB takes a significant length of time to develop. Given this, and that the autophagy system arguably represents the final line of cellular defense against the buildup of protein aggregates, the simplest explanation that could account for the presence of LB in PD is that the autophagy system has either become suboptimal in its function or is otherwise impaired altogether during the disease pathogenesis process.

4. Autophagy and PD

Morphological evidence of autophagic vacuole (AV) accumulation is certainly evident in PD as well as in several other neurodegenerative disorders (Anglade et al., 1997). However, whether the phenomenon represents attempts by the neuron to clean up its cobwebs of aggregated proteins, or a prelude to cell death, or simply a failure in AV consumption remains poorly understood. Notwithstanding this, two elegant studies conducted in 2006 aptly illustrated the importance of competent autophagy function to neuronal homeostasis (Hara et al., 2006; Komatsu et al., 2006). By means of targeted genetic disruption of essential components of the autophagy process (Atg5 or Atg7), these studies demonstrated that ablation of autophagy function in neural cells of mice results in extensive neurodegeneraion that is accompanied by widespread inclusion pathology, suggesting that autophagy failure can precipitate protein aggregation and subsequent cell death in affected neurons.

Supporting a role for failed autophagy in PD in the face of α-synuclein accumulation, α-synuclein was recently demonstrated to inhibit autophagy when over-expressed, both *in vitro* and *in vivo* (Winslow et al., 2010). The inhibition apparently occurs at a very early stage of autophagosome formation, which is likely a result of disrupted localization and mobilization of Atg9, a multi-spanning membrane protein whose associated vesicles are important sources of membranes for the synthesis of early autophagosomes (Yamamoto et al., 2012). Interesting, the reverse, i.e. autophagy enhancement, was observed when α-synuclein is depleted via RNAi-mediated knockdown (Winslow et al., 2010), suggesting that the protein might play a regulatory role in the synthesis of autophagosome. Moreover, targeted disruption of autophagy (via *Atg7* deletion) in midbrain dopaminergic neurons results in abnormal presynaptic accumulation of α-synuclein that is accompanied by dendritic and axonal dystrophy, reduced striatal DA content, and the formation of somatic and dendritic ubiquitinated inclusions (Friedman et al., 2012). Significant age-dependent loss of nigral dopaminergic neurons were also recorded in these *Atg7* conditionally knockout mice (*Atg7*-cKO[TH]), with 9 month old *Atg7*-cKO[TH] mice exhibiting about 40% reduction in the number of SN neurons that is accompanied by markedly decreased spontaneous motor activity and coordination relative to controls (Friedman et al., 2012). Together, these results suggest that failure in autophagy function precipitates inclusions formation in dopaminergic neurons that leads to their demise.

Besides macroautophagy, α-synuclein can also affect the function of CMA. For example, disease-associated α-synuclein mutants bind to the CMA lysosomal receptor with high affinity but are poorly translocated, resulting in the blockage of uptake and degradation of CMA substrates (Cuervo et al., 2004). The increase in cytosolic α-synuclein levels that ensued could favour its aggregation and concomitantly, amplify the burden of misfolded protein load for the cell. Interestingly, DA modification of α-synuclein also impairs CMA-mediated degradation by a similar mechanism (Martinez-Vicente et al., 2008). In this case, membrane-bound DA-α-synuclein monomers appear to seed the formation of oligomeric complexes, which consequently placed the translocation complex under siege. Consistent with this, CMA inhibition following L-DOPA treatment is more pronounced in ventral midbrain cultures containing dopaminergic neurons than in non-DA producing cortical neurons. Importantly, α-synuclein appears to be the principal mediator of DA-induced blockage of CMA, as ventral midbrain cultures derived from α-synuclein null mice are relatively spared from the inhibitory effects of DA on CMA (Martinez-Vicente et al., 2008). More recently, Malkus and Ischiropoulos demonstrated that CMA activity in the adult brain of A53T α-synuclein-expressing transgenic mice varies across different regions, with brain regions vulnerable to α-synuclein aggregation displaying marked deficiencies in CMA (Malkus and Ischiropoulos, 2012). Their results support an integral role for the lysosome in maintaining α-synuclein homeostasis and at the same time, provides an explanation to why certain brain regions are vulnerable to inclusion formation and cellular dysfunction while others are spared.

Perhaps the most direct evidence linking lysosomal dysfunction to PD is the demonstration that loss-of-function mutations in a gene encoding for the lysosomal P-type ATPase named ATP13A2 cause a juvenile and early-onset form of parkinsonism that is also characterized by pyramidal degeneration and dementia (Ramirez et al., 2006). In patient-derived fibroblasts as well as in ATP13A2-silenced primary mouse neurons, deficient ATPase function results in impaired lysosomal degradation capacity that concomitantly enhanced the accumulation and toxicity of α-synuclein (Usenovic et al., 2012). Importantly, silencing of endogenous α-synuclein ameliorated the toxicity in neurons depleted of ATP13A2, suggesting that ATP13A2-induced parkinsonism may be contributed by α-synuclein accumulation amid functional impairments of the lysosome. Supporting this, overexpression of wild type ATP13A2 suppresses α-synuclein-mediated toxicity in *C. elegans* while knockdown of ATP13A2 expression promotes the accumulation of misfolded α-synuclein in the animal (Rappley et al., 2009). Together, these studies demonstrate a functional link between ATP13A2-related lysosomal dysfunction and α-synuclein in promoting neurodegeneration.

Besides *α-synuclein* and *ATP13A2*, several other PD-linked genes have also been associated directly or indirectly with the autophagic process. For example, emerging evidence suggest that mutations in LRRK2 promote dysregulation in autophagy, although the role of LRRK2 in controlling autophagy-lysosome pathway is likely to be complex (discussed further in section 6). In the case of parkin, which has the ability to promote K63-linked ubiquitination, we and others have shown that the ubiquitin ligase is involved in aggresome formation and thereby their removal via autophagy (at least indirectly) (Lim et al., 2005; Olzmann et al., 2007). Consistent with its role as an "aggresome-promoter", parkin-related cases are frequently (although not exclusively) devoid of classic LBs, as revealed by a number of autopsy studies (Takahashi et al., 1994; Mori et al., 1998; Hayashi et al., 2000). In recent years, the attention to parkin-autophagy axis has however shifted towards its ability to remove damaged mitochondria via a specialized form of autophagy known as "mitophagy", a term originally coined by Lemasters (Lemasters, 2005). Accordingly, impairment in mitochondrial quality control due to failed mitophagy in parkin-deficient neurons is now thought to be a key mechanism that predisposes them to degeneration.

5. Mitophagy and PD

A role for mitochondria dysfunction in the pathogenesis of PD has long been appreciated. Through post-mortem analysis performed as early as 1989, several groups have recorded a significant reduction in the activity of mitochondrial complex I as well as ubiquinone (co-enzyme Q10) in the SN of PD brains (Schapira et al., 1989; Shults et al., 1997; Keeney et al., 2006). Moreover, mitochondrial poisoning recapitulates PD features in humans and represents a popular strategy to model the disease in animals (Dauer and Przedborski, 2003). Similarly, impairment of mitochondrial homeostasis via genetic ablation of TFAM, a mitochondrial transcription factor, in dopaminergic neurons of mice (named MitoPark mouse) results in energy crisis and neurodegeneration (Sterky et al., 2011).

Rather than being solitary and static structures as depicted in many textbooks, mitochondria are now recognized to be dynamic and mobile organelles that constantly undergo membrane remodeling through repeated cycles of fusion and fission as well as regulated turnover via mitophagy. These processes help to maintain a steady pool of healthy mitochondrial essential for energy production and beyond (e.g. calcium homeostasis). Following the seminal discovery by Youle group that identified parkin as a key mammalian regulator of mitophagy (Narendra et al., 2008), intensive research is now focused on elucidating the precise mechanism underlying parkin-mediated mitophagy and whether impaired clearance of damaged mitochondria may trigger the demise of dopaminergic neurons in the PD brain.

Mechanistically, the picture regarding parkin-mediated mitophagy that has emerged thus far is depicted in Figure 2.

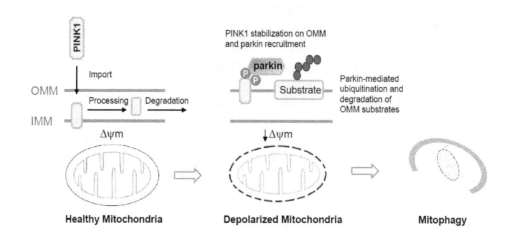

Figure 2. Model of Parkin/PINK1-mediated mitophagy

In this model, another PD-linked gene known as PINK1, which is a mitochondrial serine/ threonine kinase, collaborate closely with parkin to bring about the mitophagy process. Briefly, a key initial event that occurs upon mitochondrial depolarization is the selective accumulation of PINK1 in the outer membrane of the damaged organelle. Normally, PINK1 accumulation in healthy mitochondria is prevented by the sequential proteolytic actions of mitochondrial processing peptidase (MPP) and presenilin-associated rhomboid-like protease (PARL) that rapidly cleaves the protein to generate an unstable 53 kDa PINK1 species that is usually degraded by the proteasome or by an unknown "proteasome-like" protease (Becker et al., 2012; Greene et al., 2012). In depolarized mitochondria, PINK1 stabilization on the outer membrane enables the protein to recruit parkin to the organelle, a process that is apparently dependent on PINK1 autophosphorylation at Ser228 and Ser402 (Okatsu et al., 2012). Once recruited onto the mitochondria, parkin becomes activated and promotes the ubiquitination and subsequent degradation of many outer membrane proteins (Chan et al., 2011; Yoshii et al., 2011) including the pro-fusion mitofusin proteins (Poole et al., 2010; Ziviani et al., 2010), the elimination of which is thought to prevent unintended fusion events involving damaged mitochondria and thereby their re-entry into undamaged mitochondrial network from occurring. Mitophagy induction then occurs, which likely involves parkin-mediated K63 ubiquitination that will help recruit the autophagy adaptors HDAC6 and p62 that subse-quently lead to mitochondrial clustering around the peri-nucleus region. By virtue of their association with the autophagy process, the concerted actions of p62 and HDAC6 will presumably facilitate the final removal of damaged mitochondria by the lysosome (Ding et al., 2010; Geisler et al., 2010; Lee et al., 2010). However, a recent study from Mizushima's lab revealed that the initial cargo recognition step of mitophagy does not involves the interaction between LC3 and the adaptor molecules. Rather, parkin recruitment on the mitochondria induces the formation of ULK1 (Atg1) puncta and Atg9 structures (Itakura et al., 2012). Because ULK1 complex functions as an essential upstream nucleation step of the hierachical autophagy cascade, their results suggest that mitophagosome is generated in a de novo fashion on

damaged mitochondria. Autophagosomal LC3 is however important for the efficient incor-
poration of damaged mitochondria into the autophagosome at a later stage. Notwithstanding
this, how parkin participates in the de novo synthesis of isolation membrane awaits further
clarifications. Interestingly, the whole mitophagy process bears striking resemblance to the
formation and autophagic clearance of aggresomes. Indeed, we have termed the mitochondrial
clustering phenomenon as (formation of) "mito-aggresomes" (Lee et al., 2010). Importantly,
several groups, including ours, have demonstrated that PD-associated parkin mutants are
defective in supporting mitophagy due to distinct problem at recognition, transportation or
ubiquitination of impaired mitochondria (Lee et al., 2010; Matsuda et al., 2010), thereby
implicating dysfunctional mitophagy in the development of parkin-related parkinsonism.

Given the pivotal role of parkin/PINK1 pathway in mitochondrial quality control, it is perhaps
not surprising to note that deficiency in parkin or PINK1 function results in the accumulation
of abnormal mitochondria in several parkin/PINK1-related PD models. This defect is perhaps
most prominently observed in *Drosophila* parkin or PINK1 mutants, especially in their flight
musculature, which is plagued by pronounced mitochondrial lesions and muscle degeneration
(Greene et al., 2003; Clark et al., 2006; Park et al., 2006; Wang et al., 2007). Importantly, parkin
over expression in pink1-/- flies significantly ameliorates all the mutant phenotypes, although
the reverse, does not happen, i.e. pink1 over expression in parkin null flies does not compensate
for the loss of parkin function. These results suggest that parkin acts in the same pathway but
downstream of pink1 (Clark et al., 2006; Park et al., 2006). The hierachy is consistent with the
proposed model of parkin/PINK1 pathway in the regulation of mitochondrial quality control,
although parkin in this case can apparently do the job in the complete absence of pink1.
Notably, several other studies also suggested that mitophagy can take place in a PINK1-
deficient background (Dagda et al., 2009; Cui et al., 2010; Dagda et al., 2011). Conversely, Seibler
and colleagues found PINK1 to be essential for parkin-mediated mitophagy. They demonstrated that parkin recruitment to depolarized mitochondria is impaired in human dopaminergic neurons derived via the induced pluripotent stem cells route from PINK1-related PD
patients, a defect that can be rescued by the re-introduction of wild-type PINK1 into PINK1-
deficient neurons (Seibler et al., 2011).

As with the case with virtually all the biological models initially proposed, the parkin/PINK1
mitophagy model is currently less than perfect and clearly needs be continually updated with
each new piece of significant data. The relevance of mitophagy to sporadic PD is also debatable,
although we and others have previously shown that parkin dysfunction (presumably triggering mitophagy deficiency) may also underlie the pathogenesis of sporadic PD (Pawlyk et al.,
2003; LaVoie et al., 2005; Wang et al., 2005a). Perhaps one of most challenging tasks at hand is
to demonstrate unequivocally that mitophagy impairment, instead of a generalized impairment in the autophagy process, contributes directly to neurodegeneration *in vivo*. This would
require the genetic differentiation of targeted components that are exclusively involved in
mitophagy. Currently, key components of mitophagy and autophagy tend to overlap. Even
parkin appear to subserve both types of autophagy processes (and more). Thus, although
mitochondrial quality control is invariably important for neuronal survival, whether failure
in the removal of damaged mitochondria is in itself a driver of disease pathogenesis or is a

consequence of a progressive and general decline in autophagy function in the PD brain remains to be clarified.

6. Autophagy induction as therapeutic strategy for PD?

If failure in autophagy function were to underlie PD pathogenesis, it follows intuitively that stimulation of autophagy in the PD brain might be beneficial for the patient. Indeed, work from Rubinsztein lab and others have demonstrated that autophagy enhancement promotes beneficial outcomes in several experimental models of PD, supporting that such an approach could represent a viable therapeutic strategy (Rubinsztein et al., 2012).

Notably, most neurodegenerative disease-associated proteins, including α-synuclein, that are prone to aggregation are substrates of autophagy. Accordingly, pharmacological or genetic enhancement of autophagy can in theory help remove these aggregation-prone proteins and concomitantly reduce their associated toxicity. Rapamycin, an inducer of mTOR (mammalian Target of Rapamycin), is widely established to be a potent autophagy inducer. Expectedly, rapamycin treatment of cellular or animal models of α-synucleinopathies reduces the levels of both soluble and aggregated species of α-synuclein in an autophagy-dependent manner (Crews et al., 2010). Similarly, trehalose also accelerates the clearance of α-synuclein by means of its ability to induce autophagy, albeit in an mTOR-independent manner (Sarkar et al., 2007). Further, trehalose-treated cells are protected against subsequent pro-apoptotic insults. Together, trehalose and rapamycin exert an additive effect in the clearance of aggregate-prone proteins (Sarkar et al., 2007). Perhaps unsurprisingly, rapamycin can also rescue failed mitophagy in parkin deficient cells and result in improved mitochondrial function (Siddiqui et al., 2012), suggesting that generalized autophagy activation can help clean up all the cellular "cobwebs" be it protein aggregates or damaged organelles. More recently, Steele and colleagues showed that latrepirdine, a neuroactive compound associated with enhanced cognition and neuroprotection, also stimulates the degradation of α-synuclein and concomitantly protects against α-synuclein-induced toxicity in 3 model systems: yeast, differentiated SH-SY5Y cells and wild type mouse (Steele et al., 2012). The beneficial effects of latrepirdine again appear to be related to autophagy induction, as evident by the elevation of several autophagy markers in mouse brain following chronic administration of the compound. Using a genetic approach, Spencer and colleagues demonstrated via lentivirus-mediated gene transfer of beclin 1, a key promoter of autophagy, that genetic enhancement of autophagy in α-synuclein overexpressing mice ameliorates the synaptic and dendritic pathology in these transgenic animals and reduces the accumulation of the protein *in vivo* (Spencer et al., 2009). Taken together, these studies support the therapeutic applications of autophagy induction in PD, particularly in preventing the accumulation of α-synuclein.

Notwithstanding the above promising findings regarding the protective effects of autophagy induction, it is important to recognize that autophagy induction is a "double-edge sword" that can cut both ways, i.e. being protective or pro-death under different conditions. One therefore have to consider this caveat in considering autophagy induction as a therapeutic strategy for PD. Notably, the parkinsonian neurotoxin MPP+ that induces selective loss of dopaminergic neurons has been demonstrated by several groups to activate autophagy (Zhu et al., 2007; Xilouri et al., 2009; Wong et al., 2011), a process that appears to act through the dephosphorylation of LC3 (which enhances its recruitment into autophagosomes) (Cherra et al., 2010) and/or CDK5-mediated phosphorylation of endophilin B1 (which promotes its dimerization and recruitment of the UVRAG/Beclin 1 complex to induce autophagy) (Wong et al., 2011). In this case, autophagy induction is apparently harmful to dopaminergic neurons. Moreover, stimulation of autophagy also contributes to neuronal death induced by overexpression of α-synuclein (Xilouri et al., 2009). Conversely, inhibition of autophagy pharmacologically with 3-methylalanine (3-MA) or genetically via Atg5 or Atg12 gene silencing significantly attenuates neuronal loss associated with MPP + treatment or mutant α-synuclein expression, as is the case with knockdown of CDK5 or endophilin B1 (Wong et al., 2011). Along these lines, we found that mutant α-synuclein-associated toxicity is aggravated by the accumulation of iron, which act together to trigger autophagic cell death. The toxicity that α-synuclein-iron elicits can be ameliorated by pharmacological inhibition of autophagy (Chew et al., 2011). Interestingly, autophagy activation elicited by mutant α-synuclein overexpression can also result in excessive mitophagy and thereby unintended loss of mitochondria, which in turn promotes bioenergetics deficit and neuronal degeneration (Choubey et al., 2011). Further supporting a "pathological" role for autophagy, loss of DJ-1 function associated with recessive parkinsonism has been found to increase (instead of decrease) autophagic flux, although it is currently unclear how this relates to neuronal death in the context of DJ-1 deficiency (Irrcher et al., 2010).

Finally, mutations in LRRK2, which currently represent the most prevalent genetic contributor to PD, are also implicated in aberrant autophagy induction. For example, transgenic mice expressing disease-associated LRRK2 mutants (R1441C and G2019S) frequently exhibit increased incidence of autophagic vacuoles in their brain (Ramonet et al., 2011). Similarly, cells expressing G2019S LRRK2 mutant show increase autophagosome content and autophagy-dependent shortening of neurites (Plowey et al., 2008). Conversely, ablation of LRRK2 in mice promotes impairment of the autophagy pathway as evident by the accumulation of p62, lipofuscin granules, ubiquitinated proteins and α-synuclein-positive inclusions in their kidneys (Tong et al., 2010). The relationship between LRRK2 and autophagy is however complicated. For example, Gomez-Suaga and colleagues have recently demonstrated that LRRK2-induced accumulation of autophagosome is related to the ability of the kinase to activate a calcium-dependent protein kinase kinase-beta (CaMKK-beta)/adenosine monophosphate (AMP)-activated protein kinase (AMPK) pathway via modulation of NAADP-dependent Ca^{2+} channel on lysosomal membrane (Gomez-Suaga et al., 2012). However, they also detected at the same time a reduction in the acidification of lysosomes that can compromise autophagosome turnover and thereby autophagy (Gomez-Suaga et al., 2012), suggesting that autophagy is actually impaired rather than activated in LRRK2-expressing cells. Consistent with this, another study revealed that the expression of LRRK2 R1441C mutant leads to impaired autophagic balance that is characterized by AV accumulation containing incompletely degraded materials and increased levels of p62 (Alegre-Abarrategui et al., 2009).

Accordingly, siRNA-mediated knockdown of LRRK2 expression results in increased autophagic activity and prevented cell death caused by inhibition of autophagy in starvation
conditions. Thus, the precise role of autophagy in LRRK2-related parkinsonism is anybody's
guess at this moment, begging again caution in the proposed use of autophagy inducers as a
therapeutic recourse.

In a related development, we recently found that disease-associated LRRK2 G2019S mutant
can trigger marked mitochondrial abnormalities when overexpressed in *Drosophila*, a phenotype that can be rescued by parkin co-expression (Ng et al., 2012). Given the role of parkin in
promoting mitophagy, it is tempting to speculate that the LRRK2 mutant may retard the
clearance of damaged mitochondria via mitophagy in the absence of parkin overexpression.
Indeed, the mitochondrial phenotype LRRK2 G2019S mutant induces in the flight muscle is
reminiscent of that brought about by the loss of parkin function. Alternatively, this could also
be a result of LRRK2-induced impairment in autophagy in general. Importantly, we further
found that pharmacological or genetic activation of AMPK can effectively compensate for
parkin deficiency to bring about a significant suppression of dopaminergic and mitochondrial
dysfunction in mutant LRRK2 flies (Ng et al., 2012). Our results suggest a neuroprotective role
for AMPK that might be related to mitophagy/autophagy modulation. AMPK is an evolutio-
narily conserved cellular energy sensor that is activated by ATP depletion or glucose starvation
(Hardie, 2011). When activated, AMPK switches the cell from an anabolic to a catabolic mode
and in so doing, helps to regulate diverse cellular processes that impact on cellular energy
demands. Interestingly, like parkin, AMPK can also regulate mitophagy and also autophagy
through its ability to phosphorylate the autophagy initiator ATG1 (Egan et al., 2011; Kim et
al., 2011). Lending relevance to our findings, a recent report demonstrated that AMPK is
activated in mice treated with MPTP and that inhibition of AMPK function by compound C
enhances MPP(+)-induced cell death (Choi et al., 2010). More recently, a PD cohort-based study
revealed that Metformin-inclusive sulfonylurea therapy reduces the risk for the disease
occurring with Type 2 diabetes in a Taiwanese population (Wahlqvist et al., 2012). Metformin
is a direct activator of AMPK. Together, these findings suggest that AMPK activation may
protect against the development of PD, presumably via its ability to maintain energy balance
via the modulation of autophagy as well as a range of other cellular processes. Given that
caveats associated with direct autophagy induction, and that excessive autophagy can result
in energy crisis especially in the aged brain, perhaps AMPK activation, through its ability to
maintain both protein and energy homeostasis, would represent a better approach than direct
autophagy induction as a therapeutic strategy for PD.

7. Conclusion

In essence, the case for autophagy dysfunction as a contributor to the pathogenesis of PD is
rather compelling. As evident from the above discussion, virtually all the major PD-associated
gene products have some direct or indirect relationship with the autophagy-lysosome axis.
What is less clear is whether autophagy induction is neuroprotective or is a key driver of
neurodegeneration. One can envisage that the activation of autophagy may be beneficial in

the short term (particularly when the induction is transient and timely), but deleterious when it is becomes chronic or excessive. Finding the tipping autophagy threshold point between neuroprotection and neurodegeneration would therefore be an important endeavour, the clarification of which has important implications for the future development of autophagy-related therapeutics for the PD patient.

Acknowledgements

This work was supported by grants from Singapore Millennium Foundation, National Medical Research Council and A*STAR Biomedical Research Council (LKL). G.L. is supported by a graduate scholarship from the Singapore Millennium Foundation.

Author details

Grace G.Y. Lim[1], Chengwu Zhang[2] and Kah-Leong Lim[1,2,3]

1 Department of Physiology, National University of Singapore, Singapore

2 National Neuroscience Institute, Singapore

3 Duke-NUS Graduate Medical School, Singapore

References

[1] Alegre-abarrategui, J, Christian, H, Lufino, M. M, Mutihac, R, Venda, L. L, Ansorge, O, & Wade-martins, R. (2009). LRRK2 regulates autophagic activity and localizes to specific membrane microdomains in a novel human genomic reporter cellular model. Hum Mol Genet , 18, 4022-4034.

[2] Anglade, P, Vyas, S, Javoy-agid, F, Herrero, M. T, Michel, P. P, Marquez, J, Mouatt-prigent, A, Ruberg, M, Hirsch, E. C, & Agid, Y. (1997). Apoptosis and autophagy in nigral neurons of patients with Parkinson's disease. Histol Histopathol , 12, 25-31.

[3] Becker, D, Richter, J, Tocilescu, M. A, Przedborski, S, & Voos, W. (2012). Pink1 kinase and its membrane potential (Deltapsi)-dependent cleavage product both localize to outer mitochondrial membrane by unique targeting mode. J Biol Chem , 287, 22969-22987.

[4] Bjorkoy, G, Lamark, T, Brech, A, Outzen, H, Perander, M, Overvatn, A, Stenmark, H, & Johansen, T. forms protein aggregates degraded by autophagy and has a protec-tive effect on huntingtin-induced cell death. J Cell Biol , 171, 603-614.

[5] Braak, H. Del Tredici K, Rub U, de Vos RA, Jansen Steur EN, Braak E ((2003). Staging of brain pathology related to sporadic Parkinson's disease. Neurobiol Aging , 24, 197-211.

[6] Chan, N. C, Salazar, A. M, Pham, A. H, Sweredoski, M. J, Kolawa, N. J, Graham, R. L, Hess, S, & Chan, D. C. (2011). Broad activation of the ubiquitin-proteasome system by Parkin is critical for mitophagy. Hum Mol Genet , 20, 1726-1737.

[7] Cherra, S. J. rd, Kulich SM, Uechi G, Balasubramani M, Mountzouris J, Day BW, Chu CT ((2010). Regulation of the autophagy protein LC3 by phosphorylation. J Cell Biol , 190, 533-539.

[8] Chew, K. C, Ang, E. T, Tai, Y. K, Tsang, F, Lo, S. Q, Ong, E, Ong, W. Y, Shen, H. M, Lim, K. L, Dawson, V. L, Dawson, T. M, & Soong, T. W. (2011). Enhanced autophagy from chronic toxicity of iron and mutant A53T alpha-synuclein: implications for neuronal cell death in Parkinson disease. J Biol Chem , 286, 33380-33389.

[9] Choi, J. S, Park, C, & Jeong, J. W. (2010). AMP-activated protein kinase is activated in Parkinson's disease models mediated by 1-methyl-4-phenyl-1,2,3,6-tetrahydropyridine. Biochem Biophys Res Commun , 391, 147-151.

[10] Choubey, V, Safiulina, D, Vaarmann, A, Cagalinec, M, Wareski, P, Kuum, M, Zharkovsky, A, & Kaasik, A. induces neuronal death by increasing mitochondrial autophagy. J Biol Chem , 286, 10814-10824.

[11] Clark, I. E, Dodson, M. W, Jiang, C, Cao, J. H, Huh, J. R, Seol, J. H, Yoo, S. J, Hay, B. A, & Guo, M. (2006). Drosophila pink1 is required for mitochondrial function and interacts genetically with parkin. Nature , 441, 1162-1166.

[12] Conway, K. A, Lee, S. J, Rochet, J. C, Ding, T. T, Williamson, R. E, & Lansbury, P. T. Jr. ((2000). Acceleration of oligomerization, not fibrillization, is a shared property of both alpha-synuclein mutations linked to early-onset Parkinson's disease: implications for pathogenesis and therapy. Proc Natl Acad Sci U S A , 97, 571-576.

[13] Crews, L, Spencer, B, Desplats, P, Patrick, C, Paulino, A, Rockenstein, E, Hansen, L, Adame, A, Galasko, D, & Masliah, E. (2010). Selective molecular alterations in the autophagy pathway in patients with Lewy body disease and in models of alpha-synucleinopathy. PLoS One 5:e9313.

[14] Cuervo, A. M, Stefanis, L, Fredenburg, R, Lansbury, P. T, & Sulzer, D. (2004). Impaired degradation of mutant alpha-synuclein by chaperone-mediated autophagy. Science , 305, 1292-1295.

[15] Cui, M, Tang, X, Christian, W. V, Yoon, Y, & Tieu, K. (2010). Perturbations in mitochondrial dynamics induced by human mutant PINK1 can be rescued by the mitochondrial division inhibitor mdivi-1. J Biol Chem , 285, 11740-11752.

[16] Dagda, R. K, & Cherra, S. J. rd, Kulich SM, Tandon A, Park D, Chu CT ((2009). Loss of PINK1 function promotes mitophagy through effects on oxidative stress and mito-chondrial fission. J Biol Chem , 284, 13843-13855.

[17] Dagda, R. K, Gusdon, A. M, Pien, I, Strack, S, Green, S, Li, C, Van Houten, B, & Cher-ra, S. J. rd, Chu CT ((2011). Mitochondrially localized PKA reverses mitochondrial pathology and dysfunction in a cellular model of Parkinson's disease. Cell Death Dif-fer , 18, 1914-1923.

[18] Dauer, W, & Przedborski, S. (2003). Parkinson's disease: mechanisms and models. Neuron , 39, 889-909.

[19] Ding, W. X, Ni, H. M, Li, M, Liao, Y, Chen, X, Stolz, D. B, & Dorn, G. W. nd, Yin XM ((2010). Nix is critical to two distinct phases of mitophagy, reactive oxygen species-mediated autophagy induction and Parkin-ubiquitin-mitochondrial priming. J Biol Chem 285:27879-27890., 62.

[20] Dorsey, E. R, Constantinescu, R, Thompson, J. P, Biglan, K. M, Holloway, R. G, Kie-burtz, K, Marshall, F. J, Ravina, B. M, Schifitto, G, Siderowf, A, & Tanner, C. M. (2007). Projected number of people with Parkinson disease in the most populous na-tions, 2005 through 2030. Neurology , 68, 384-386.

[21] Egan, D. F, Shackelford, D. B, Mihaylova, M. M, Gelino, S, Kohnz, R. A, Mair, W, Vasquez, D. S, Joshi, A, Gwinn, D. M, Taylor, R, Asara, J. M, Fitzpatrick, J, Dillin, A, Viollet, B, Kundu, M, Hansen, M, & Shaw, R. J. (2011). Phosphorylation of ULK1 (hATG1) by AMP-activated protein kinase connects energy sensing to mitophagy. Science , 331, 456-461.

[22] Fortun, J, & Dunn, W. A. Jr., Joy S, Li J, Notterpek L ((2003). Emerging role for au-tophagy in the removal of aggresomes in Schwann cells. J Neurosci , 23, 10672-10680.

[23] Friedman, L. G, Lachenmayer, M. L, Wang, J, He, L, Poulose, S. M, Komatsu, M, Hol-stein, G. R, & Yue, Z. (2012). Disrupted autophagy leads to dopaminergic axon and dendrite degeneration and promotes presynaptic accumulation of alpha-synuclein and LRRK2 in the brain. J Neurosci , 32, 7585-7593.

[24] Geisler, S, Holmstrom, K. M, Skujat, D, Fiesel, F. C, Rothfuss, O. C, Kahle, P. J, & Springer, W. (2010). PINK1/Parkin-mediated mitophagy is dependent on VDAC1 and SQSTM1. Nat Cell Biol 12:119-131., 62.

[25] Giasson, B. I, Uryu, K, Trojanowski, J. Q, & Lee, V. M. (1999). Mutant and wild type human alpha-synucleins assemble into elongated filaments with distinct morpholo-gies in vitro. J Biol Chem , 274, 7619-7622.

[26] Gomez-suaga, P, Luzon-toro, B, Churamani, D, Zhang, L, Bloor-young, D, Patel, S, Woodman, P. G, Churchill, G. C, & Hilfiker, S. (2012). Leucine-rich repeat kinase 2 regulates autophagy through a calcium-dependent pathway involving NAADP. Hum Mol Genet , 21, 511-525.

[27] Greene, A. W, Grenier, K, Aguileta, M. A, Muise, S, Farazifard, R, Haque, M. E, Mcbride, H. M, & Park, D. S. Fon EA ((2012). Mitochondrial processing peptidase regulates PINK1 processing, import and Parkin recruitment. EMBO Rep , 13, 378-385.

[28] Greene, J. C, Whitworth, A. J, Kuo, I, Andrews, L. A, Feany, M. B, & Pallanck, L. J. (2003). Mitochondrial pathology and apoptotic muscle degeneration in Drosophila parkin mutants. Proc Natl Acad Sci U S A , 100, 4078-4083.

[29] Hara, T, Nakamura, K, Matsui, M, Yamamoto, A, Nakahara, Y, Suzuki-migishima, R, Yokoyama, M, Mishima, K, Saito, I, Okano, H, & Mizushima, N. (2006). Suppression of basal autophagy in neural cells causes neurodegenerative disease in mice. Nature , 441, 885-889.

[30] Hardie, D. G. (2011). AMP-activated protein kinase: an energy sensor that regulates all aspects of cell function. Genes Dev , 25, 1895-1908.

[31] Hayashi, S, Wakabayashi, K, Ishikawa, A, Nagai, H, Saito, M, Maruyama, M, Taka-hashi, T, Ozawa, T, Tsuji, S, & Takahashi, H. (2000). An autopsy case of autosomal-recessive juvenile parkinsonism with a homozygous exon 4 deletion in the parkin gene. Mov Disord , 15, 884-888.

[32] Irrcher, I, et al. (2010). Loss of the Parkinson's disease-linked gene DJ-1 perturbs mi-tochondrial dynamics. Hum Mol Genet , 19, 3734-3746.

[33] Itakura, E, Kishi-itakura, C, Koyama-honda, I, & Mizushima, N. (2012). Structures containing Atg9A and the ULK1 complex independently target depolarized mito-chondria at initial stages of Parkin-mediated mitophagy. J Cell Sci , 125, 1488-1499.

[34] Iwata, A, Riley, B. E, Johnston, J. A, & Kopito, R. R. and microtubules are required for autophagic degradation of aggregated huntingtin. J Biol Chem , 280, 40282-40292.

[35] Johnston, J. A, Ward, C. L, & Kopito, R. R. (1998). Aggresomes: a cellular response to misfolded proteins. J Cell Biol , 143, 1883-1898.

[36] Kawaguchi, Y, Kovacs, J. J, Mclaurin, A, Vance, J. M, Ito, A, & Yao, T. P. (2003). The deacetylase HDAC6 regulates aggresome formation and cell viability in response to misfolded protein stress. Cell , 115, 727-738.

[37] Keeney, P. M, Xie, J, Capaldi, R. A, & Bennett, J. P. Jr. ((2006). Parkinson's disease brain mitochondrial complex I has oxidatively damaged subunits and is functionally impaired and misassembled. J Neurosci , 26, 5256-5264.

[38] Kim, J, Kundu, M, Viollet, B, & Guan, K. L. (2011). AMPK and mTOR regulate au-tophagy through direct phosphorylation of Ulk1. Nat Cell Biol , 13, 132-141.

[39] Kirkin, V, Lamark, T, Sou, Y. S, Bjorkoy, G, Nunn, J. L, Bruun, J. A, Shvets, E, Mce-wan, D. G, Clausen, T. H, Wild, P, Bilusic, I, Theurillat, J. P, Overvatn, A, Ishii, T, Ela-zar, Z, Komatsu, M, Dikic, I, & Johansen, T. (2009). A role for NBR1 in autophagosomal degradation of ubiquitinated substrates. Mol Cell , 33, 505-516.

[40] Klionsky, D. J, et al. (2011). A comprehensive glossary of autophagy-related molecules and processes (2nd edition). Autophagy , 7, 1273-1294.

[41] Komatsu, M, Waguri, S, Chiba, T, Murata, S, Iwata, J, Tanida, I, Ueno, T, Koike, M,
Uchiyama, Y, Kominami, E, & Tanaka, K. (2006). Loss of autophagy in the central
nervous system causes neurodegeneration in mice. Nature , 441, 880-884.

[42] LaVoie MJOstaszewski BL, Weihofen A, Schlossmacher MG, Selkoe DJ ((2005). Dopamine covalently modifies and functionally inactivates parkin. Nat Med , 11,
1214-1221.

[43] Lee, J. Y, Nagano, Y, Taylor, J. P, Lim, K. L, & Yao, T. P. (2010). Disease-causing mutations in Parkin impair mitochondrial ubiquitination, aggregation, and HDAC6-de-
pendent mitophagy. J Cell Biol , 189, 671-679.

[44] Lemasters, J. J. (2005). Selective mitochondrial autophagy, or mitophagy, as a targeted defense against oxidative stress, mitochondrial dysfunction, and aging. Rejuvena-
tion Res , 8, 3-5.

[45] Lewy, F. H. (1912). Paralysis agitans. I. Pathologische Anatomie Ed. M Lewandow-
ski:, 920-933.

[46] Liberek, K, Lewandowska, A, & Zietkiewicz, S. (2008). Chaperones in control of protein disaggregation. Embo J , 27, 328-335.

[47] Lim, K. L, & Ng, C. H. (2009). Genetic models of Parkinson disease. Biochim Biophys
Acta , 1792, 604-615.

[48] Lim, K. L, Dawson, V. L, & Dawson, T. M. (2006). Parkin-mediated lysine 63-linked
polyubiquitination: a link to protein inclusions formation in Parkinson's and other
conformational diseases? Neurobiol Aging , 27, 524-529.

[49] Lim, K. L, Chew, K. C, Tan, J. M, Wang, C, Chung, K. K, Zhang, Y, Tanaka, Y, Smith,
W, Engelender, S, Ross, C. A, Dawson, V. L, & Dawson, T. M. (2005). Parkin mediates
nonclassical, proteasomal-independent ubiquitination of synphilin-1: implications
for Lewy body formation. J Neurosci , 25, 2002-2009.

[50] Mak, S. K, Mccormack, A. L, Manning-bog, A. B, & Cuervo, A. M. Di Monte DA
((2010). Lysosomal degradation of alpha-synuclein in vivo. J Biol Chem , 285,
13621-13629.

[51] Malkus, K. A, & Ischiropoulos, H. (2012). Regional deficiencies in chaperone-mediated autophagy underlie alpha-synuclein aggregation and neurodegeneration. Neurobiol Dis , 46, 732-744.

[52] Manning-bog, A. B, Mccormack, A. L, Li, J, Uversky, V. N, & Fink, A. L. Di Monte
DA ((2002). The herbicide paraquat causes up-regulation and aggregation of alpha-
synuclein in mice: paraquat and alpha-synuclein. J Biol Chem , 277, 1641-1644.

[53] Martin, I, Dawson, V. L, & Dawson, T. M. (2011). Recent advances in the genetics of Parkinson's disease. Annu Rev Genomics Hum Genet , 12, 301-325.

[54] Martinez-vicente, M, Talloczy, Z, Kaushik, S, Massey, A. C, Mazzulli, J, Mosharov, E. V, Hodara, R, Fredenburg, R, Wu, D. C, Follenzi, A, Dauer, W, Przedborski, S, Ischir-opoulos, H, Lansbury, P. T, Sulzer, D, & Cuervo, A. M. (2008). Dopamine-modified alpha-synuclein blocks chaperone-mediated autophagy. J Clin Invest , 118, 777-788.

[55] Matsuda, N, Sato, S, Shiba, K, Okatsu, K, Saisho, K, Gautier, C. A, Sou, Y. S, Saiki, S, Kawajiri, S, Sato, F, Kimura, M, Komatsu, M, Hattori, N, & Tanaka, K. (2010). PINK1 stabilized by mitochondrial depolarization recruits Parkin to damaged mitochondria and activates latent Parkin for mitophagy. J Cell Biol , 189, 211-221.

[56] Mori, H, Kondo, T, Yokochi, M, Matsumine, H, Nakagawa-hattori, Y, Miyake, T, Su-da, K, & Mizuno, Y. (1998). Pathologic and biochemical studies of juvenile parkinson-ism linked to chromosome 6q. Neurology , 51, 890-892.

[57] Narendra, D, Tanaka, A, Suen, D. F, & Youle, R. J. (2008). Parkin is recruited selec-tively to impaired mitochondria and promotes their autophagy. J Cell Biol , 183, 795-803.

[58] Narhi, L, Wood, S. J, Steavenson, S, Jiang, Y, Wu, G. M, Anafi, D, Kaufman, S. A, Martin, F, Sitney, K, Denis, P, Louis, J. C, Wypych, J, Biere, A. L, & Citron, M. (1999). Both familial Parkinson's disease mutations accelerate alpha-synuclein aggregation. J Biol Chem , 274, 9843-9846.

[59] Ng, C. H, Guan, M. S, Koh, C, Ouyang, X, Yu, F, Tan, E. K, Neill, O, Zhang, S. P, Chung, X, & Lim, J. KL ((2012). AMP Kinase Activation Mitigates Dopaminergic Dys-function and Mitochondrial Abnormalities in Drosophila Models of Parkinson's Dis-ease. J Neurosci , 32, 14311-14317.

[60] Okatsu, K, Oka, T, Iguchi, M, Imamura, K, Kosako, H, Tani, N, Kimura, M, Go, E, Koyano, F, Funayama, M, Shiba-fukushima, K, Sato, S, Shimizu, H, Fukunaga, Y, Ta-niguchi, H, Komatsu, M, Hattori, N, Mihara, K, Tanaka, K, & Matsuda, N. (2012). PINK1 autophosphorylation upon membrane potential dissipation is essential for Parkin recruitment to damaged mitochondria. Nat Commun 3:1016.

[61] Olanow, C. W, Perl, D. P, Demartino, G. N, & Mcnaught, K. S. (2004). Lewy-body for-mation is an aggresome-related process: a hypothesis. Lancet Neurol , 3, 496-503.

[62] Olzmann, J. A, Li, L, Chudaev, M. V, Chen, J, Perez, F. A, Palmiter, R. D, & Chin, L. S. linked polyubiquitination targets misfolded DJ-1 to aggresomes via binding to HDAC6. J Cell Biol , 178, 1025-1038.

[63] Opazo, F, Krenz, A, Heermann, S, Schulz, J. B, & Falkenburger, B. H. (2008). Accu-mulation and clearance of alpha-synuclein aggregates demonstrated by time-lapse imaging. J Neurochem , 106, 529-540.

[64]   Pankiv, S, Clausen, T. H, Lamark, T, Brech, A, Bruun, J. A, Outzen, H, Overvatn, A, Bjorkoy, G, & Johansen, T. Binds Directly to Atg8/LC3 to Facilitate Degradation of Ubiquitinated Protein Aggregates by Autophagy. J Biol Chem , 282, 24131-24145.

[65]   Park, J, Lee, S. B, Lee, S, Kim, Y, Song, S, Kim, S, Bae, E, Kim, J, Shong, M, Kim, J. M, & Chung, J. (2006). Mitochondrial dysfunction in Drosophila PINK1 mutants is complemented by parkin. Nature , 441, 1157-1161.

[66]   Pawlyk, A. C, Giasson, B. I, Sampathu, D. M, Perez, F. A, Lim, K. L, Dawson, V. L, Dawson, T. M, Palmiter, R. D, Trojanowski, J. Q, & Lee, V. M. (2003). Novel monoclonal antibodies demonstrate biochemical variation of brain parkin with age. J Biol Chem , 278, 48120-48128.

[67]   Peng, J, Schwartz, D, Elias, J. E, Thoreen, C. C, Cheng, D, Marsischky, G, Roelofs, J, Finley, D, & Gygi, S. P. (2003). A proteomics approach to understanding protein ubiquitination. Nat Biotechnol , 21, 921-926.

[68]   Pickart, C. M. (2000). Ubiquitin in chains. Trends Biochem Sci , 25, 544-548.

[69]   Pickart, C. M, & Cohen, R. E. (2004). Proteasomes and their kin: proteases in the machine age. Nat Rev Mol Cell Biol , 5, 177-187.

[70]   Plowey, E. D, & Cherra, S. J. rd, Liu YJ, Chu CT ((2008). Role of autophagy in G2019S-LRRK2-associated neurite shortening in differentiated SH-SY5Y cells. J Neurochem , 105, 1048-1056.

[71]   Poole, A. C, Thomas, R. E, Yu, S, Vincow, E. S, & Pallanck, L. (2010). The mitochondrial fusion-promoting factor mitofusin is a substrate of the PINK1/parkin pathway. PLoS One 5:e10054.

[72]   Ramirez, A, Heimbach, A, Grundemann, J, Stiller, B, Hampshire, D, Cid, L. P, Goebel, I, Mubaidin, A. F, Wriekat, A. L, Roeper, J, Al-din, A, Hillmer, A. M, Karsak, M, Liss, B, Woods, C. G, Behrens, M. I, & Kubisch, C. (2006). Hereditary parkinsonism with dementia is caused by mutations in ATP13A2, encoding a lysosomal type 5 P-type ATPase. Nat Genet , 38, 1184-1191.

[73]   Ramonet, D, et al. (2011). Dopaminergic neuronal loss, reduced neurite complexity and autophagic abnormalities in transgenic mice expressing G2019S mutant LRRK2. PLoS One 6:e18568.

[74]   Rappley, I, Gitler, A. D, & Selvy, P. E. LaVoie MJ, Levy BD, Brown HA, Lindquist S, Selkoe DJ ((2009). Evidence that alpha-synuclein does not inhibit phospholipase D. Biochemistry , 48, 1077-1083.

[75]   Rubinsztein, D. C, Codogno, P, & Levine, B. (2012). Autophagy modulation as a potential therapeutic target for diverse diseases. Nat Rev Drug Discov , 11, 709-730.

[76] Sarkar, S, Davies, J. E, Huang, Z, Tunnacliffe, A, & Rubinsztein, D. C. (2007). Treha-lose, a novel mTOR-independent autophagy enhancer, accelerates the clearance of mutant huntingtin and alpha-synuclein. J Biol Chem , 282, 5641-5652.

[77] Schapira, A. H, Cooper, J. M, Dexter, D, Jenner, P, Clark, J. B, & Marsden, C. D. (1989). Mitochondrial complex I deficiency in Parkinson's disease. Lancet 1:1269.

[78] Seibler, P, Graziotto, J, Jeong, H, Simunovic, F, Klein, C, & Krainc, D. (2011). Mito-chondrial Parkin Recruitment Is Impaired in Neurons Derived from Mutant PINK1 Induced Pluripotent Stem Cells. J Neurosci , 31, 5970-5976.

[79] Sherer, T. B, Kim, J. H, Betarbet, R, & Greenamyre, J. T. (2003). Subcutaneous rote-none exposure causes highly selective dopaminergic degeneration and alpha-synu-clein aggregation. Exp Neurol , 179, 9-16.

[80] Shults, C. W, Haas, R. H, Passov, D, & Beal, M. F. levels correlate with the activities of complexes I and II/III in mitochondria from parkinsonian and nonparkinsonian subjects. Ann Neurol , 42, 261-264.

[81] Siddiqui, A, Hanson, I, & Andersen, J. K. (2012). Mao-B elevation decreases parkin's ability to efficiently clear damaged mitochondria: protective effects of rapamycin. Free Radic Res , 46, 1011-1018.

[82] Spencer, B, Potkar, R, Trejo, M, Rockenstein, E, Patrick, C, Gindi, R, Adame, A, Wyss-coray, T, & Masliah, E. (2009). Beclin 1 gene transfer activates autophagy and amelio-rates the neurodegenerative pathology in alpha-synuclein models of Parkinson's and Lewy body diseases. J Neurosci , 29, 13578-13588.

[83] Steele, J. W, et al. (2012). Latrepirdine stimulates autophagy and reduces accumula-tion of alpha-synuclein in cells and in mouse brain. Mol Psychiatry.

[84] Sterky, F. H, Lee, S, Wibom, R, Olson, L, & Larsson, N. G. (2011). Impaired mitochon-drial transport and Parkin-independent degeneration of respiratory chain-deficient dopamine neurons in vivo. Proc Natl Acad Sci U S A , 108, 12937-12942.

[85] Takahashi, H, Ohama, E, Suzuki, S, Horikawa, Y, Ishikawa, A, Morita, T, Tsuji, S, & Ikuta, F. (1994). Familial juvenile parkinsonism: clinical and pathologic study in a family. Neurology , 44, 437-441.

[86] Tan, J. M, Wong, E. S, & Lim, K. L. (2009). Protein misfolding and aggregation in Par-kinson's disease. Antioxid Redox Signal , 11, 2119-2134.

[87] Tan, J. M, Wong, E. S, Dawson, V. L, Dawson, T. M, & Lim, K. L. linked polyubiqui-tin potentially partners with to promote the clearance of protein inclusions by au-tophagy. Autophagy 4:251-253., 62.

[88] Tan, J. M, Wong, E. S, Kirkpatrick, D. S, Pletnikova, O, Ko, H. S, Tay, S. P, Ho, M. W, Troncoso, J, Gygi, S. P, Lee, M. K, Dawson, V. L, Dawson, T. M, & Lim, K. L. linked

ubiquitination promotes the formation and autophagic clearance of protein inclusions associated with neurodegenerative diseases. Hum Mol Genet , 17, 431-439.

[89] Tong, Y, Yamaguchi, H, Giaime, E, Boyle, S, Kopan, R, & Kelleher, R. J. rd, Shen J ((2010). Loss of leucine-rich repeat kinase 2 causes impairment of protein degradation pathways, accumulation of alpha-synuclein, and apoptotic cell death in aged mice. Proc Natl Acad Sci U S A , 107, 9879-9884.

[90] Usenovic, M, Tresse, E, Mazzulli, J. R, Taylor, J. P, & Krainc, D. (2012). Deficiency of ATP13A2 leads to lysosomal dysfunction, alpha-synuclein accumulation, and neurotoxicity. J Neurosci , 32, 4240-4246.

[91] Uversky, V. N. (2007). Neuropathology, biochemistry, and biophysics of alpha-synuclein aggregation. J Neurochem , 103, 17-37.

[92] Uversky, V. N, Li, J, Bower, K, & Fink, A. L. (2002). Synergistic effects of pesticides and metals on the fibrillation of alpha-synuclein: implications for Parkinson's disease. Neurotoxicology , 23, 527-536.

[93] Wahlqvist, M. L, Lee, M. S, Hsu, C. C, Chuang, S. Y, Lee, J. T, & Tsai, H. N. (2012). Metformin-inclusive sulfonylurea therapy reduces the risk of Parkinson's disease occurring with Type 2 diabetes in a Taiwanese population cohort. Parkinsonism Relat Disord.

[94] Wakabayashi, K, Tanji, K, Odagiri, S, Miki, Y, Mori, F, & Takahashi, H. (2012). The Lewy Body in Parkinson's Disease and Related Neurodegenerative Disorders. Mol Neurobiol.

[95] Wang, C, Lu, R, Ouyang, X, Ho, M. W, Chia, W, Yu, F, & Lim, K. L. (2007). Drosophila overexpressing parkin R275W mutant exhibits dopaminergic neuron degeneration and mitochondrial abnormalities. J Neurosci , 27, 8563-8570.

[96] Wang, C, Ko, H. S, Thomas, B, Tsang, F, Chew, K. C, Tay, S. P, Ho, M. W, Lim, T. M, Soong, T. W, Pletnikova, O, Troncoso, J, Dawson, V. L, Dawson, T. M, & Lim, K. L. alterations in parkin solubility promote parkin aggregation and compromise parkin's protective function. Hum Mol Genet , 14, 3885-3897.

[97] Webb, J. L, Ravikumar, B, Atkins, J, Skepper, J. N, & Rubinsztein, D. C. (2003). Alpha-Synuclein is degraded by both autophagy and the proteasome. J Biol Chem , 278, 25009-25013.

[98] Winslow, A. R, Chen, C. W, Corrochano, S, Acevedo-arozena, A, Gordon, D. E, Peden, A. A, Lichtenberg, M, Menzies, F. M, Ravikumar, B, Imarisio, S, Brown, S, Kane, O, Rubinsztein, C. J, & Alpha-synuclein, D. C. impairs macroautophagy: implications for Parkinson's disease. J Cell Biol , 190, 1023-1037.

[99] Wong, A. S, Lee, R. H, Cheung, A. Y, Yeung, P. K, Chung, S. K, Cheung, Z. H, & Ip, N. Y. (2011). Cdk5-mediated phosphorylation of endophilin B1 is required for induced autophagy in models of Parkinson's disease. Nat Cell Biol , 13, 568-579.

[100] Wong, E, & Cuervo, A. M. (2010). Autophagy gone awry in neurodegenerative diseases. Nat Neurosci , 13, 805-811.

[101] Wong, E. S, Tan, J. M, Soong, W. E, Hussein, K, Nukina, N, Dawson, V. L, Dawson, T. M, Cuervo, A. M, & Lim, K. L. (2008). Autophagy-mediated clearance of aggresomes is not a universal phenomenon. Hum Mol Genet , 17, 2570-2582.

[102] Xilouri, M, Vogiatzi, T, Vekrellis, K, Park, D, & Stefanis, L. (2009). Abberant alpha-synuclein confers toxicity to neurons in part through inhibition of chaperone-mediated autophagy. PLoS One 4:e5515.

[103] Yamamoto, H, Kakuta, S, Watanabe, T. M, Kitamura, A, Sekito, T, Kondo-kakuta, C, Ichikawa, R, Kinjo, M, & Ohsumi, Y. (2012). Atg9 vesicles are an important membrane source during early steps of autophagosome formation. J Cell Biol , 198, 219-233.

[104] Yoshii, S. R, Kishi, C, Ishihara, N, & Mizushima, N. (2011). Parkin mediates proteasome-dependent protein degradation and rupture of the outer mitochondrial membrane. J Biol Chem.

[105] Zhu, J. H, Horbinski, C, Guo, F, Watkins, S, Uchiyama, Y, & Chu, C. T. (2007). Regulation of autophagy by extracellular signal-regulated protein kinases during 1-methyl-4-phenylpyridinium-induced cell death. Am J Pathol , 170, 75-86.

[106] Ziviani, E, Tao, R. N, & Whitworth, A. J. (2010). Drosophila parkin requires PINK1 for mitochondrial translocation and ubiquitinates mitofusin. Proc Natl Acad Sci U S A , 107, 5018-5023.

10

Mutations of PARK Genes and Alpha-Synuclein and Parkin Concentrations in Parkinson's Disease

Anna Oczkowska, Margarita Lianeri,
Wojciech Kozubski and Jolanta Dorszewska

1. Introduction

Parkinson's disease (PD) is a chronic and progressive neurological disorder characterized by resting tremor, rigidity, and bradykinesia, affecting at least 2% of individuals above the age of 65 years. Parkinson's disease is a result of degeneration of the dopamine-producing neurons of the *substantia nigra*. Available therapies in PD will only improve the symptoms but not halt progression of disease. The most effective treatment for PD patients is therapy with L-3,4-dihydroxy-phenylalanine (L-dopa) [Olanow, 2008].

It is now believed that the cause of PD, are both environmental and genetic factors. During the last two decades, there has been breakthrough progress in genetics of PD. It is known that genetic background of PD is in mutations a number of pathogenic genes PARK, e.g. *SNCA, PRKN, UCHL1, DJ-1, PINK1, ATP13A2*, and *LRRK2* (Polrolniczak et a., 2011, 2012). In 2001, Shimura et al. first described the presence in the human brain complex containing Parkin with the glycosylated form of the alpha-synuclein (ASN, alpha-SP22). Moreover, the study by Dorszewska et al. (2012) has been shown, that in the PD patients increased plasma level of ASN was associated by the decreased of Parkin plasma level. It has also shown that configuration: increased plasma level of ASN and decreased of Parkin concentration was associated with earlier onset of PD. It seems that in PD genotypic testing of PARK mutations and analysis of their phenotypes (e.g. ASN, Parkin) may be diagnostic agents for these patients.

2. Mutations in *PRKN*, *SPR* and *HTRA2* genes and polymorphism of NACP-Rep1 region of *SNCA* promoter in the patients with Parkinson's disease

During the last two decades, there has been breakthrough progress in genetics of PD. Currently it is known that genetic background of PD is heterogeneous and mutations in a number of pathogenic genes (e.g. *SNCA*, *PRKN*, *UCHL1*, *DJ-1*, *PINK1*, *ATP13A2*, and *LRRK2*) have been described as associated with familial (FPD) or as genetic risk factors increasing the risk to develop of sporadic PD (SPD). Some of these genes (like *SNCA* and *PRKN)* are fairly well understood while the others (like *SPR* and *HTRA2*) are still little known (Corti et al., 2011).

Monogenic forms, caused by a single mutation in a dominantly or recessively inherited gene, are well-established. Nevertheless, they are relatively rare types of PD and account for about 30% of the FPD and 3–5% of the SPD cases. Although 18 specific chromosomal locus (called *PARK* and numbered in chronological order of their identification) have been reported as more or less convincingly related to FPD (Klein & Westenberger, 2012), the majority of PD cases are SPD (only about 10% of patients report a positive family history) [Thomas & Beal, 2007] while the results of the studies of SPD genetic are still ambiguous and divergent in different ethnic origin (Klein & Schlossmacher, 2007; Lesage & Brice, 2009). Few studies (e.g. Abbas et al., 1999; Gilks et al., 2005; Guo et al., 2010; Mellick et al., 2005; Trotta et al., 2012) suggest a strong correlation of genetic factors with an increased risk of SPD development, while the other reports are contradictory (Chung et al., 2011; Spadafora et al., 2003). However, genome-wide association studies have provided convincing evidence that polymorphic variants in some genes contribute to higher risk of SPD (Gao et al., 2009). Moreover, it is suggested that the etiology of PD is multifactorial, which probably results from coocurence of genetic and environmental factors (Klein & Westenberger, 2012).

Summarizing, from the existing studies reported, it is not yet clear how common mutations in few genes, including: *PRKN*, *HTRA2*, *SPR* and *SNCA* genes contribute to idiopathic PD (Nuytemans et al., 2010). Finally despite previous reports, significance of these genes mutation and polymorphism in pathogenesis of PD (especially SPD) is not clear and is still debated, mainly because of discrepancy of studies results and variance between different ethnic populations. To clarify these issues, more data of genetic analysis are needed while there were only a few reports of genetic studies of PD in Polish populations (Bialecka et al., 2005; Koziorowski et al., 2010). Moreover, little is understood about putative director functional interactions between the genes that cause PD, and a single pathway unifying these factors has not been confirmed (Bras et al., 2008; Brooks et al., 2009; Klein et al., 2005).

2.1. Polymorphism of NACP-Rep1 region of *SNCA* promoter in the patients with Parkinson's disease

SNCA gene, encoding ASN, was first gene describing as related with PD. Missence mutations and multiplications of this gene, generally have been described as related with FPD (Kruger et al., 1998), however *SNCA* duplications were also reported in SPD (Abeliovich et al., 2000;

Ahn et al., 2008; Liu et al., 2004; Nishioka et al., 2009; Nuytemans et al., 2009). Therefore, it have been suspected that not only mutations in the *SNCA* gene, but also other factors affecting the expression of ASN may contribute to the PD manifestation including, SPD.

The study by Chiba-Falek et al. (2006) has shown that the region NACP-Rep1 of *SNCA* gene promoter, there is the polymorphic region differenting in dinucleotide repeats count and affecting the level of ASN expression. Moreover, it has been shown that polymorphism of NACP-Rep1 region in promoter of *SNCA*, are associated with an increased risk of SPD in some population like: German, Australian, American and Polish, but the other multi-population studies have observed no association or reported an inverse association between the risk allele and PD (Farrer et al., 2001; Kruger et al., 1999; Maraganore et al., 2006; Polrolniczak et al., 2012; Tan et al., 2003).

Region NACP-Rep1 contains dinucleotide repeats (TC)x(T)2(TC)y(TA)2(CA)z, which may vary both the number of repeats, and include substitutions of nucleotides. However, it has been proven, that a change in the length of the NACP-Rep1 region more than substitutions, affects the regulation of the expression of ASN (Fuchs et al., 2008; Mellick et al., 2005; Tan et al., 2003). As the most common in humans it has been described five alleles of NACP-Rep1 of the *SNCA* gene promoter: -1, 0, +1, +2, +3. Generally in the European population the most frequently was allele +1 of NACP-Rep1. It has been also shown, that the allele 0 of NACP-Rep1 region in *SNCA* promoter is two pairs shorter than allele +1, allele -1 respectively, shorter by 4 bp however alleles 2 and 3 are longer by 2 and 4 bp.

Functional analysis on the two most common NACP-Rep1 alleles +1 and +2 suggested that the +2 allele is associated with an up-regulation of *SNCA* expression, whereas the +1 variant shows reduced gene expression (Chiba Falek & Nussbaum, 2001; Cronin et al., 2009). In addition, allele +1 of the region NACP-Rep1 of *SNCA* promoter, containing 259 bp, significantly reduces the risk of PD in the population of Europe, America and Australia (Fuchs et al., 2008; Maraganore et al., 2006; Tan et al., 2000) while another study failed to replicate the finding in population of Japan, Singapore and Italy (Spadafora et al., 2003; Tan et al., 2003).

Nerveless, although protective effect of allele +1 rather not currently subject to discussion, but for alleles 0, +2 and +3 it has been suggested both no impact, as well as increasing the risk of PD, and even sometimes the protective action (Maraganore et al., 2006; Spadafora et al., 2003; Tan et al., 2000; Trotta et al., 2012). The following studies by Tan et al. (2000) and Myhre et al. (2008) observed a higher frequency of the +3 allele in PD cases compared with healthy controls while in the study by both Tan et al. (2003) and Spadafora et al. (2003) no significant differences of the various genotypes between PD and controls were found in population of Singapore and Italy. However, the study in Italy population, have also shown evidence of association for allele +2 on NACP-Rep1 (Trotta et al., 2012). In 2006, a meta-analysis of 11 study populations provided strong evidence that the 263bp allele was more frequent in PD cases increasing risk of this disease while the 261bp allele did not differ between PD cases and unaffected controls but the authors suggested, that the lack of association of the +2 allele in the meta-analysis could be due to the large fluctuation in its frequencies observed in the analyzed populations (Maraganore et al., 2006). Therefore the aim of the study was analysis of NACP-Rep1 region in PD patients and in controls in Polish population.

2.1.1. Patients

The studies were conducted on 90 patients with PD [SPD patients, 10 with early onset of PD, EOPD, and 80 with late onset of PD, LOPD patients), including 42 women and 47 men aging 34-82 years. Control group included 113 individuals, 79 women and 34 men, 39-83 years of age. Demographic data of all groups summarized in Table 1.

Patients with PD were diagnosed using the criteria of UK Parkinson's Disease Society Brain Bank (Litvan et al., 2003), however stage of disease according to the scale of Hoehn and Yahr (Hoehn & Yahr, 1967).

None of the control subjects had verifiable symptoms of dementia or any other neurological disorders. All subjects had negative family history of PD. All patients were recruited from the Neurology Clinic of Chair and Department of Neurology, University of Medical Sciences, Poznan in Poland. Only Caucasian, Polish subjects were included in this study. A Local Ethical Committee approved the study and the written consent of all patients or their caregivers was obtained.

Factor	Controls	Patients with PD
Individuals	113	90
Age	39-83	34-82
Mean age ±SD	55.5±9.5	61.9±10.1
F/M	79/34	42/47

Table 1. Demographic data of patients with PD and control subjects analyzed for NACP-Rep1 region in *SNCA* promoter. SD – standard deviation, F – female, M – male.

2.1.2. Genetic investigations

Isolation of DNA. DNA was isolated from peripheral blood lymphocytes by fivefold centrifugation in a lytic buffer, containing 155 mM NH_4Cl, 10 mM $KHCO_3$, 0.1 mM Na_2EDTA, pH 7.4, in the presence of buffer containing 75 mM NaCl, 9 mM Na_2EDTA, pH 8.0, and sodium dodecyl sulfate and proteinase K (Sigma, St. Louis, MO). Subsequently, NaCl was added, the lysate was centrifuged, and DNA present in the upper layer was precipitated with 98% ethanol. Extracted genomic DNA was stored at -80°C.

Analysis of G88C mutation of SNCA gene. For exon 3 of *SNCA* analysis, a total of 20 ng gDNA was amplified in 25 µl PCR reactions using specific primers (5′-AAGTGTATTT-TATGTTTTCC-3′; 5′-AACTGACATTTGGGGTTTACC-3′) [Lin et al., 1999] and empirically defined reaction conditions. The PCR product was digested with MvaI (Fermentas, Canada) according to Kruger et al. (1998) method for screening c.88 G>C mutation in *SNCA* gene.

Analysis of NACP-Rep1 polymorphism of SNCA promoter region. For analysis of NACP-Rep1 region of *SNCA* promoter, analyzed region was amplified using described previously primers

(5'-GACTGGCCCAAGATTAACCA-3'; 5'- CCTGGCATATTTGATTGCAA-3') under the conditions: (95°C 30'', 64°C 45'', 72°C 30'') [Tan et al., 2003]. One of the primers was labeled with fluorescent marker – FAM. Sizing of the PCR products was performed by capillary electrophoresis on the 3130xl Genetic Analyzer (Applied Biosystems HITACHI, USA) using GeneScan Size Standard 600LIZ (Applied Biosystems, USA) and controls. The results of electrophoresis were analyzed using Peak Scanner Software v.1.0 (Applied Biosystems, USA). Genotypes were differentiated according to the length of the PCR product. Designations of alleles was followed those previously described (Farrer et al., 2001; Xia et al., 2001).

Moreover, random duplicate samples (10%) were genotyped for all assays for quality control with 100% reproducibility.

Statistical analysis. Statistical analysis was performed using Statistica for Windows Software. The level of significance was set at 5%. Chi-square test and Fisher's exact probability test, test for the two components of the structure, univariate odds ratio (ORs) and logistic regression analysis were used to compare the categorical variables and distribution of alleles and genotypes. The allele frequencies of PD patients and controls were evaluated with regards to Hardy-Weinburg equilibrium using standardized formula.

2.1.3. Results

Screening for mutation c.88 G>C of *SNCA* gene in patients with PD and neurologically healthy controls detected no mutations in both group allow the exclusion of FPD determined by this mutation.

Using PCR amplification and capillary electrophoresis five previously described polymorphic alleles of NACP-Rep1 region in *SNCA* promoter were identified (designated -1, 0, +1, +2, +3) [Farrer et al., 2001; Xia et al., 2001]. Alleles and genotypes frequencies were in Hardy-Weinburg equilibrium in both groups: PD and controls with the exception of alleles +1 and +2, which frequencies in PD patients differed significantly from the expected frequencies calculated from Hardy-Weinburg equilibrium (exact test; $p=0.032$ and $p=0.006$ respectively). The frequency of allele +1 (Table 2) was significantly higher in healthy controls as compared to PD patients ($p<0.001$). In contrast to the allele +1, the frequency of alleles +2 and +3 were significantly higher in PD patients as compared to controls ($p<0.01$; $p<0.05$ respectively). However, the frequency of allele 0 was similar between PD and controls. Moreover, presence of allele -1 was detected only in control subjects (Polrolniczak et al., 2012).

The frequency of +1/+1 genotype was almost fourfold higher in control group than in PD patients ($p<0.001$) whereas the frequency of the genotype +1/+2 was similar in both groups (Table 3). Comparisons of +2/+2 genotype frequencies between PD patients and control group revealed no significant differences but the frequency of this genotype was almost twofold higher in PD patients as compared to controls ($p=0.056$). It has been also detected, that the frequency of +2/+3 was significantly higher in PD patients compared to controls and was almost threefold higher in PD patients ($p<0.05$). Moreover, genotype +1/+3 has been detected only in one PD patient while genotype -1/+1 occurred only in controls (Table 3).

Allele	Controls	Patients with PD
-1	1%	0%
0	5%	6%
+1	53%	33%***
+2	40%	54%**
+3	2%	7%*
Total subjects number	226	180

Table 2. NACP-Rep1 alleles frequency in PD patients and controls. Results are expressed as a percentage. Test for two components of the structure was used. Differences significant at: *$p<0.05$; **$p<0.01$; ***$p<0.001$, as compared to the controls.

Genotypes	Controls	Patients with PD
-1/+1	2%	0%
0/+1	7%	7%
0/+2	3%	4%
+1/+1	23%	6%***
+1/+2	50%	47%
+1/+3	0%	1%
+2/+2	12%	22%
+2/+3	4%	13%*
Total subjects number	113	90

Table 3. NACP-Rep1 genotype frequencies in PD patients and in controls. Results are expressed as a percentage. Test for two components of the structure was used. Differences significant at: *$p<0.05$; ***$p<0.001$, as compared to the controls.

Logistic regression analysis have shown, that PD risk (as measured by OR, Table 4) has been reduced in presence of allele +1 and reduces with increasing dose of +1 allele. Moreover, OR pointed to the association the presence of allele +2 with increased risk of PD manifestation in dose dependent manner. Influence of the presence of allele +3 of the increase PD risk has been detected only in heterozygous variant. Genotype +3/+3 have not been detected in any person in both control and PD patient group.

Allele	Heterozygous model		Homozygous model		Common odds ratio	
OR (95% CI)	p	OR (95% CI)	p	OR	p
-1	-	>0,05	-	>0.05	-	>0.05 (F)
0	-	>0,05	-	>0.05	-	>0.05 (C)
+1	0.406 (0.210-0.785)**	<0.01	0.107 (0.035-0.322)***	<0.001	0.342***	<0.001 (C)
+2	2.719 (1.292-5.719)**	<0.01	4.615 (1.774-12.009)**	<0.001	2.163***	<0.001 (C)
+3	4.601 (1.445-14.647)**	<0.01	-	>0.05	4.601**	<0.01 (F)

Table 4. Modulation of PD risk manifestation by NACP-Rep1 variants measured by odds ratio. Logistic regression analysis, Fisher's exact test and Chi square test were used. OR – odds ratio; CI – confidence interval; F-Fisher's exact test; C-Chi square test. Differences significant at: **p<0.01; ***p<0.001, as compared to the controls.

Our results similarly to studies in the European, Australian and American populations indicated that, the presence of genotype +1/+1 may reduce PD risk while another study failed to replicate the finding in population of Italy (Fuchs et al., 2008; Maraganore et al., 2006; Mellick et al., 2005; Polrolniczak et al., 2012; Spadafora et al., 2003; Tan et al., 2003; Trotta et al., 2012). It is suggested, that reduction of PD risk by genotype +1/+1 may be related with decreasing ASN expression (Chiba-Falek et al., 2006; Fuchs et al., 2008). In the study in Polish population it has been also observed, in PD patient with genotype +1/+1 tendency to slower progression of the disease and better response to pharmacotherapy at using low doses of the L-dopa treatment compared the other genotypes of NACP-Rep1 (Polrolniczak et al., 2012). It seems, that in PD patients with genotype +1/+1 reduced ASN level, due to reduce ASN aggregation and maintenance of dopamine homeostasis in the central nervous system (CNS) probably leads to milder course of disease compared to patients with other genotypes of NACP-Rep1 (Maguire-Zeiss et al., 2005).

Although the study in Singapore and Italian populations shown no association for alleles +2 and +3 with PD our results confirming the study in populations: German, Italian, Japanese, and multipopulation research detected higher frequency of those alleles in PD patients compared with controls and indicated association of genotypes +2/+2 and +2/+3 with increased risk of PD in Polish population (Maraganore et al., 2006; Mellick et al., 2005; Polrolniczak et al., 2012; Spadafora et al., 2003; Tan et al., 2003; Trotta et al., 2012). It is believed that the influence of genotype +2/+2 and +2/+3 on the risk of PD most likely may be associated with over-expression of ASN, leading to increased aggregation of ASN and the severity of the neurotoxic effect (Chiba-Falek et al., 2006; Cronin et al., 2009; Fuchs et al., 2008). Furthermore in our study in patients with genotypes +2/+2 and +2/+3 we observed tendency to faster progression of the disease but no association with response to therapy (Polrolniczak et al., 2012). This observations seems corresponding with the results of the study by Ritz et al. (2012) shoved that risk of faster decline of motor function was increased four-fold in carriers of the +3 allele of NACP-Rep1 promoter variant. Moreover, the study by Kay et al. (2008) have indicated a trend of decreasing onset age with increasing allele size while the other study have shown, that age at onset of carriers of at least one allele +2 was earlier compared to noncarriers (Hadjigeorgiou et al., 2006).

However, in contrast to the results of Kay et al. (2008) in Polish population it has not indicated any association of allele 0 with risk of PD, however presence of this genetic variant was correlated in Spearman correlation test (p=0,019; r=-0,507) with decrease in stage of disease in patients suffering for PD over 10 years compared patients with the other genotypes of NACP-Rep1 (Polrolniczak et al., 2012).

It seems that examination of genotypes of region NACP-Rep1 of *SNCA* promoter may help to explain the pathogenesis of PD, as well as facilitate early diagnosis and determine the degree of risk for this neurodegenerative disease.

2.2. Mutations in *PRKN* in the patients with Parkinson's disease

Mutations of *PRKN* were first identified in Japanese families with autosomal recessive juvenile Parkinsonism and since then more than 100 mutations in this gene have been found. Mutation in *PRKN* gene encoding Parkin, have been found both in the EOPD (<40 years) and in the LOPD (>40 years) forms of PD (Bardien et al., 2009; Kitada et al., 1998). Although *PRKN* mutations have been identified in all 12 exons of this gene, the most common seem to be mutations in exons 2, 4, 7, 8, 10 and 11. The vast majority, FPD conditioned by *PRKN* mutation is inherited as an autosomal recessive but it has been also reported heterozygous mutations related with PD manifestation.

Furthermore, it has been shown that mutations in the gene *PRKN* occur at different frequencies both in Caucasians and in populations of African and Asian countries (Kitada et al., 1998; Lucking & Briece, 2000). However, the literature on the prevalence of mutations in *PRKN* and their involvement in the modulation of PD risk are very diverse and have a wide variation depending on the studied population, and the age of subjects included in the study.

It is suggested, that mutations in *PRKN*, including homo- and heterozygous mutations are detected in about 40-50% of early-onset FPD and in about 1.3-20% of SPD patients (Choi et al., 2008; Herdich et al., 2004; Kann et al., 2002; Mellick et al., 2009; Sironi et al., 2008).

The study by Abbas et al. (1999), point mutations of *PRKN* in the European population were approximately twice as common as homozygous exonic deletions. In the European population it has been reported *PRKN* mutations in about 19% of SPD and 50% of early-onset FPD (Lucking & Briece, 2000). Further the study by Lucking et al. (2001) in the sporadic cases revealed that 77% with age of disease onset below 20 years had mutations in *PRKN* gene, but in cases with age of disease onset between 31 and 45 years mutations were found only in 3% in European population. The larger cases studies have confirmed reports of Lucking et al. (2001) and it has shown *PRKN* mutations in 67% of cases with age of onset below 20 years and in 8% of cases with an age of onset between 30–45 years. In another study involving 363 affected subjects from 307 families it has identified *PRKN* mutations in 2% of all late-onset families screened, thereby directly implicating the *PRKN* gene in LOPD (Oliveira et al., 2003). In population of Korea it has been detected *PRKN* mutations in EOPD in 5% frequency while in Japanse population in 11% (Hattori et al., 1998). In Italian population mutations of *PRKN* occurred in frequency 8-13%, in French in 16%, in German in 9% and in Americans in 4% while in North African in 21%, and in Brazilian in about 8% (Chen et al., 2003; Klein et al., 2005; Lucking & Briece, 2000; Periquet et al., 2003).

The observation, that mutations in the *PRKN* gene are common in juvenile- (JPD) and EOPD and increasing evidence supporting a direct role for Parkin in LOPD make this gene a particularly compelling candidate for intensified investigation. However, despite previous reports, significance of *PRKN* mutation and polymorphism in pathogenesis of PD is still not clear.

The aim of the study was to estimate the frequency of *PRKN* mutation in Polish PD patients and controls.

2.2.1. Patients

According to the inclusion and exclusion criteria a total of 199 subjects were included in this study: 87 SPD patients (10 EOPD patients, and 77 sporadic LOPD patients), including 41 women and 45 men aging 34-82 years. Control group included 112 individuals, 78 women and 34 men, 39-83 years of age. Demographic data of all groups summarized in Table 5. Patients with PD were diagnosed using the criteria of UK Parkinson's Disease Society Brain Bank (Litvan et al., 2003), however stage of disease according to the scale of Hoehn and Yahr (Hoehn & Yahr, 1967). None of the control subjects had verifiable symptoms of dementia or any other neurological disorders. All subjects had negative family history of PD. All patients were recruited from the Neurology Clinic of Chair and Department of Neurology, University of Medical Sciences, Poznan in Poland. Only Caucasian, Polish subjects were included in the study. A Local Ethical Committee approved the study and the written consent of all patients or their caregivers was obtained.

Factor	Controls	Patients with PD
Individuals	112	87
Age	39-83	34-82
Mean age ±SD	55.6±9.5	61.4±9.9
F/M	78/34	41/45

Table 5. Demographic data of patients with PD and control subjects analyzed for *PRKN* mutation. SD – standard deviation, F – female, M – male.

2.2.2. Genetic investigations

Isolation of DNA. See point 2.1.2

Analysis of deletion of exon 2 and 4 of PRKN gene. Exon deletion in *PRKN* was examined by amplifying exon 2 and 4 using internal and external specific primers previously described (5'-ATGTTGCTATCACCATTTAAG-3'; 5'-AGATTGGCAGCGCAGGCGGCA-3' for exon 2)

[Choi et al., 2008] or generated using the online software Pimer3 (http://www-ge-nome.wi.mit.edu/cgibin/primer/primer3_www.cgi) based on the published genomic se-quence of the *PRKN* gene (5'-TTTCCCAAATATTGCTCTA-3'; 5'-GCAGTGTGGAGTAAAGTTCAAGG-3' for exon 2 and 5'-GCATTATTAGCCACTTCTTCTGC-3'; 5'-TGCTGACACTGCATTTCCTT-3'; 5'-AGATTTCACTCTTGGAGCATAAA-3'; 5'-CAAAGGCGCATAAACGAAA-3' for exon 4). PCR cycling conditions were empirically defined (Polrolniczak et al., 2012).

Analysis of exon 4, 7 and 11 of PRKN gene. High resolution melting (HRM) were used for mutation screening in exon 4, 7 and 11 of *PRKN*. HRM was performed with the LightCycler 480 Real-Time PCR system (Roche, USA) and High Resolution Master Mix (Roche, USA). Reactions were performed on 96-well plates, using 5 ng of template DNA, 1x Master Mix, 2.5 mM MgCl2, and 10 pmol primers (on request) in a 10 μl reaction volume. PCR cycling conditions comprised of an initial denaturation step of 95°C for 5 min, 30 cycles of denaturation at 95°C for 15 s, annealing at 64°C (or 63°C for exon 4) for 15 s, extension at 72°C C for 15 s, and a final extension step of 72°C for 7 min. HRM analysis was performed from 55°C to 95°C (Polrolniczak et al., 2012). Melting curves and difference plots were analyzed by 3 investigators blinded to phenotype. For the samples with shifted melting curves, PCR products were cleaned and sequenced in the forward and reverse directions. Sequencing was performed using the 3130xl Genetic Analyzer (Applied Biosystems HITACHI, USA) and reads were aligned to the human reference genome with BioEdit Software (Tom Hall Ibis Biosciences, Canada). Coding DNA mutation numbering is relative to NM_004562.2.

Analysis of c.930 G>C substitution in exon 8 of PRKN gene. For exon 8 of *PRKN* analysis 20 ng gDNA was amplified in 25 μl using PCR reaction with specific primers (5'- CTAAA-GAGGTGCGGTTGGAG-3'; 5'- GGAGCCCAAACTGTCTCATT-3') generated using the online software Pimer3 based on the published genomic sequence of the *PRKN* gene. PCR cycling conditions were empirically defined. Screening for the c.930 G>C mutation of *PRKN* was performed by a RFLP analysis on 2% agarose gels using Mva I (Fermentas, Canada) as restriction enzyme. All detected mutations were confirmed by sequencing of PCR product.

Moreover, random duplicate samples (10%) were genotyped for all assays for quality control with 100% reproducibility.

Statistical analysis. Statistical analyses were performed using Statistica for Windows Software. The level of significance was set at 5%. Chi-square test and Fisher's exact probability test, univariate odds ratio (ORs) and logistic regression analysis were used to compare the catego-rical variables and distribution of alleles. The allele frequencies of PD patients and controls were evaluated with regards to Hardy-Weinburg equilibrium using standardized formula.

2.2.3. Results

Analysis of deletions of exons 2 and 4 *PRKN* has detected no genetic changes both in PD patients and control group. However, point mutation screening in patients with PD and healthy controls identified 5 missence substitutions which were almost fourfold more frequent in PD patients as compared with controls (p<0.001) [Table 6]. We also showed, that the presence of *PRKN* substitution increased risk of PD over six-fold (p<0.001; OR=6.059). All substitutions were non-synonymous and were in heterozygous state.

	Controls	Patients with PD	OR	95% CI	p
PRKN mutations	8%	31%***	6.059	2.188-11.207	<0.001 (C)
Total subjects number	112	87	-	-	-

Table 6. Total *PRKN* point mutations frequencies in PD patients and controls. Results are expressed as a percentage. Chi square test was used. OR – odds ratio; CI – confidence interval; C - Chi square test. Differences significant at: ***p<0.001, as compared to the controls.

In exon 4 of *PRKN* two mutations were detected: c.500 G>A transition leads to S167A substitution (with frequency sevenfold higher in PD than in control group; p<0.05) and a novel heterozygous mutation c.520 C>T resulting L174F substitution and occurring only in PD patients. Furthermore, first time in Polish population we detected c.823 C>T (exon 7, R275T; only in PD) and c.930 G>C (exon 8, E310D) substitutions (over threefold more frequently in PD than in controls; p<0.01). Moreover, we detected also a transition c.1180 G>A in exon 11 of *PRKN*. It has been also shown, that c.500 G>A, c.930 G>C and c.1180 G>A substitutions significantly increased PD risk (Table 7). Simultaneously analysis of the amino acid sequence of the Parkin (encoded by *PRKN* gene) revealed that the substitution E310D and L174F are located in conserved region whereas substitution R275T and D394N in a limited conserved region of this protein (Polrolniczak et al., 2012).

Mutation/ polymorphism	c.500 G>A	c.520 C>T	c.823 C>T	c.930 G>C	c.1180 G>A
Controls	1%	0%	0%	5%	2%
PD patients	7%*	2%	1%	18%**	11%**
OR	8.000	-	-	3.926	6.938
95% CI	0.945-67.712	-	-	1.436-10.735	1.480-32.528
p	<0.05 (F)	>0.05 (F)	>0.05 (F)	<0.01 (C)	<0.01 (C)

Table 7. *PRKN* point mutations frequencies in PD patients and controls. Results are expressed as a percentage. Logistic regression analysis, Fisher's exact test and Chi square test were used. OR – odds ratio; CI – confidence interval; F - Fisher's exact test; C - Chi square test. Differences significant at: *p<0.05; **p<0.01 as compared to the controls.

Additionally in 5% PD patients it has been detected more than one mutation in *PRKN* gene while all control subjects who had substitution in *PRKN*, had only one mutation (Table 8).

Coexistence of substitutions in *PRKN* gene	Percentage of PD patients
c.823 C>T , c.1180 G>A	1%
c.500 G>A, c.520 C>T	1%
c.930 G>C, c.1180 G>A	2%
c.500 G>A, c.930 G>C, c.1180 G>A	1%

Table 8. Coexistence more than one *PRKN* point mutations in PD patients in Polish population (Polrolniczak et al., 2012).

It is suggested, that single or multiple exon deletions and duplications occur with a frequency of 15.8% and account for about 50% of all mutations of *PRKN* gene (Nuytemans et al., 2010). Nevertheless, although many reports indicated important role of *PRKN* exons 2 and 4 deletions in pathogenesis of idiopatic PD (Choi et al., 2008; Guo et al., 2010; Macedo et al., 2009; Pankratz et al., 2009) in the study in Polish population it has not detected any deletion of exon 2 and 4 in *PRKN* gene as opposed to the German and Japan population, as well as the results obtained in the multipopulation study (Cookson et al., 2008; Nishioka et al., 2009; Polrolniczak et al., 2011; 2012; Shapira et al., 2002). On the other hand, our results were consistent with the study by Kruger et al. (1999), Sinha et al. (2005), as well Barsottini et al. (2011). However, it not be ruled out, that Polish patients have deletion of other not tested exons. Oliveri et al. (2001) suggested that deletion mutations of *PRKN* were not as common in LOPD as in EOPD. Therefore, it seems that copy number variation of *PRKN* is most probably related with EOPD (Wang et al., 2004).

However, point mutations in *PRKN* gene although they are characteristic for EOPD, currently it is suggested that it can be also involved in the pathogenesis of LOPD. However, studies utilizing common mutations and polymorphisms in tests for association with LOPD have produced mixed results (Hu et al., 2000; Oliveri et al., 2001; Satoh & Kuroda, 1999; Wang et al., 1999).

Furthermore there is no question that Parkin-associated parkinsonism is recessive; that is, both alleles are mutant, but despite previous reports whether a heterozygous mutation can cause or increase the risk for PD remains an issue of debate (Farrer et al., 2001; Klein et al., 2000; Lucking et al., 2001; Maruyama et al., 2000).

In the German population the frequency of *PRKN* mutations was 9% (Kann et al., 2002), in Brazilian population 8% (Periquet et al., 2001), and in the American population reached value of less than 4% (Chen et al., 2003) while in the Japanese population reached 66% (Hattori et al., 1998). In Polish population it has been showed small share of *PRKN* mutation in the patho-genesis of EOPD (Dawson & Dawson, 2003) while our study in LOPD have shown, that *PRKN* mutation in Polish population occurred with frequency 20,6% (Polrolniczak et al., 2011; 2012) what was similar to SPD in European population (Nishioka et al., 2009).

Moreover, we showed, that in the Polish population the most frequently were polymorphisms c.500 G>A, c.1180 G>A and c.930 G>C of *PRKN*. Simultaneously, it appears that these poly-morphisms may have incomplete penetration or lead to preclinical changes in the CNS and increased risk LOPD probably in combination with other genetic or environmental factors, as evidenced by Bardien et al. reports (2009). The other two identified *PRKN* mutations (c.823 C> T, c.520 C> T) were detected only in PD patients, what may indicate a high penetration of these substitutions (Sinha et al., 2005), while novel mutation c.520 C>T was identified in two patients and led to a relatively early onset of disease before age 40.

It is suggested, that haploinsufficiency may be considered as a reduction of normal gene expression accompanied by a loss of normal protein activity. Moreover, a lot of reports indicate to the existence of a second, undetected mutation in these patients, perhaps in the promoter or intronic regions (Giasson & Lee, 2001).

Our results, also suggests that the presence more than one heterozygous mutation in the *PRKN* gene may be necessary to PD manifestation. This hypothesis was first proposed by Abbas et al. (1999) moreover, later reviews generally assume the existence of a second, undetected mutation (Giasson & Lee, 2001). In our study also it is probably that patient who had one mutation in *PRKN* may have more genetic changes in not tested region of the gene so extension the studies of the other region of *PRKN* gene is necessary to clarify this issue. On the other hand it can not be ruled that one heterozygous mutation in *PRKN* may be sufficient to increase risk of PD and induce preclinical changes in *substantia nigra* (Khan et al., 2005).

Finally, it seems that clinically, PD patients with *PRKN* substitution generally are characterized by slower progression of the disease compared with PD patients without mutation. Moreover, it has been also observed, that in PD patients with *PRKN* mutations response to L-dopa therapy has been better than in PD patients without substitutions. This observation are generally consistent with the typical descriptions of *PRKN* patients which present slow disease progression (Abbas et al., 1999; Lucking & Briece, 2000) and good response to L-dopa treatment although it have been showed that patients with *PRKN* mutation were more likely to develop treatment-induced motor complications earlier in the treatment (Khan et al., 2005; Lucking & Briece, 2000).

It seems, that point mutation in *PRKN* gene may be involved in the pathogenesis of LOPD and modulate clinical futures in this disease. It is also probably, that analysis of mutations in *PRKN* gene may be useful for diagnostic and prognostic process in PD.

2.3. Mutations in *HTRA2* and *SPR* in the patients with Parkinson's disease

It seems that presence of mutation in the other genes involved in the pathogenesis of PD like *SPR* (involved in dopamine biosynthesis) and *HTRA2* (involved with mitochondrial pathway of PD) probably may additionally affect the levels of ASN and Parkin through interaction with these proteins (Bogaerts et al., 2008; Karamohamed et al., 2003; Sharma et al., 2006; Sharma et al., 2011; Strauss et al., 2005). However, role of those genes in pathogenesis of PD is not enough known. The serine protease HTRA2 is localized to the inner membrane space of mitochondria (Suzuki et al., 2001). Mitochondrial dysfunction as well as ubiquitin–proteasome system damage has been proposed as possible mechanisms leading to dopaminergic neuronal degeneration (Lin & Beal, 2006; Malkus et al., 2009; Rubinsztein, 2006). Therefore *HTRA2* likewise *PRKN* may be included in mitochondrial pathway of PD independently of *PRKN* but that does not exclude the effects of dysfunction of *HTRA2* and *PRKN* may be additive.

Locus of *HTRA2* gene was recently assigned the PARK13 name, but the association of HTRA2 mutations and PD has not been confirmed in independent studies yet. In the study by Strauss et al. (2005) a single heterozygous *HTRA2* substitution (c.1195 G>A, Gly399Ser) was detected in four German patients with sporadic PD while another substitution (c.421 G>T, Ala141Ser) was more frequently found in PD than in controls. However, in a recent study by Simin-Sanchez & Singleton (2008) both variations were not associated with PD while in Belgian population it have been detected another substitution of *HTRA2* (c.1210 C>T, R404W) in sporadic PD (Bogaerts et al., 2008). These inconsistent findings raise a question about the role of mitochondrial *HTRA2* in PD susceptibility.

SPR gene is located in region covered by the locus PARK3 on chromosome 2p13 (Gasser et al., 1998), but the gene responsible for PD in PARK3 families has not yet been identified. One of the candidates is *SPR* gene. The study of Karamohamed et al. (2003) refined association to a region containing the *SPR* gene with PD, and it have been confirmed in further reports, but the study by Sharma et al. (2011) have not shown the association *SPR* and PD risk (Karamo-hamed et al., 2003; Sharma et al., 2006; 2011). However, authors emphasize varied genetic distributions between different populations (Sharma et al., 2011). It is known, that SPR is involved in dopamine synthesis and likewise ASN probably may be responsible for distur-bances in methabolisme of dopamine. The study of Tobin et al. (2007) has shown that expres-sion of *SPR* was significantly increased in PD patient compared with controls. However mutations in *SPR* in PD have not been analyzed so far. Moreover, it is known that phosphor-ylation of *SPR* increase sensitivity for protease activity and that in human SPR protein phosphorylated is only Ser213 (Fujimoto et al., 2002). Therefore, we decided to search for mutation in codon 213 of *SPR* in PD cases.

2.3.1. Patients

The studies were conducted on 89 patients with PD (10 EOPD patients, and 79 sporadic LOPD patients), including 41 women and 47 men aging 34-82 years. Control group included 113 individuals, 79 women and 34 men, 39-83 years of age. Demographic data of all groups summarized in Table 9.

Patients with PD were diagnosed using the criteria of UK Parkinson's Disease Society Brain Bank (Litvan et al., 2003), however stage of disease according to the scale of Hoehn and Yahr (Hoehn & Yahr, 1967).

None of the control subjects had verifiable symptoms of dementia or any other neurological disorders. All subjects had negative family history of PD. All patients were recruited from the Neurology Clinic of Chair and Department of Neurology, University of Medical Sciences, Poznan in Poland. Only Caucasian, Polish subjects were included in the study. A Local Ethical Committee approved the study and the written consent of all patients or their caregivers was obtained.

Factor	Controls	Patients with PD
Individuals	113	89
Age	39-83	34-82
Mean age ±SD	55.5±9.5	62.0±10.1
F/M	79/34	41/47

Table 9. Demographic data of patients with PD and control subjects analyzed for *HTRA2* and *SPR* mutations. SD – standard deviation, F – female, M – male.

2.3.2. Genetic investigations

Isolation of DNA. See point 2.1.2

Analysis of HTRA2 gene. Exons 1 and 7 of *HTRA2* were amplified in 25 µl by PCR under the empirically defined conditions. Primers to amplify (on request) were generated using the online software Pimer3 based on the published genomic sequence of the *HTRA2* gene. PCR products were digested with MboII, MvaI and MspI restriction enzymes (Fermentas, Canada) for screening for c.421 G>T, c.1195 G>A and c.1210 C>T mutations (respectively) and analyzed on 2.5% agarose gels.

Analysis of SPR gene. Exon 3 of *SPR* gene were amplified using PCR with specific primers (5'-TCCATGTTCAGTGGGCTTTT-3'; 5'- TTTCTGGGCTGACACCTTG-3') generated with Primer3 software under the empirically defined conditions. Screening for the c.637 T>A and c.637 T>G mutations of *SPR* was performed by a RFLP analysis on 2.5% agarose gels using TaaI and SsiI (Fermentas, Canada) as restriction enzymes. All detected mutations were confirmed by sequencing of PCR product. Moreover, random duplicate samples (10%) were genotyped for all assays for quality control with 100% reproducibility.

Statistical analysis. See point 2.2.2.

2.3.3. Results

In Polish population the presence of *HTRA2* point mutation was detected in 3% of PD patients (in 2% - c.1195 G>A resulting A141S substitution and in 1% c.421 G>T leads to G399S substitution) and none of controls (Table 10). However, c.1210 C>T mutation of *HTRA2* has not occurred both in PD patients and controls.

Mutation/polymorphism	c.421 G>T	c.1195 G>A	c.1210 C>T	Total substitutions
Controls	0%	0%	0%	0%
PD patients	1%	2%	0%	3%
OR	-	-	-	9.080
95% CI	-	-	-	-
p	>0.05 (F)	>0.05 (F)	>0.05 (F)	=0.05 (F)

Table 10. *HTRA2* point mutations frequencies in PD patients and in controls. Results are expressed as a percentage. Logistic regression analysis and Fisher's exact test were used. OR – odds ratio; CI – confidence interval; F-Fisher's exact test.

In 213 codon of *SPR* gene novel mutation c.637 T>A was identified in 4% patients with PD and 2% controls (Table 11). This substitution is non-synonymous and leads to S213T changes in amino acid chain. However, we did not detected the second analyzed substitution c.637 C>G *SPR* in any of the subjects.

Mutation/polymorphism	c.637 T>A	c.637 C>G
Controls	2%	0%
PD patients	4%	0%
OR	-	-
95% CI	-	-
p	>0.05 (F)	>0.05 (F)

Table 11. *SPR* point mutations frequencies in PD patients and in controls. Results are expressed as a percentage. Logistic regression analysis and Fisher's exact test were used. OR – odds ratio; CI – confidence interval; F-Fisher's exact test.

In PD patients with substitutions in *HTRA2* gene it have been observed slower progression of the disease wherein there was statistically significant association (Spearman correlation test) transition c.1195 G>A with decrease stage of disease (p=0.029; r=-0.237) but association of c.421 G>T substitution have not been significant and have remained at the level of trend. Furthermore it have been shown, that using in PD patients with *HTRA2* mutations doses of L-dopa were lower than in patients without mutations and the response to therapy was better in presence of substitution. Finally, it seems that identified *HTRA2* mutations may be one of PD risk factor, especially since Strauss et al. (2005) demonstrated the presence of olfactory dysfunction in asymptomatic *HTRA2* mutation carrier.

Moreover, it seems that mutation c.637 T>A, because of localization, probably may affect phosphorylation of SR and thereby its activity and finally regulate biosynthesis of DA and serotonin (5-HT). However, analysis of expression and functional testing are necessary to explain importance and role of this mutation. Nevertheless, what is important, in our study c. 637 T>A *SPR* mutation has been significantly associated in Spearman correlation test, with the presence of depressive symptoms in PD patients (p<0.0001; r=0.371) probably by regulating the level of 5-HT (McHugh et al., 2009). Simultaneously, the presence of c.637 T>A of *SPR* mutation in PD patients have not been associated with differences in progression of the disease, response to L-dopa therapy, amount using L-dopa dose or presence of dementia compared to PD patients without *SPR* mutation.

2.4. Coexistence of mutations in more than one gene (*SNCA, PRKN, HTRA2* and *SPR*) in the patients with Parkinson's disease

Our study indicated, that in PD patients as well as in controls in the Polish population, *PRKN* mutations most frequently accompanied by the presence of genotype +1/+2. Interesting the coexistence of mutations *PRKN* with genotypes +2/+2 and +2/+3 have been demonstrated only in patients with PD (Fig. 1). It seems that co-occurrence of point mutation of *PRKN* and polymorphism of *SNCA* promoter region may in additive manner increase risk of PD manifestation.

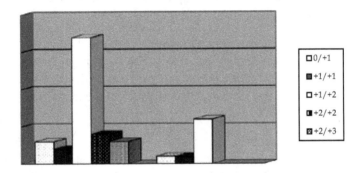

Figure 1. The frequency of NACP-Rep1 region of *SNCA* promoter variants in subjects with *PRKN* mutations (PD patients and controls).

Furthermore, in the patients with PD we demonstrated coexistence of point mutations in *PRKN* and *SPR* or *PRKN* and *HTRA2* genes (Table 12). However, in controls, coexistence of mutations *PRKN* and *SPR* have been observed also in one person. Therefore it seems that in patients with mutation of *PRKN* and *HTRA2* genes, simultaneous incorrect function of two proteins involved in the mitochondria proper functioning (HTRA2 and Parkin) may additionally increase risk of PD manifestation.

Probe number	Group	Substitutions		
		PRKN	*HTRA2*	*SPR*
25	PD patient	c.500 G>A	-	c.637 T>A
114	PD patient	c.930 G>C	c.1195 G>A	-
202	PD patient	c.930 G>C	c.421 G>T	-
18	Control	c.930 G>C	-	c.637 T>A

Table 12. Coexistence of mutations in more than one analyzed gene in PD patients and controls.

3. Role of alpha-synuclein in pathogenesis of Parkinson's disease

Alpha-synuclein is a protein composed of 140 amino acids and is a part of family of proteins with the β- and γ-synuclein (Clayton & George, 1998). For many years, the structure of ASN was determined as the "not-folded" chain of amino acids, taking the helical form only in conjunction with the lipids of cell membranes. It was thought that the ASN is a monomer form but the recent studies have shown that under physiological conditions ASN largely takes the form of tetramers, and may take the helical form without connection to the lipid membrane (Bartels et al., 2011).

Immunohistochemical studies have shown that in the cells, there is essentially ASN bonded to both the nuclear membrane, and in the synaptic vesicles (Totterdel & Meredith, 2005). To a lesser extent, ASN occurs in the free form in the cytoplasm.

Functions of ASN are not fully understood, however, due to cellular location of this protein it is suggested, that function of ASN may be related with the synaptic transport (Alim et al., 2002). There are also reports indicating that ASN participate in the process of differentiation and survival of the dopaminergic neuron progenitor cells of the mouse and human (Michell et al., 2007; Schneider et al., 2007).

Under pathological conditions ASN may change the structure and take the form of beta harmonica, what may lead to aggregation of ASN and formation of soluble oligomers, and then the insoluble filaments and deposits in the nerve cells (Bodles et al., 2001). As it have been shown, ASN is one of the main components of Lewy's bodies (LB), pathology, round or polymorphonuclear cellular inclusions in the cytoplasm of nerve cells. Moreover, it is suggested, that the formation of insoluble deposits of ASN and the aggregation process may give rise to the formation of LB (Halliday et al., 2006).

It is obvious that the process of aggregation of the ASN is a negative phenomenon for neural cells not only because of the high toxicity of the resulting aggregates, but also because of the ASN physiological function disorders caused by the reduction of bioavailability of this protein (Conway et al., 2000). It has been shown, that in PD, the process of ASN aggregation may be modulated by a number factors (Fig. 2) [Haggerty et al., 2011; Li et al., 2008; Ren et al., 2009; Sherer et al., 2002].

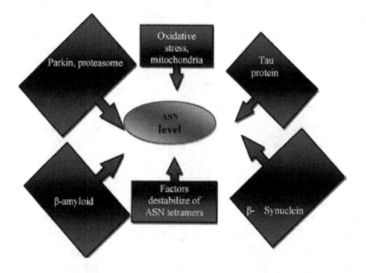

Figure 2. Selected factors affect alpha-synuclein (ASN) level.

3.1. Alpha-synuclein concentration in Parkinson's disease

It has been shown that aggregation of the ASN may be caused among others by multiplication of *SNCA* gene. Furthermore, it has been shown that triplication of *SNCA* gene leads to two-fold increase of ASN level, while duplication of *SNCA* gene increases the level of this protein one and a half-fold (Farrer et al., 2001; Singleton et al., 2003). Therefore it is believed that increased level of ASN may be related with PD manifestation (Farrer et al., 2001; Mata et al., 2004). It is also known that over-expression of ASN in neuron facilitates aggregation of this protein even in the presence of the correct structure of ASN. Moreover, elevated expression of *SNCA*-mRNA levels have been found in the affected regions of PD brain (Chiba-Falek et al., 2006). Increased of ASN level has been also associated with progress and worsening of the disease symptoms (Singleton et al., 2003). However, there are only few reports investigating the level of ASN in the blood of PD patients (Bialek et al., 2011; Fuchs et al., 2008; Lee et al., 2006).

The aim of the study was to estimate the concentration of ASN in plasma of patients with PD and in control group.

3.1.1. Patients

The studies were conducted on 32 patients with PD, including 18 women and 14 men aging 35-82 years. Control group included 24 individuals, 20 women and 4 men, 40-69 years of age. Demographic data of all groups summarized in Table 13.

Patients with PD were diagnosed using the criteria of UK Parkinson's Disease Society Brain Bank (Litvan et al., 2003), however stage of disease according to the scale of Hoehn and Yahr (Hoehn & Yahr, 1967). None of the control subjects had verifiable symptoms of dementia or any other neurological disorders.

All patients were recruited from the Neurology Clinic of Chair and Department of Neurology, University of Medical Sciences, Poznan in Poland. Only Caucasian, Polish subjects were included in the study.

A Local Ethical Committee approved the study and the written consent of all patients or their caregivers was obtained.

Factor	Controls	Patients with PD
Individuals	24	32
Age	40-69	35-82
Mean age ±SD	55.3±6.8	62.5±10.5
F/M	20/4	18/14

Table 13. Demographic data of patients with PD and control subjects analyzed for ASN concentrations. SD – standard deviation, F – female, M – male.

3.1.2. Analysis of ASN concentrations

Preparation of samples. Blood samples from these subjects were drawn using EDTA as an anticoagulant in the morning after an overnight fast and the samples were centrifuge for 15 min at 1000xg at 4° C within 30 min and plasma was frozen at −80° C for later use.

Determination of ASN concentration. ASN ELISA was performed using the Enzyme-linked Immunosorbent Assay Kit for Human Synuclein Alpha (Uscn Life Science Inc., China) according to the manufacturer's protocol. The minimal detection limits in this assay is typically less than 4.8 pg/ml. The standard curve concentrations used were 1000; 5000; 250; 125; 62.5; 31.2 and 15.6 pg/ml. The intra- and interassay precision of coefficiences of variation were <10% and <12% respectively. After completion of each assay the plate(s) were read at 450 nm on an EPOCH Multi-Volume Spectrophotometer (BioTek, USA) and the results were analyzed using Gen5 2.1 Software (BioTek, USA).

3.1.3. Results

Detectable concentrations of ASN have been detected in higher percentage of controls than in PD patients. However, in patients with PD has been shown higher concentration of ASN (Table 14).

Parameter	Controls	Patients with PD
Detectable concentrations of ASN, n [%]	4 [17%]	4 [12%]
ASN concentrations [pg/ml]	[68.19-645.57]	[55.2-1294.9]

Table 14. ASN concentrations in the patients with PD and in control group. Results are expressed as an interval between the minimum and maximum measurement, n – number, % - of subjects; detectable concentrations of ASN – above 0.058 pg/ml in ELISA test.

In PD patients, the highest concentrations of ASN were present in two first stages of disease progress (Hoehn and Yahr scale) [Table 15] and in the first ten years of the disease (Table 16).

Stage of disease according to the scale of Hoehn and Yahr	ASN concentrations in PD patients [pg/ml]
1	[55.2]
2	[60.94-1294.9]
3	-

Table 15. Detectable (above 0.058 pg/ml in ELISA test) concentrations of ASN in PD patients depending on stage of disease in Hoehn and Yafr scale. Results are expressed as an interval between the minimum and maximum measurement/single result.

Duration of disease	ASN concentrations in PD patients [pg/ml]
< 5 years	[55.2-293.67]
5-10 years	[1294.9]
>10 years	-

Table 16. Detectable (above 0.058 pg/ml in ELISA test) concentrations of ASN in PD patients depending on duration of the disease. Results are expressed as an interval between the minimum and maximum measurement/single result.

In this study and Bialek et al. (2011) have been shown higher concentration of plasma ASN level in PD patients as compared to controls. However, it seems that aggregation of the ASN in the nerve cells may reduce ASN ability to pass through the blood-brain barrier, which in turn may result in significantly reduced levels of this protein in the peripheral blood. Moreover, a high concentration of ASN has been detected only in the initial period of PD (in two first stages of PD progress in Hoehn and Yahr scale, and in the first ten years of the disease), probably even before the accumulation of deposits in the form of LB in the brain of PD patients. However, in the study by Pchelina et al. (2011) the level of ASN was significantly lower in patients with *LRRK2*-associated PD compared with SPD and controls what may be caused also by severed ASN aggregation in this group.

4. Role of Parkin in pathogenesis of Parkinson's disease

Parkin is a cytoplasmic protein which plays a vital role in the proper functioning of the mitochondria and functions as an E3 ligase ubiquitin stimulating protein binding (directed to degradation in the proteasome) with ubiquitin, consequently preventing the cell apoptosis (Zhang et al., 2000). Ubiquitination is a vital cellular quality control mechanism that prevents accumulation of misfolded and damaged proteins in the cell. It is thought that substrates of Parkin include among others synphilin-1, ASN, CDC-rel1, cyclin E, p38 tRNA synthase, Pael-R and synaptotagmin XI. It has been shown in the study by Zhang et al, [2000] Parkin is also responsible for their own ubiquitination and degradation in the proteasome.

Recent studies have shown that Parkin may play a role in decision-making, choosing between two systems of degradation: the proteasome activity (through its ability to promote ubiquitination K48 associated with the proteasome) and macroautophagy (through K63 ubiquitination related to cell signaling and the formation of LB) [Henn et al., 2007; Lim et al., 2006].

4.1. Parkin concentration in Parkinson's disease

The aim of the study was to estimate the concentration of Parkin in plasma of patients with PD and in control group.

Patients (see point 3.1.1.)

Analysis of Parkin concentrations

Preparation of samples. Blood samples from these subjects were drawn using EDTA as an anticoagulant in the morning after an overnight fast and the samples were centrifuge for 20 min at 1000xg at 4° C within 30 min and plasma was frozen at −80° C for later use.

Determination of Parkin concentration. Parkin ELISA was performed using the Enzyme-linked Immunosorbent Assay Kit for Human Parkinson Disease Protein 2 (Uscn Life Science Inc., China) according to the manufacturer's protocol. The minimal detection limits in this assay is typically less than 0.058 ng/ml. The standard curve concentrations used were 10; 5; 2.5; 1.25; 0.625; 0.312; and 0.156 ng/ml. The intra- and interassay precision of coefficients of variation were <10% and <12% respectively. After completion of each assay the plate(s) were read at 450 nm on an EPOCH Multi-Volume Spectrophotometer (BioTek, USA) and the results were analyzed using Gen5 2.1 Software (BioTek, USA).

4.1.1. Results

Detectable concentrations of Parkin have been detected in similar percentage of controls and PD patients. However, in patients with PD has been shown lower concentration of Parkin (Table 17).

Parameter	Controls	Patients with PD
Detectable concentrations of Parkin, n [%]	5 [21%]	7 [22%]
Parkin concentrations [ng/ml]	[0.036-4.436]	[0.076-2.123]

Table 17. Parkin concentrations in the patients with PD and control group. Results are expressed as an interval between the minimum and maximum measurement. n – number, % - of subjects; detectable concentrations of Parkin – above 0.058 ng/ml in ELISA test.

In PD patients, the highest concentration of Parkin occurred in 2 stage of disease progress with tendency to reduce the concentration in the 3 stage of the disease (Hoehn and Yahr scale) [Table 18] and in the first ten years of the disease (Table 19).

Stage of disease according to the scale of Hoehn and Yahr	Parkin concentrations in PD patients [ng/ml]
1	-
2	[0.158-2.123]
3	[0.076-0.409]

Table 18. Detectable (above 0.058 ng/ml in ELISA test) concentrations of Parkin in PD patients depending on stage of disease in Hoehn and Yahr scale. Results are expressed as an interval between the minimum and maximum measurement/single result.

Duration of disease	Parkin concentrations in PD patients [ng/ml]
< 5 years	[0.549-2.123]
5-10 years	[0.158-2.054]
>10 years	[0.076] mutation in 11 exon of *PRKN*

Table 19. Detectable (above 0.058 ng/ml in ELISA test) concentrations of Parkin in PD patients depending on duration of the disease. Results are expressed as an interval between the minimum and maximum measurement/single result.

It is known that dysfunction of Parkin may lead to manifestation of PD in several mechanism including mitochondrial and ubiquitination disturbances. It also seems that expression and cellular level of Parkin may be essential factor for proper function of this protein. However, the presence of Parkin protein has been demonstrated in human serum using Western blotting, there is few analysis of the level of this protein in the blood of PD patients (Dorszewska et al., 2012; Kasap et al., 2009). In the study by Dorszewska et al. (2012) has been detected lower plasma Parkin concentration in PD patients than in controls. Moreover, increased levels of the Parkin have been detected in PD patients in the early stages of PD (Hoehn and Yahr scale) and decreasing with the progress and duration of this disease. It seems that in the early stages of PD development may occur to increase of Parkin expression through the ongoing degenerative process and to the accumulation of pathological proteins-Parkin substrates. However, as the disease progresses, probably, resources of the Parkin running out and occurs weaken its neuroprotective function.

5. Relationship between alpha-synuclein and Parkin levels in Parkinson's disease

In 2001, Shimura et al. first described the presence in the human brain complex containing Parkin with the glycosylated form of the ASN (alpha-SP22), thus indicating the involvement of Parkin in ASN degradation in ubiquitin-proteasome system [Shimura et al., 2001; Chung et al., 2004]. It has been also shown that dysfunction of the Parkin can lead to ineffective elimination of ASN and the aggregation of this protein [Haass & Kahle, 2001]. In addition, according to the reports, the Parkin may also interact with the dopamine and indirectly influence the aggregation of the ASN in the nerve cell (Oyama et al., 2010). Therefore, it seems that the levels of these two proteins may be related and dependent on each other.

Patients (see point 3.1.1.)

Analysis of ASN (see point 3.1.2.), and Parkin (see point 4.1.2.) concentrations

5.1. Results

In patients with PD detectable levels of Parkin occurred in a nearly two-fold higher incidence than the ASN (Tables 14, 17).

Parameter	Controls	Patients with PD
ASN concentration [pg/ml]	[68.19-645.57]	[55.2-1294.9]
Parkin concentration [pg/ml]	[36.0-4436.0]	[76.0-2123.0]

Table 20. ASN and Parkin concentrations in the patients with PD and control group. Detectable concentrations of ASN and Parkin – above 0.058 pg/ml in ELISA test. Results are expressed as an interval between the minimum and maximum measurement.

Stage of disease according to the scale of Hoehn and Yahr	ASN concentrations in PD patients [pg/ml]	Parkin concentrations in PD patients [pg/ml]
1	[55.2]	-
2	[60.94-1294.9]	[158.0-2123.0]
3	-	[76.0-409.0]

Table 21. Detectable (above 0.058 pg/ml in ELISA test) concentrations of ASN and Parkin in PD patients depending on stage of disease in Hoehn and Yahr scale. Results are expressed as an interval between the minimum and maximum measurement/single result.

Duration of disease	ASN concentrations in PD patients [pg/ml]	Parkin concentrations in PD patients [pg/ml]
< 5 years	[55.2-293.67]	[549.0-2123.0]
5-10 years	[1294.9]	[158.0-2054.0]
>10 years	-	[76.0] mutation in 11 exon of *PRKN*

Table 22. Detectable (above 0.058 pg/ml in ELISA test) concentrations of ASN and Parkin in PD patients depending on duration of the disease. Results are expressed as an interval between the minimum and maximum measurement/single result.

In this study and studies by Bialek et al. (2011) and Dorszewska et al. (2012) have been shown, that in PD patients increased level of ASN was associated with the decreased level of Parkin in contrast to control group (Tables 20-22). Independently for the analyzed group, the highest levels of ASN have been observed in the subjects who had very low Parkin levels. It suggested that low concentration of Parkin may contribute to increased ASN level in the nerve cells and combined with over-expression of ASN intensify or accelerate neurodegenerative process. Moreover, it has been also shown that configuration: increased plasma level of ASN and decreased of Parkin was associated with earlier onset of this disease.

6. Mutations in PARK (*PRKN, SPR, HTRA2, SNCA*) genes and ASN and Parkin concentrations in Parkinson's disease

Our study on Polish population shown that in PD patients *PRKN* (exons 4, 8, 11) mutations were more than four times frequency as compared to controls. Moreover, in PD patients more frequently occurred genotypes +2/+2 and +2/+3 of the promoter region *SNCA* gene than in controls. In patients with PD shown higher concentration of ASN while higher Parkin level in controls. In PD patients without mutations in PARK, highest concentration of ASN and Parkin was present in two first stages of disease progress (Hoehn and Yahr scale) and in the first ten years of the disease. However, only in PD patient with mutation in 11 exon of *PRKN* gene shown presence of Parkin without ASN after ten years of disease duration (Table 19, 22).

It seems that analysis of these pathological proteins with PARK gene mutations may be useful in the diagnostic and monitoring of the PD progress in the future.

7. Conclusion

In Polish population, in *PRKN* gene point mutations occur few times more often in PD patients than controls. Control subjects tend to show higher level of plasma Parkin whereas patients suffering from PD tend to generate higher level of plasma ASN. In PD patients without point mutations in PRKN gene Parkin and ASN plasma levels increase until 2nd stage of disease in Hoehn and Yahr scale and during first 10 years of disease.

Analysis of the variations of PARK gene as well as plasma levels of ASN and Parkin may consist an additional diagnostic factor for PD.

Author details

Anna Oczkowska[1], Margarita Lianeri[1], Wojciech Kozubski[2] and Jolanta Dorszewska[1]

1 Poznan University of Medical Sciences, Laboratory of Neurobiology Department of Neurology, Poznan, Poland

2 Poznan University of Medical Sciences, Chair and Department of Neurology, Poznan, Poland

References

[1] Alim, M.A., Hossain, M.S., Arima, K., Takeda, K., Izumiyama, Y., Nakamura, M., Kaji, H., Shinoda, T., Hisanaga, S., & Ueda, K. (2002). Tubulin seeds alpha-synuclein fi-

bril formation. *Journal of Biological Chemistry*, Vol.277, No.3, (January 2002), pp. 2112-2117, ISSN 0021-9258

[2] Abbas, N., Lucking, C.B., Ricard, S., Dürr, A., Bonifati, V., De Michele, G., Bouley, S., Vaughan, J.R., Gasser, T., Marconi, R., Broussolle, E., Brefel-Courbon, C., Harhangi, B.S., Oostra, B.A., Fabrizio, E., Böhme, G.A., Pradier, L., Wood, N.W., Filla, A., Meco, G., Denefle, P., Agid, Y., & Brice, A. (1999). A wide variety of mutations in the parkin gene are responsible for autosomal recessive parkinsonism in Europe. *Human Molecular Genetics*, Vol.8, No.4, (April 1999), pp. 567-574, ISSN 0964-6906

[3] Abeliovich, A., Schmitz, Y., Fariñas, I., Choi-Lundberg, D., Ho, W.H., Castillo, P.E., Shinsky, N., Verdugo, J.M., Armanini, M., Ryan, A., Hynes, M., Phillips, H., Sulzer, D., & Rosenthal, A. (2000). Mice lacking alpha-synuclein display functional deficits in the nigrostriatal dopamine system. Neuron, Vol.25, No1., (January 2000), pp. 239-252, ISSN 0896-6273

[4] Ahn, T.B., Kim, S.Y., Kim, J.Y., Park, S.S., Lee, D.S., Min, H.J., Kim, Y.K., Kim, S.E., Kim, J.M., Kim, H.J., Cho, J., & Jeon, B.S. (2008). alpha Synuclein gene duplication is present in sporadic Parkinson disease. *Neurology*, Vol.70, No.1, (January 2008), pp. 43-49, ISSN 0896-6273

[5] Bardien, S., Keyser, R., Yako, Y., Lombard, D., & Carr, J. (2009). Molecular analysis of the parkin gene in South African patients diagnosed with Parkinson's disease. *Parkinsonism and Related Disorders*, Vol.15, No.2, (February 2009), pp. 116-121, ISSN 1353-8020

[6] Barsottini, O.G., Felício, A.C., de Carvalho Aguiar, P., Godeiro-Junior, C., Pedroso, J.L., de Aquino, C.C., Bor-Seng-Shu, E., & de Andrade, L.A. (2011). Heterozygous exon 3 deletion in the Parkin gene in a patient with clinical and radiological MSA-C phenotype. *Clinical Neurology and Neurosurgery*, Vol.113, No.5, (June 2011), pp. 404-406, ISSN *0303-8467*

[7] Bartels, T., Choi, J.G., & Selkoe, D.J. (2011). α-Synuclein occurs physiologically as a helically folded tetramer that resists aggregation. *Nature*, Vol.477, No.7362, (August 2011), pp. 107-110, ISSN 0028-0836

[8] Bialecka, M., Hui, S., Klodowska-Duda, G., Opala, G., Tan, E.K., & Drozdzik, M. (2005). Analysis of LRRK 2 G 2019 S and I 2020 T mutations in Parkinson's disease. *Neuroscience Letters*, Vol.390, No.1, (December 2005), pp. 1-3, ISSN 0304-3940

[9] Bialek, P., Półrolniczak, A., Dorszewska, J., Florczak-Wyspiańska, J., Owecki, M., Skibinska, M., & Kozubski W. (2011). Mutations of the SNCA gene and alpha- synuclein level in the patients with diseases of the extrapyramidal system. Pharmacological Reports, 63, 5, 1285, ISSN 1734-1140, Neurochemical Conference 2011. Abstracts of the Days of Neurochemistry Genetic and molecular mechanisms of neurological diseases. Progress in diagnosis and therapy. Warsaw, Poland, October 20-21, 2011

[10] Bodles, A.M., Guthrie, D.J., Greer, B., & Irvine, G.B. (2001). Identification of the region of non-Abeta component (NAC) of Alzheimer's disease amyloid responsible for

its aggregation and toxicity. *Journal of Neurochemistry*, Vol.78, No.2, (July 2001), pp. 384-395, ISSN 1471-4159

[11] Bogaerts, V., Nuytemans, K., Reumers, J., Pals, P., Engelborghs, S., Pickut, B., Corsmit, E., Peeters, K., Schymkowitz, J., De Deyn, P.P., Cras, P., Rousseau, F., Theuns, J., & Van Broeckhoven, C. (2008). Genetic variability in the mitochondrial serine protease HTRA2 contributes to risk for Parkinson disease. *Human Mutation*, Vol.29, No. 6, (June 2008), pp. 832-840, ISSN 1059-7794

[12] Bras, J., Guerreiro, R., Ribeiro, M., Morgadinho, A., Januario, C., Dias, M., Calado, A., Semedo, C., Oliveira, C., Hardy, J., & Singleton, A. (2008). Analysis of Parkinson disease patients from Portugal for mutations in SNCA, PRKN, PINK1 and LRRK2. *BMC Neurology*, Vol.22, No.8, (January 2008), pp. 1, ISSN 1471-2377

[13] Brooks, J., Ding, J., Simon-Sanchez, J., Paisan-Ruiz, C., Singleton, A.B., & Scholz, S.W. (2009). Parkin and PINK1 mutations in early-onset Parkinson's disease: comprehensive screening in publicly available cases and control. *Journal of Medical Genetics*, Vol. 46, No.6, (June 2009), pp. 375-381, ISSN 1552-4833

[14] Chen, R., Gosavi, N.S., Langston, J.W., & Chan, P. (2003). Parkin mutations are rare in patients with young-onset parkinsonism in a US population. Parkinsonism & Related Disorders, Vol.9, No.5, (June 2003), pp. 309-312, ISSN 1353-8020

[15] Chiba-Falek, O., & Nussbaum, R.L. (2001). Effect of allelic variation at the NACP-Rep1 repeat upstream of the alpha-synuclein gene (SNCA) on transcription in a cell culture luciferase reporter system. *Human Molecular Genetics*, Vol.10, No.26, (December 2001), pp. 3101-3109, ISSN 0964-6906

[16] Chiba-Falek, O., Lopez, G.J., & Nussbaum, R.L. (2006). Levels of alpha-synuclein mRNA in sporadic Parkinson disease patients. *Movement Disorders*, Vol.21, No.10, (October 2006), pp. 1703-1708, ISSN 0885-3185

[17] Choi, J.M., Woo, M.S., Ma, H.I., Kang, S.Y., Sung, Y.H., Yong, S.W., Chung, S.J., Kim, J.S., Shin, H.W., Lyoo, C.H., Lee, P.H., Baik, J.S., Kim, S.J., Park, M.Y., Sohn, Y.H., Kim, J.H., Kim, J.W., Lee, M.S., Lee, M.C., Kim, D.H., & Kim, Y.J. (2008). Analysis of PARK genes in a Korean cohort of early-onset Parkinson disease. Neurogenetics, Vol. 9, No.4, (October 2008), pp. 263-269, ISSN 1563-5260

[18] Chung, K.K., Thomas, B., Li, X., Pletnikova, O., Troncoso, J.C., Marsh, L., Dawson, V.L., & Dawson, T.M. (2004). S-nitrosylation of parkin regulates ubiquitination and compromises parkin's protective function. *Science*, Vol.304, No.5675, (May 2004), pp. 1328-1331, ISSN 0036-8075

[19] Chung, S.J., Armasu, S.M., Biernacka, J.M., Lesnick, T.G., Rider, D.N., Lincoln, S.J., Ortolaza, A.I., Farrer, M.J., Cunningham, J.M., Rocca, W.A., & Maraganore, D.M. (2011). Common variants in PARK loci and related genes and Parkinson's disease. *Movement Disorders*, Vol.26, No.2, (February 2011), pp. 280-288, ISSN 0885-3185

[20] Clayton, D.F., & George, J.M. (1998). The synucleins: a family of proteins involved in synaptic function, plasticity, neurodegeneration and disease. *Trends in Neuroscience*, Vol.21, No.6, (January 1998), pp. 249-254, ISSN 0166-2236

[21] Conway, K.A., Lee, S.J., Rochet, J.C., Ding, T.T., Williamson, R.E., & Lansbury, P.T.Jr. (2000). Acceleration of oligomerization, not fibrillization, is a shared property of both α-synuclein mutations linked to early-onset Parkinson's disease: implications for pathogenesis and therapy. Proceedings of the National Academy of Sciences of the United States, Vol.97, No.2, (January 2000), pp. 571-576, ISSN 0027-8424

[22] Cookson, M.R., Hardy, J., & Lewis, P.A. (2008). Genetic Neuropathology of Parkinson's Disease. *International Journal of Clinical and Experimental Pathology*, Vol.1, No.3, (January 2008), pp. 217-231, ISSN 1936-2625

[23] Corti, O., Lesage, S., & Brice, A. (2011). What genetics tells us about the causes and mechanisms of Parkinson's disease. *Physiological Reviews*, Vol.91, No.4, (October 2011), pp. 1161–1218, ISSN 0031-9333

[24] Cronin, K.D., Ge, D., Manninger, P., Linnertz, C., Rossoshek, A., Orrison, B.M., Bernard, D.J., El-Agnaf, O.M., Schlossmacher, M.G., Nussbaum, R.L., & Chiba-Falek, O. (2009) Expansion of the Parkinson disease-associated SNCA-Rep1 allele upregulates human alpha-synuclein in transgenic mouse brain. *Human Molecular Genetics*, Vol.18, No.17, (September 2009), pp. 3274-3285, ISSN 0964-6906

[25] Dawson, T.M., & Dawson, V.L. (2003). Molecular pathways of neurodegeneration in Parkinson's disease. *Science*, Vol.302, No.5646, (October 2003), pp. 819-822, ISSN 0036-8075

[26] Dorszewska, J., Debek, A., Oczkowska, A., Florczak-Wyspiańska J., Owecki M., & Kozubski W. (2012). Polymorphism of the PARK2 gene and Parkin protein levels in patients with Parkinson Disease. Acta Neurobiologie Experimentalis, 70, 1, P53, 191, ISSN 0065-1400. Abstracts of the 11th International Symposium on Molecular Basis of Pathology and Therapy in Neurological Disorders. Warsaw, Poland, November 22-23, 2012

[27] Farrer, M., Chan, P., Chen, R., Tan, L., Lincoln, S., Hernandez, D., Forno, L., Gwinn-Hardy, K., Petrucelli, L., Hussey, J., Singleton, A., Tanner, C., Hardy, & J., Langston, J.W. (2001). Lewy bodies and parkinsonism in families with parkin mutations. *Annals Neurology*, Vol.50, No.3, (September 2001), pp. 293-300, ISSN 0364-5134

[28] Fuchs, J., Tichopad, A., Golub, Y., Munz, M., Schweitzer, K.J., Wolf, B., Berg, D., Mueller, J.C., & Gasser, T. (2008). Genetic variability in the SNCA gene influences alpha-synuclein levels in the blood and brain. *FASEB Journal*, Vol.22, No.5, (May 2008), pp. 1327-1334, ISSN 0892-6638

[29] Fujimoto, K., Takahashi, S.Y., & Katoh S. (2002). Mutational analysis of sites in sepiapterin reductase phosphorylated by Ca2./calmodulin-dependent protein kinase II.

Biochimica et Biophysica Acta, Vol.1594, No.1, (January 2002), pp. 191-198, ISSN 0006-3002

[30] Gao, X., Martin, E.R., Liu, Y., Mayhew, G., Vance, J.M., & Scott, W.K. (2009). Genome-wide linkage screen in familial Parkinson disease identifies loci on chromosomes 3 and 18. *American Journal of Human Genetics*, Vol.84, No.4, (April 2009), pp. 499–504, ISSN 0002-9297

[31] Gasser, T., Müller-Myhsok, B., Wszolek, Z.K., Oehlmann, R., Calne, D.B., Bonifati, V., Bereznai, B., Fabrizio, E., Vieregge, P., & Horstmann, R.D. (1998). A susceptibility locus for Parkinson's disease maps to chromosome 2p13. *Nature Genetics*, Vol.18, No.3, (March 1998), pp. 262-265, ISSN 1061-4036

[32] Giasson, B.I., & Lee, V.M. (2001). Parkin and the molecular pathways of Parkinson's disease. Neuron, Vol.31, No.6, (September 2001), pp. 885-888, ISSN 0896-6273

[33] Gilks, W.P., Abou-Sleiman, P.M., Gandhi, S., Jain, S., Singleton, A., Lees, A.J., Shaw, K., Bhatia, K.P., Bonifati, V., Quinn, N.P., Lynch, J., Healy, D.G., Holton, J.L., Revesz, T., & Wood, N.W. (2005). A common LRRK2 mutation in idiopathic Parkinson's disease. *Lancet*, Vol.365, No.9457, (February 2005), pp. 415–416, ISSN 0140-6736

[34] Guo, J.F., Zhang, X.W., Nie, L.L., Zhang, H.N., Liao, B., Li, J., Wang, L., Yan, X.X., & Tang, B.S. (2010). Mutation analysis of Parkin, PINK1 and DJ-1 genes in Chinese patients with sporadic early onset parkinsonism. *Journal of Neurology*, Vol.257, No.7, (July 2010), pp. 1170-1175, ISSN 0340-5354

[35] Haass, C., & Kahle, P.J. (2001). Neuroscience. Parkin and its substrates. *Science*, Vol. 293, No.5528, (July 2001), pp. 224-225, ISSN 0036-8075

[36] Hadjigeorgiou, G.M., Xiromerisiou, G., & Gourbali, V. (2006). Association of alpha-synuclein Rep1 polymorphism and Parkinson's disease: influence of Rep1 on age at onset. Movement Disorders, Vol.21, No.4, (April 2006), pp. 534-539, ISSN 0885-3185

[37] Haggerty, T., Credle, J., Rodriguez, O., Wills, J., Oaks, A.W., Masliah, E., & Sidhu, A. (2011). Hyperphosphorylated Tau in an α-synuclein-overexpressing transgenic model of Parkinson's disease. *European Journal of Neuroscience*, Vol.33, No.9, (May 2011), pp. 1598-1610, ISSN 1460-9568

[38] Halliday, G.M., Del Tredici, K., & Braak, H. (2006). Critical appraisal of brain pathology staging related to presymptomatic and symptomatic cases of sporadic Parkinson's disease. Journal of Neural Transmission, Vol.70, pp. 99-103, ISSN 0300-9564

[39] Hattori, N., Kitada, T., Matsumine, H., Asakawa, S., Yamamura, Y., Yoshino, H., Kobayashi, T., Yokochi, M., Wang, M., Yoritaka, A., Kondo, T., Kuzuhara, S., Nakamura, S., Shimizu, N., & Mizuno, Y. (1998). Molecular genetic analysis of a novel parkin gene in Japanese families with autosomal recessive juvenile parkinsonism: evidence for variable homozygous deletions in the parkin gene in affected individuals. *Annals Neurology*, Vol.44, No.6, (December 1998), pp. 935-941, ISSN 0364-5134

[40] Hedrich, K., Eskelson, C., Wilmot, B., Marder, K., Harris, J., Garrels, J., Meija-Santana, H., Vieregge, P., Jacobs, H., Bressman, S.B., Lang, A.E., Kann, M., Abbruzzese, G., Martinelli, P., Schwinger, E., Ozelius, L.J., Pramstaller, P.P., Klein, & C., Kramer, P. (2004). Distribution, type, and origin of Parkin mutations: review and case studies. Movement Disorders, Vol.19, No.10, (October 2004), pp. 1146-1157, ISSN 0885-3185

[41] Henn, I.H., Bouman, L., Schlehe, J.S., Schlierf, A., Schramm, J.E., Wegener, E., Nakaso, K., Culmsee, C., Berninger, B., Krappmann, D., Tatzelt, J., & Winklhofer, K.F. (2007). Parkin mediates neuroprotection through activation of IkappaB kinase/nuclear factor-kappaB signaling. Journal of Neuroscience, Vol.27, No.8, (February 2007), pp. 1868-1878, ISSN 0270-6474

[42] Hoehn, M.M., & Yahr M.D. (1967). Parkinsonism: onset, progression and mortality. Neurology, Vol.17, No.5, (May 1967), pp. 427-442, ISSN 0896-6273

[43] Hu, C.J., Sung, S.M., Liu, H.C., Lee, C.C., Tsai, C.H., & Chang, J.G. (2000). Polymorphisms of the parkin gene in sporadic Parkinson's disease among Chinese in Taiwan. European Neurology, Vol.44, No.2, pp. 90-93, ISSN 0014-3022

[44] Kann, M., Jacobs, H., Mohrmann, K., Schumacher, K., Hedrich, K., Garrels, J., Wiegers, K., Schwinger, E., Pramstaller, P.P., Breakefield, X.O., Ozelius, L.J., Vieregge, P., & Klein, C. (2002). Role of parkin mutations in 111 community-based patients with early-onset parkinsonism. Annals Neurology, Vol.51, No.5, (May 2002), pp. 621-625, ISSN 0364-5134

[45] Karamohamed, S., DeStefano, A.L., Wilk, J.B., Shoemaker, C.M., Golbe, L.I., Mark, M.H., Lazzarini, A.M., Suchowersky, O., Labelle, N., Guttman, M., Currie, L.J., Wooten, G.F., Stacy, M., Saint-Hilaire, M., Feldman, R.G., Sullivan, K.M., Xu, G., Watts, R., Growdon, J., Lew, M., Waters, C., Vieregge, P., Pramstaller, P.P., Klein, C., Racette, B.A., Perlmutter, J.S., Parsian, A., Singer, C., Montgomery, E., Baker, K., Gusella, J.F., Fink, S.J., Myers, R.H., Herbert, A, GenePD study. (2003). A haplotype at the PARK3 locus influences onset age for Parkinson's disease: the GenePD study. Neurology, Vol.61, No.11, (December 2003), pp. 1557-1561, ISSN 0896-6273

[46] Kasap, M., Akpinar, G., Sazci, A., Idrisoglu, H.A., & Vahaboğlu, H. (2009). Evidence for the presence of full-length PARK2 mRNA and Parkin protein in human blood. Neuroscience Letters, Vol.460, No.3, (September 2009), pp. 196-200, ISSN 0304-3940

[47] Kay, D.M., Factor, S.A., Samii, A., Higgins, D.S., Griffith, A., Roberts, J.W., Leis, B.C., Nutt, J.G., Montimurro, J.S., Keefe, R.G., Atkins, A.J., Yearout, D., Zabetian, C.P., & Payami, H. (2008). Genetic association between alpha-synuclein and idiopathic Parkinson's disease. American Journal of Medical Genetics Part B: Neuropsychiatric Genetics, Vol.147B, No.7, (October 2008), pp. 1222-1230, ISSN 1552-4841

[48] Khan, N.L., Scherfler, C., Graham, E., Bhatia, K.P., Quinn, N., Lees, A.J., Brooks, D.J., Wood, N.W., & Piccini, P. (2005). Dopaminergic dysfunction in unrelated, asympto-

matic carriers of a single parkin mutation. *Neurology*, Vol.64, No.1, (January 2005), pp. 134-136, ISSN 0896-6273

[49] Kitada, T., Asakawa, S., Hattori, N., Matsumine, H., Yamamura, Y., & Minoshima, S. (1998). Mutations in the parkin gene cause autosomal recessive juvenile parkinsonism. *Nature*, Vol.392, No.6676, (April 1998), pp. 605-608, ISSN 0028-0836

[50] Klein, C., Schumacher, K., Jacobs, H., Hagenah, J., Kis, B., Garrels, J., Schwinger, E., Ozelius, L., Pramstaller, P., Vieregge, P., & Kramer, P.L. (2000). Association studies of Parkinson's disease and parkin polymorphisms. *Annals Neurology*, Vol.48, No.1, (July 2000), pp. 126-127, ISSN 0364-5134

[51] Klein, C., Djarmati, A., Hedrich, K., Schafer, N., Scaglione, C., Marchese, R., Kock, N., Schule, B., Hiller, A., Lohnau, T., Winkler, S., Wiegers, K., Hering, R., Bauer, P., Riess, O., Abbruzzese, G., Martinelli, P., & Pramstaller, P.P. (2005). PINK1, Parkin, and DJ-1 mutations in Italian patients with early-onset parkinsonism. *European Journal of Human Genetics*, Vol.13, No.9, (September 2005), pp. 1086-1093, ISSN 1018-4813

[52] Klein, C., & Schlossmacher, M.G. (2007). Parkinson disease, 10 years after its genetic revolution: multiple clues to a complex disorder. *Neurology*, Vol.69, No.22, (November 2007), pp. 2093-2104, ISSN 0896-6273

[53] Klein, C., & Westenberger, A. (2012). Genetics of Parkinson's disease. *Cold Spring Harbor Perspectives in Medicine*, Vol.2, No.1, (January 2012), pp. e1-16, ISSN 2157-1422

[54] Koziorowski, D., Hoffman-Zacharska, D., Sławek, J., Szirkowiec, W., Janik, P., Bal, J., & Friedman, A. (2010). Low frequency of the PARK2 gene mutations in Polish patients with the early-onset form of Parkinson disease. Parkinsonism & Related Disorders, Vol.16, No.2, (February 2010), pp. 136-138, ISSN 1353-8020

[55] Krüger, R., Kuhn, W., Müller, T., Woitalla, D., Graeber, M., Kösel, S., Przuntek, H., Epplen, J.T., Schöls, L., & Riess, O. (1998). Ala30Pro mutation in the gene encoding alpha-synuclein in Parkinson's disease. *Nature Genetics*, Vol.18, No.2, (February 1998), pp. 106-108, ISSN 1061-4036

[56] Krüger, R., Vieira-Säcker, A.M., Kuhn, W., Müller, T., Woitalla, D., Schöls, L., Przuntek, H., Epplen, J.T., & Riess, O. (1999). Analysis of the parkin deletion in sporadic and familial Parkinson's disease. Journal of Neural Transmission, 1999, Vol.106, No. 2, pp. 159-163, ISSN 0300-9564

[57] Lee, P.H., Lee, G., Park, H.J., Bang, O.Y., Joo, I.S., & Huh, K. (2006). The plasma alpha-synuclein levels in patients with Parkinson's disease and multiple system atrophy. Journal of Neural Transmission, Vol.113, No.10, (October 2006), pp. 1435-1439, ISSN 0300-9564

[58] Lesage, S., & Brice, A. (2009). Parkinson's disease: from monogenic forms to genetic susceptibility factors. *Human Molecular Genetics*, Vol.18, No.R1, (April 2009), pp. R48-59, ISSN 0964-6906

[59] Li, J.Y., Englund, E., Holton, J.L., Soulet, D., Hagell, P., Lees, A.J., Lashley, T., Quinn, N.P., Rehncrona, S., Björklund, A., Widner, H., Revesz, T., Lindvall, O., & Brundin, P. (2008). Lewy bodies in grafted neurons in subjects with Parkinson's disease suggest host-to-graft disease propagation. *Nature Medicine*, Vol.14, No.5, (May 2008), pp. 501-503, ISSN 1078-8956

[60] Lim, K.L., Dawson, V.L., & Dawson, T.M. (2006). Parkin-mediated lysine 63-linked polyubiquitination: a link to protein inclusions formation in Parkinson's and other conformational diseases? Neurobiology of Aging, Vol.27, No.4, (April 2006), pp. 524-529, ISSN 0197-4580

[61] Lin, J.J., Yueh, K.C., Chang, D.C., & Lin, S.Z. (1999). Absence of G209A and G88C mutations in the alpha- synuclein gene of Parkinson's disease in a Chinese population. *European Neurology*, Vol.42, No.4, pp. 217-220, ISSN 0014-3022

[62] Lin, M.T., & Beal, M,F. (2006). Mitochondrial dysfunction and oxidative stress in neurodegenerative diseases. *Nature*, Vol.443, No.7113, (October 2006), pp. 787-795, ISSN 0028-0836

[63] Litvan, I., Bhatia, K.P., Burn, D.J., Goetz, C.G., Lang, A.E., McKeith, I., Quinn, N., Sethi, K.D., Shults, C., & Wenning, G.K. (2003). Movement Disorders Society Scientific Issues Committee report: SIC Task Force appraisal of clinical diagnostic criteria for Parkinsonian disorders. *Movement Disorders*, Vol.18, No.5, (May 2003), pp. 467-486, ISSN 0885-3185

[64] Liu, Q., Xie, F., Siedlak, S.L., Nunomura, A., Honda, K., Moreira, P.I., Zhua, X., Smith, M.A., & Perry, G. (2004). Neurofilament proteins in neurodegenerative diseases. *Cellular and Molecular Life Sciences*, Vol.61, No.24, (December 2004), pp. 3057-3075, ISSN 1420-682X

[65] Lucking, C.B., & Briece, A. (2000). Alpha-synuclein and Parkinson's disease. *Cellular and Molecular Life Sciences*, Vol.57, No.13-14, (December 2000), pp. 1894-1908, ISSN 1420-682X

[66] Lucking, C.B., Bonifati, V., Periquet, M., Vanacore, N., Brice, A., & Meco, G. (2001). Pseudo-dominant inheritance and exon 2 triplication in a family with parkin gene mutations. *Neurology*, Vol.57, No.5, (September 2001), pp. 924-927, ISSN 0896-6273

[67] Macedo, M.G., Verbaan, D., Fang, Y., van Rooden, S.M., Visser, M., Anar, B., Uras, A., Groen, J.L., Rizzu, P., van Hilten, J.J., & Heutink, P. (2009). Genotypic and phenotypic characteristics of Dutch patients with early onset Parkinson's disease. *Movement Disorders*, Vol.24, No.2, (January 2009), pp. 196-203, ISSN 0885-3185

[68] Maguire-Zeiss, K.A., Short, D.W., & Federoff, H.J. (2005). Synuclein, dopamine and oxidative stress: co-conspirators in Parkinson's disease? *Molecular Brain Research*, Vol. 134, No.1, (March 2005), pp. 18-23, ISSN 0169-328X

[69] Malkus, K.A., Tsika, E., & Ischiropoulos, H. (2009). Oxidative modifications, mitochondrial dysfunction, and impaired protein degradation in Parkinson's disease:

how neurons are lost in the Bermuda triangle. *Molecular Neurodegeneration*, Vol.4, No. 24, (June 2009), pp. e1-16, ISSN 1750-1326

[70] Maraganore, D.M., de Andrade, M., & Elbaz, A. (2006). Genetic Epidemiology of Parkinson's Disease (GEO-PD) Consortium. Collaborative analysis of alpha-synuclein gene promoter variability and Parkinson disease. JAMA, Vol.296, No.6, (August 2006), pp. 661-670, ISSN 0098-7484

[71] Maruyama, M., Ikeuchi, T., Saito, M., Ishikawa, A., Yuasa, T., Tanaka, H., Hayashi, S., Wakabayashi, K., Takahashi, H., & Tsuji, S. (2000). Novel mutations, pseudo-dominant inheritance, and possible familial affects in patients with autosomal recessive juvenile parkinsonism. *Annals Neurology*, Vol.48, No.2, (August 2000), pp. 245-250, ISSN 0364-5134

[72] Mata, I.F., Lockhart, P.J., & Farrer, M.J. (2004). Parkin genetics: one model for Parkinson's disease. *Human Molecular Genetics*, Vol.13, No.1, (April 2004), pp. R127-133, ISSN 0964-6906

[73] McHugh, P.C., Joyce, P.R., & Kennedy, M.R. (2009). Polymorphisms of sepiapterin reductase gene alter promoter activity and may influence risk of bipolar disorder. *Pharmacogenetics and Genomics*, Vol.19, No.5, (May 2009), pp. 330-337, ISSN 1744-6872

[74] Mellick, G.D., Maraganore, D.M., & Silburn, P.A. (2005). Australian data and meta-analysis lend support for alpha-synuclein (NACP-Rep1) as a risk factor for Parkinson's disease. *Neuroscience Letters*, 375, No.2, (February 2005), pp. 112-116, ISSN 0304-3940

[75] Mellick, G.D., Siebert, G.A., Funayama, M., Buchanan, D.D., Li, Y., Imamichi, Y., Yoshino, H., Silburn, P.A., & Hattori, N. (2009). Screening PARK genes for mutations in early-onset Parkinson's disease patients from Queensland, Australia. Parkinsonism & Related Disorders, 2009, Vol.15, No.2, (February 2009), pp. 105-109, ISSN 1353-8020

[76] Michell, A.W., Tofaris, G.K., Gossage, H., Tyers, P., Spillantini, M.G., & Barker, R.A. (2007). The effect of truncated human alpha-synuclein (1-120) on dopaminergic cells in a transgenic mouse model of Parkinson's disease. *Cell Transplantation*, Vol.16, No. 5, pp. 461-474, ISSN 0963-6897

[77] Myhre, R., Toft, M., Kachergus, J., Hulihan, M.M., Aasly, J.O., Klungland, H., & Farrer, M.J. (2008). Multiple alpha-synuclein gene polymorphisms are associated with Parkinson's disease in a Norwegian population. Acta Neurologica Scandinavica, Vol. 118, No.5, (November 2008), pp. 320-327, ISSN 0001-6314

[78] Nishioka, K., Ross, O.A., Ishii, K., Kachergus, J.M., Ishiwata, K., Kitagawa, M., Kono, S., Obi, T., Mizoguchi, K., Inoue, Y., Imai, H., Takanashi, M., Mizuno, Y., Farrer, M.J., & Hattori, N. (2009). Expanding the clinical phenotype of SNCA duplication carriers. *Movement Disorders*, Vol.24, No.12, (September 2009), pp. 1811-1819, ISSN 0885-3185

[79] Nuytemans, K., Meeus, B., Crosiers, D., Brouwers, N., Goossens, D., Engelborghs, S., Pals, P., Pickut, B., Van den Broeck, M., Corsmit, E., Cras, P., De Deyn, P.P., Del-Favero, J., Van Broeckhoven, C., & Theuns, J. (2009). Relative contribution of simple mutations vs. copy number variations in five Parkinson disease genes in the Belgian population. *Human Mutation*, Vol.30, No.7, (July 2009), pp. 1054-1061, ISSN 1059-7794

[80] Nuytemans, K., Theuns, J., Cruts, M., & Van Broeckhoven, C. (2010). Genetic Etiology of Parkinson Disease Associated with Mutations in the SNCA, PARK2, PINK1, PARK7, and LRRK2 Genes: A Mutation Update. *Human Mutation*, Vol.31, No.7, (July 2010), pp. 763-780, ISSN 1059-7794

[81] Olanow, C.W. (2008). Levodopa/dopamine replacement strategies in Parkinson's disease: future directions. *Movement Disorders*, Vol.23, Suppl. 3, pp. S613-622, ISSN 0885-3185

[82] Oliveri, R.L., Zappia, M., Annesi, G., Bosco, D., Annesi, F., Spadafora, P., Pasqua, A.A., Tomaino, C., Nicoletti, G., Pirritano, D., Labate, A., Gambardella, A., Logroscino, G., Manobianca, G., Epifanio, A., Morgante, L., Savettieri, G., Quattrone, A. (2001). The parkin gene is not involved in late-onset Parkinson's disease. *Neurology*, Vol.57, No.2, (July 2001), pp. 359-362, ISSN 0896-6273

[83] Oliveira, S.A., Scott, W.K., Martin, E.R., Nance, M.A., Watts, R.L., Hubble, J.P., Koller, W.C., Pahwa, R., Stern, M.B., Hiner, B.C., Ondo, W.G., Allen, F.H. Jr., Scott, B.L., Goetz, C.G., Small, G.W., Mastaglia, F., Stajich, J.M., Zhang, F., Booze, M.W., Winn, M.P., Middleton, L.T., Haines, J.L., Pericak-Vance, M.A., & Vance, J.M. (2003). Parkin mutations and susceptibility alleles in late-onset Parkinson's disease. *Annals Neurology*, Vol.53, No.5, (May 2003), pp. 624-629, ISSN 0364-5134

[84] Oyama, G., Yoshimi, K., Natori, S., Chikaoka, Y., Ren, Y.R., Funayama, M., Shimo, Y., Takahashi, R., Nakazato, T., Kitazawa, S., & Hattori, N. (2010). Impaired in vivo dopamine release in parkin knockout mice. *Brain Research*, Vol.1352, (September 2010), pp. 214-222, ISSN 0006-8993

[85] Pankratz, N., Kissell, D.K., Pauciulo, M.W., Halter, C.A., Rudolph, A., Pfeiffer, R.F., Marder, K.S., Foroud, T., Nichols, W.C. Parkinson Study Group-PROGENI Investigators. (2009). Parkinson Study Group-PROGENI Investigators Parkin dosage mutations have greater pathogenicity in familial PD than simple sequence mutations. Neurology, Vol.73, No.4, (July 2009), pp. 279-286, ISSN 0896-6273

[86] Periquet, M., Lücking, C., Vaughan, J., Bonifati, V., Dürr, A., De Michele, G., Horstink, M., Farrer, M., Illarioshkin, S.N., Pollak, P., Borg, M., Brefel-Courbon, C., Denefle, P., Meco, G., Gasser, T., Breteler, M.M., Wood, N., Agid, Y., & Brice, A. French Parkinson's Disease Genetics Study Group. The European Consortium on Genetic Susceptibility in Parkinson's Disease. (2001). Origin of mutations in the parkin gene in Europe: exon rearrangements are independent recurrent events, whereas point mutations may result from founder effects. *American Journal of Human Genetics*, Vol. 68, No.3, (March 2001), pp. 617-626, ISSN 0002-9297

[87] Periquet, M., Latouche, M., Lohmann, E., Rawal, N., De, M.G., Ricard, S., Teive, H., Fraix, V., Vidailhet, M., Nicholl, D., Barone, P., Wood, N.W., Raskin, S., Deleuze, J.F., Agid, Y., Durr, A., & Brice, A. French Parkinson's Disease Genetics Study Group; European Consortium on Genetic Susceptibility in Parkinson's Disease. (2003). Parkin mutations are frequent in patients with isolated early-onset parkinsonism. *Brain*, Vol. 126, No.Pt 6, (June 2003), pp. 1271-1278, ISSN 0006-8950

[88] Pchelina, S.N., Emelyanov, A.K., Yakimovskii, A.F., Miller, D.W., Shabalina, I.G., Drozdova, A.S., Schwarzman, A.L. (2011). Reduced content of α-synuclein in peripheral blood leukocytes of patients with LRRK2-associated Parkinson's disease. *Bulletin of Experimental Biology and Medicine*, Vol.150, No.6, (April 2011), pp. 679-681, ISSN 0007-4888

[89] Polrolniczak (Oczkowska), A., Dorszewska, J., Bialek, P., Florczak-Wyspianska, J., Owecki, M., & Kozubski, W. (2012). Analysis of the frequency of mutations in genes important for molecular diagnostics of Parkinson disease. *Acta Biochimica Polonica*, 59, Suppl. 3, 16, ISSN 1734-154X, Abstracts of the 47th Congress of the Polish Biochemical Society and Polish-German Biochemical Societies Joint Meeting. Poznan, Poland, September 11th-14th, 2012

[90] Polrolniczak (Oczkowska), A., Dorszewska, J., Florczak, J., Owecki, M., Rozycka, A., Jagodzinski, P., & Kozubski, W. (2011). Analysis of SNCA and PARK2 mutations in sporadic parkinson's disease. *Neurodegenerative disease*, 8, Suppl. 1, P1, ISSN 1758-2032, Abstracts of the 10th International Conference on Alzheimer's and Parkinson's Diseases. Barcelona, Spain, March 9-13, 2011

[91] Ren, J.P., Zhao, Y.W., & Sun, X.J. (2009). Toxic influence of chronic oral administration of paraquat on nigrostriatal dopaminergic neurons in C57BL/6 mice. *Chinese Medical Journal (English Edition)*, Vol.122, No.19, (October 2009), pp. 2366-2371, ISSN 0366-6999

[92] Ritz, B., Rhodes, S.L., Bordelon, Y., & Broinstein, J. (2012). α-Synuclein Genetic Variants Predict Faster Motor Symptom Progression in Idiopathic Parkinson Disease. *PLoS ONE*, Vol.7, No.5, (May 2012), pp. 1-8, ISSN 1932-6203

[93] Rubinsztein, DC. (2006). The roles of intracellular protein-degradation pathways in neurodegeneration. *Nature*, Vol.443, No.7113, (October 2006), pp. 780-786, ISSN 0028-0836

[94] Satoh, J., & Kuroda, Y. (1999). Association of codon 167 Ser/Asn heterozygosity in the parkin gene with sporadic Parkinson's disease. Neuroreport, Vol.10, No.13, (September 1999), pp. 2735-2739, ISSN 0959-4965

[95] Schapira, A.H. (2002). Dopamine agonists and neuroprotection in Parkinson's disease. *European Journal of Neurology*, 2002, Vol.9, Suppl. 3, (November 2002), pp. 7-14, ISSN 1351-5101

[96] Schneider, B.L., Seehus, C.R., Capowski, E.E., Aebischer, P., Zhang, S.C., & Svendsen, C.N. (2007). Overexpression of alpha-synuclein in human neural progenitors leads to

specific changes in fate and differentiation. *Human Molecular Genetics*, 2007, Vol.16, No.6, (May 2007), pp. 651-666, ISSN 0964-6906

[97] Sharma, M., Mueller, J.C., Zimprich, A., Lichtner, P., Hofer, A., Leitner, P., Maass, S., Berg, D., Dürr, A., Bonifati, V., De Michele, G., Oostra, B., Brice, A., Wood, N.W., Muller-Myhsok, B., & Gasser, T, European Consortium on Genetic Susceptibility in Parkinson's Disease (GSPD). (2006). The sepiapterin reductase gene region reveals association in the PARK3 locus: analysis of familial and sporadic Parkinson's disease in European populations. *Journal of Medical Genetics*, Vol.43, No.7, (July 2006), pp. 557-562, ISSN 0022-2593

[98] Sharma, M., Maraganore, D.M., Ioannidis, J.P., Riess, O., Aasly, J.O., Annesi, G., Abahuni, N., Bentivoglio, A.R., Brice, A., Van Broeckhoven, C., Chartier-Harlin, M.C., Destée, A., Djarmati, A., Elbaz, A., Farrer, M., Ferrarese, C., Gibson, J.M., Gispert, S., Hattori, N., Jasinska-Myga, B., Klein, C., Lesage, S., Lynch, T., Lichtner, P., Lambert, J.C., Lang, A.E., Mellick, G.D., De Nigris, F., Opala, G., Quattrone, A., Riva, C., Rogaeva, E., Ross, O.A., Satake, W., Silburn, P.A., Theuns, J., Toda, T., Tomiyama, H., Uitti, R.J., Wirdefeldt, K., Wszolek, Z., Gasser, T., & Krüger, R., Genetic Epidemiology of Parkinson's Disease Consortium. (2011). Genetic Epidemiology of Parkinson's Disease Consortium. Role of sepiapterin reductase gene at the PARK3 locus in Parkinson's disease. *Neurobiology of Aging*, Vol.32, No.11, (November 2011), pp. 2108 e1-5, ISSN 0197-4580

[99] Sherer, T.B., Betarbet, R., Stout, A.K., Lund, S., Baptista, M., Panov, A.V., Cookson, M.R., & Greenamyre, J.T. (2002). An in vitro model of Parkinson's disease: linking mitochondrial impairment to altered α-synuclein metabolism and oxidative damage. *Journal of Neuroscience*, Vol.22, No.16, (August 2002), pp. 7006-7015, ISSN 0270-6474

[100] Shimura, H., Schlossmacher, M.G., Hattori, N., Frosch, M.P., Trockenbacher, A., Schneider, R., Mizuno, Y., Kosik, & K.S., Selkoe, D.J. (2001). Ubiquitination of a new form of alpha-synuclein by parkin from human brain: implications for Parkinson's disease. *Science*, Vol.293, No.5528, (July 2001), pp. 263-269, ISSN 0036-8075

[101] Simon-Sanchez, J., & Singleton, A.B. (2008). Sequencing analysis of OMI/HTRA2 shows previously reported pathogenic mutations in neurologically normal controls. *Human Molecular Genetics*, Vol.17, No.13, (July 2008), pp. 1988-1993, ISSN 0964-6906

[102] Singleton, A.B., Farrer, M., Johnson, J., Singleton, A., Hague, S., Kachergus, J., Hulihan, M., Peuralinna, T., Dutra, A., Nussbaum, R., Lincoln, S., Crawley, A., Hanson, M., Maraganore, D., Adler, C., Cookson, M.R., Muenter, M., Baptista, M., Miller, D., Blancato, J., Hardy, J., & Gwinn-Hardy, K. (2003). Alpha-Synuclein locus triplication causes Parkinson's disease. *Science*, Vol.302, No.5646, (October 2003), pp. 841, ISSN 0036-8075

[103] Sinha, R., Racetteb, B., Perlmutterb, J.S., & Parsian, A. (2005). Prevalence of parkin gene mutations and variations in idiopathic Parkinson's disease. Parkinsonism & Related Disorders, Vol.11, No.6, (September 2005), pp. 341-347, ISSN 1353-8020

[104] Sironi, F., Primignani, P., Zini, M., Tunesi, S., Ruffmann, C., Ricca, S., Brambilla, T., Antonini, A., Tesei, S., Canesi, M., Zecchinelli, A., Mariani, C., Meucci, N., Sacilotto, G., Cilia, R., Isaias, I.U., Garavaglia, B., Ghezzi, D., Travi, M., Decarli, A., Coviello, D.A., Pezzoli, G., Goldwurm, S. (2008). Parkin analysis in early onset Parkinson's disease. Parkinsonism & Related Disorders, Vol.14, No.4, pp. 326-333, ISSN 1353-8020

[105] Spadafora, P., Annesi, G., Pasqua, A.A., Serra, P., Cirò Candiano, I.C., Carrideo, S., Tarantino, P., Civitelli, D., De Marco, E.V., Nicoletti, G., Annesi, F., & Quattrone, A. (2003). NACP-REP1 polymorphism is not involved in Parkinson's disease: a case-control study in a population sample from southern Italy. Neuroscience Letters, Vol. 351, No.2, (November 2003), pp. 75-78, ISSN 0304-3940

[106] Strauss, K.M., Martins, L.M., Plun-Favreau, H., Marx, F.P., Kautzmann, S., Berg, D., Gasser, T., Wszolek. Z., Müller, T., Bornemann, A., Wolburg, H., Downward, J., Riess, O., Schulz, J.B., & Krüger, R. (2005). Loss of function mutations in the gene encoding Omi/HtrA2 in Parkinson's disease. Human Molecular Genetics, Vol.14, No.15, (August 2005), pp. 2099-2111, ISSN 0964-6906

[107] Suzuki, Y., Imai, Y., Nakayama, H., Takahashi, K., Takio, K., & Takahashi, R. (2001). A serine protease, HtrA2, is released from the mitochondria and interacts with XIAP, inducing cell death. Molecular Cell, Vol.8, No.3, (September 2001), pp. 613-621, ISSN 1097-2765

[108] Tan, E.K., Matsuura, T., Nagamitsu, S., Khajavi, M., Jankovic, J., & Ashizawa, T. (2000). Polymorphism of NACP-Rep1 in Parkinson's disease: an etiologic link with essential tremor? Neurology, Vol.54, No.5, (March 2000), pp. 1195-1198, ISSN 0896-6273

[109] Tan, E.K., Tan, C., Shen, H., Chai, A., Lum, S.Y., Teoh, M.L., Yih, Y., Wong, M.C., & Zhao, Y. (2003). Alpha synuclein promoter and risk of Parkinson's disease: microsatellite and allelic size variability. Neuroscience Letters, Vol.336, No.1, (January 2003), pp. 70-72, ISSN 0304-3940

[110] Thomas, B., & Beal, M.F. (2007). Parkinson's disease. Human Molecular Genetics, Vol. 16, Spec No.2, (October 2007), pp. R183–194, ISSN 0964-6906

[111] Tobin, J.E., Cui, J., Wilk, J.B., Latourelle, J.C., Laramie, J.M., McKee, A.C., Guttman, M., Karamohamed, S., DeStefano, A.L., & Myers, R.H. (2007). Sepiapterin reductase expression is increased in Parkinson's disease brain tissue. Brain Research, Vol. 30, No.1139, (March 2007), pp. 42-47, ISSN 0006-8993

[112] Totterdell, S., & Meredith, G.E. (2005). Localization of alpha-synuclein to identified fibers and synapses in the normal mouse brain. Neuroscience, Vol.135, No.3, pp. 907-913, ISSN 0306-4522

[113] Trotta, L., Guella, I., Soldà, G., Sironi, F., Tesei, S., Canesi, M., Pezzoli, G., Goldwurm, S., Duga, S., & Asselta, R. (2012). SNCA and MAPT genes: Independent and joint ef-

fects in Parkinson disease in the Italian population. Parkinsonism & Related Disorders, Vol.18, No.3, (March 2012), pp. 257-262, ISSN 1353-8020

[114] Wang, M., Hattori, N., Matsumine, H., Kobayashi, T., Yoshino, H., Morioka, A., Kitada, T., Asakawa, S., Minoshima, S., Shimizu, N., & Mizuno, Y. (1999). Polymorphism in the parkin gene in sporadic Parkinson's disease. *Annals Neurology*, Vol.45, No.5, (May 1999), pp. 655-658, ISSN 0364-5134

[115] Wang, T., Liang, Z., Sun, S., Cao, X., Peng, H., Liu, H., & Tong, E. (2004). Exon deletions of parkin gene in patients with Parkinson disease. *Journal* of *Huazhong University of Science and Technology* [*Medical Sciences*], Vol.24, No.3, pp. 262-265, ISSN 1672-0733

[116] Xia, Y., Saitoh, T., Uéda, K., Tanaka, S., Chen, X., Hashimoto, M., Hsu, L., Conrad, C., Sundsmo, M., Yoshimoto, M., Thal, L., Katzman, & R., Masliah. E. (2001). Characterization of the human alpha-synuclein gene: Genomic structure, transcription start site, promoter region and polymorphisms. *Journal of Alzheimer's Disease*, Vol.3, No.5, (October 2001), pp. 485-494, ISSN 1387-2877

[117] Zhang, Y., Gao, J., Chung, K.K., Huang, H., Dawson, V.L., & Dawson, T.M. (2000). Parkin functions as an E2-dependent ubiquitin- protein ligase and promotes the degradation of the synaptic vesicle-associated protein, CDCrel-1. *Proceedings of the National Academy of Sciences USA*, Vol.97, No.24, (November 2000), pp. 13354-13359, ISSN 0027-8424

Permissions

List of Contributors

Sacnité Albarran Bravo and Benjamín Florán Garduño
Departamento de Fisiología, Biofísica y Neurociencias, Centro de Investigación y de Estudios Avanzados del Instituto Politécnico Nacional, Mexico

Claudia Rangel-Barajas
Department of Pharmacology & Neuroscience, University of North Texas Health Science Center, Fort Worth, USA

F.Y. Ho
Department of Biochemistry, University of Groningen, Groningen, The Netherlands

K.E. Rosenbusch and A. Kortholt
Department of Cell Biochemistry, University of Groningen, Groningen, The Netherlands

Peter Podgorny and Cory Toth
University of Calgary, Canada

L.T.B. Gobbi, F.A. Barbieri, R. Vitório, M.P. Pereira, C. Teixeira-Arroyo, P.C.R. Santos, L.C. Morais, P.H.S. Pelicioni, L. Simieli, D. Orcioli-Silva, J. Lahr, F. Stella, M.J.D. Caetano and P.M. Formaggio
UNESP Univ Estadual Paulista, Rio Claro, Brazil

A.Y.Y. Hamanaka, A.C. Salles, A.P.T. Alves, C.B. Takaki, E. Lirani-Silva, F.A. Cezar, M.D.T.O. Ferreira, N.M. Rinaldi, R.A. Batistela and V. Raile
The PROPARKI Group, Brazil

Grace G.Y. Lim
Department of Physiology, National University of Singapore, Singapore

Kah-Leong Lim
Department of Physiology, National University of Singapore, Singapore
National Neuroscience Institute, Singapore
Duke-NUS Graduate Medical School, Singapore

Keisuke Suzuki, Masayuki Miyamoto, Ayaka Numao, Hideki Sakuta, Hiroaki Fujita, Yuji Watanabe and Koichi Hirata
Department of Neurology, Dokkyo Medical University, Japan

Tomoyuki Miyamoto and Masaoki Iwanami
Department of Neurology, Dokkyo Medical University Koshigaya Hospital, Japan

Naoki Tani
Department of Neurosurgery, Otemae Hospital, Osaka, Japan

Ryoma Morigaki and Satoshi Goto
Department of Motor Neuroscience and Neurotherapeutics, Institute of Health Biosciences, Graduate School of Medical Sciences, University of Tokushima, Tokushima, Japan

Ryuji Kaji
Department of Clinical Neuroscience, Institute of Health Biosciences, Graduate School of Medical Sciences, University of Tokushima, Tokushima, Japan

Alessia Carocci and Alessia Catalano
Department of Pharmacy-Drug Sciences, University of Bari "Aldo Moro", Bari, Italy

Maria Stefania Sinicropi, Graziantonio Lauria and Giuseppe Genchi
Department of Pharmacy, Health and Nutritional Sciences, University of Calabria, Cosenza, Italy

Chengwu Zhang
National Neuroscience Institute, Singapore

Anna Oczkowska, Margarita Lianeri and Jolanta Dorszewska
Poznan University of Medical Sciences, Laboratory of Neurobiology Department of Neurology, Poznan, Poland

Wojciech Kozubski
Poznan University of Medical Sciences, Chair and Department of Neurology, Poznan, Poland

Index

Printed in the USA
CPSIA information can be obtained
at www.ICGtesting.com
JSHW050724090124
54998JS00021B/35

9 798887 403625